The Inner Physician

Roger Neighbour

The Inner Physician

Why and how to practise 'big picture medicine'

Roger Neighbour OBE MA DSc FRCGP

Illustrations by
Jamie Hynes MB ChB MRCGP

Foreword by
Iona Heath CBE FRCP FRCGP

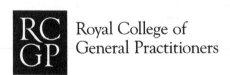

Royal College of
General Practitioners

Distributed by

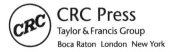

CRC Press
Taylor & Francis Group
Boca Raton London New York

CRC Press is an imprint of the
Taylor & Francis Group, an **informa** business

CRC Press
Taylor & Francis Group
6000 Broken Sound Parkway NW, Suite 300
Boca Raton, FL 33487-2742

Visit the Taylor & Francis Web site at
http://www.taylorandfrancis.com

and the CRC Press Web site at
http://www.crcpress.com

Only connect the prose and the passion, and both will
be exalted … Live in fragments no longer.

E.M. Forster (1879–1970)
English novelist
From *Howards End* (1910), Chapter 22

Contents

About the author

Roger Neighbour OBE MA MB BChir DSc FRCP FRCGP FRACGP
Roger qualified from King's College, Cambridge, and St Thomas' Hospital. After vocational training in Watford, he was a principal in general practice in Abbot's Langley, Hertfordshire, from 1974 to 2003. He was a trainer and course organiser with the Watford Vocational Training Scheme (VTS) for many years, an MRCGP examiner for 20 years, and Convener of the RCGP's Panel of Examiners from 1997 to 2002. In 2003 he was elected President of the Royal College of General Practitioners for a 3-year term, and in 2011 was awarded an OBE for services to medical education.

An interest in the psychology of the doctor–patient relationship and of the teacher–learner relationship in vocational training led Roger to write *The Inner Consultation* (1987)[1] and *The Inner Apprentice* (1992).[2] A collection of his medico-philosophical writings, *I'm Too Hot Now*, was published in 2005.[3]

Now retired from clinical practice, Roger continues to write, teach and lecture in the UK and worldwide on consulting skills and medical education. He plays the violin to semi-professional standard, and enjoys spending time at his apartment in Normandy. He also plays golf badly, but not quite badly enough to give up.

---

1   Neighbour R. *The Inner Consultation*, 2nd edn. Oxford: Radcliffe Publishing, 2004.

2   Neighbour R. *The Inner Apprentice*, 2nd edn. Oxford: Radcliffe Publishing, 2004.

3   Neighbour R. *I'm Too Hot Now*. Oxford: Radcliffe Publishing, 2005.

About the illustrator

Jamie Hynes MB ChB MRCGP DRCOG PGCertMedEd
Jamie is an enthusiastic and fulfilled GP, committed husband and father to two boys. Qualified from Birmingham in 2002, he is currently a Training Programme Director for City VTS in Birmingham. He recalls that when as a medical student he was questioned about his CV's mention of artistic interests, he described the practice of medicine as an art. He is delighted to keep utilising the creativity from life before training in this book, as well as in his practice and VTS websites. Jamie's video-poem extolling the virtues and privileges of general practice, *The National Health* (2015), won the RCGP Midland Faculty's 'Inspiration' competition.

About the foreword writer

Iona Heath CBE FRCP FRCGP
Iona worked as an inner city GP in Kentish Town in London from 1975 until 2010. She is a Past President of the Royal College of General Practitioners.

Iona has written regularly for the *British Medical Journal* and has contributed essays to many other medical journals across the world. She has been particularly interested in exploring the nature of general practice, the importance of medical generalism, issues of justice and liberty in relation to health care, the corrosive influence of the medical industrial complex and the commercialisation of medicine, as well as the challenges posed by disease-mongering, the care of the dying, and violence within families. Her book *Matters of Life and Death* was published in 2008.[4]

---

4   Heath I. *Matters of Life and Death: key writings.* Oxford: Radcliffe Publishing, 2008.

Acknowledgements

All the time I was contemplating and writing this book I drew encouragement from my 40 years of friendship with Dr John Horder CBE, sadly now deceased. John was the Renaissance man of general practice. He was, in the old-fashioned sense of the phrase, a wonderful doctor – skilled, perceptive, courageous and modest in equal measure. He was a pioneer in vocational training, a friend of the Balints, and a former President of the Royal College of General Practitioners. As if this wasn't enough, John was a fine painter in watercolours, and an accomplished organist and pianist with whom I spent many hours playing violin sonatas. I offer this book as a tribute to his memory.

Iona Heath, too, has been a good friend for more years than either of us cares to remember. She is wonderfully articulate about the core ideas and values of general practice, managing to be both champion and maverick, traditionalist and iconoclast. There is no one I should have preferred to write the foreword for this book, and I am so pleased that she agreed. Thank you, Iona.

I love Jamie Hynes' line drawings. It has been a pleasure to have this excuse to get to know him and (if he'll forgive me for saying so) to watch him develop as a fine GP and teacher. Thanks, Jamie.

I am very grateful to the late Michael Crichton, with whom I corresponded shortly before his death in 2008, for permission to quote from his book *Travels*, and for agreeing to lend his name to Crichton's switch.

The following friends generously sent me their own Crichton's switch stories: Tom Boyd, Andrew Carter, Xanthe Cross, Dan Edgecumbe, David Haslam, Julian Howells, Patrick Hutt, Jamie Hynes, Carol McKenzie, Paul McKenzie, Margaret Murray, Gunnar Nordgren, Duncan Shrewsbury, David Warriner and Tom Wiggall. I was moved and enlightened by their frankness. It was reassuring to me, and I hope that it will be to readers, to have it confirmed that we all wrestle similar demons and protect ourselves in similar ways. Thank you all very much.

I acknowledge with gratitude the Royal Literary Fund for permission to quote Henry Reed's poem *Judging Distances*; Professor Carl Heneghan of Oxford University for permission to refer in detail to his and his colleagues' work on the diagnostic process; and Professor Jenny Doust for permission to use data from her 2009 *British Medical Journal* paper on using probabilistic reasoning.

I offer my sincere thanks to Helen Farrelly and her colleagues in the RCGP Publications Department, and particularly to Gillian Nineham, for their help and encouragement (and, in Gill's case, for not losing patience every time I told her I'd nearly finished the writing). It has also been a real pleasure to work with the team at Prepress Projects, notably Gillian Whytock. Gillian is everything I dared hope for in a copy-editor: painstaking and thorough, yet sensitive and tactful.

But most especially – and I don't care if it's trite to say so – I want to thank the countless patients who, over the years, have taught me that the best way of helping them isn't necessarily the way I learned at medical school. Medicine would be easier without them, but they do make it the best job in the world.

Roger Neighbour
Bedmond, UK
rogerneighbour@gmail.com

Foreword

Following *The Inner Consultation* and *The Inner Apprentice*, this is the third of Roger Neighbour's brilliant series of 'Inner' books. The first appeared in 1987, at a time when its author could still, by medical standards, be described as a bright young thing; the second came 5 years later; but we have had to wait more than 20 years for *The Inner Physician*. It has been worth the wait, because this book is the distillation of an extraordinarily thoughtful career in general practice: consulting, learning and teaching. Roger Neighbour has spent a lifetime exploring and seeking to explain the inner: the hidden, the implicit and the assumed.

A few weeks ago a rather shabby parcel arrived at my house. It contained my own copy of *The Inner Consultation*, with my name and the date of November 1989 written inside the front cover, but there was no covering letter or other hint of the identity of the sender. The spine, originally a shade of pink and still pink when I had last seen it, had faded to a pale but undeniable green. I had lent it, years ago, to a trainee: who, I cannot recall. And, despite the lack of a confession, I was very grateful and happy to have the book back. Better late than never, and I feel sure that it must have been appreciated in the interim. That book had been my introduction to Roger, whom I have since had the pleasure of coming to know as a friend and colleague.

I remember very clearly reading *The Inner Consultation* for the first time and feeling slightly irritated by being asked to remember the five checkpoints of the consultation by staring at my left hand. As so often, my first impression was wrong: Roger Neighbour is a teacher of genius, and I have never forgotten those five checkpoints of connecting, summarising, handing over, safety netting and housekeeping, and have gone on to teach them to generations of students and trainees while solemnly counting off the fingers of my left hand.

This latest book, *The Inner Physician*, is less didactic than its predecessors but is constantly inviting its readers to think about what it is to be a doctor or a patient. In essence it is a gentle, careful explanation of the fundamental importance of the doctor's subjective self: the inner physician. It recognises that, if the subjectivity of the doctor is denied or suppressed, the subjectivity of the patient will be similarly marginalised and unrecognised, to the detriment of the interactions and outcomes of care. When both physicians and patients are reduced to interchangeable units within industrialised, bureaucratic systems of health care, each is no longer able, in Roger's words, 'to authenticate the humanity of the other'.

He defines diagnosis as 'insight on the verge of action', and describes the diagnostic process as 'best understood as bringing meaning to a predicament that was hitherto mysterious'. I have never read a better description, and it challenges doctors everywhere to beware the reductionist labelling that bedevils so much of what passes for diagnosis. His formulation sent me back to W.H. Auden's famous introduction to *The Poet's Tongue*, the anthology he compiled in 1935 with John Garrett. Auden wrote:

> *Poetry is not concerned with telling people what to do, but with extending our knowledge of good and evil, perhaps making the necessity for action more urgent and its nature more clear, but only leading us to the point where it is possible for us to make a rational moral choice.*

Today, doctors find themselves surrounded by guidelines, diktats and incentives, all telling them what to do. Roger Neighbour quotes both poets and poetry; his description of diagnosis is evocative of Auden's view of poetry and so leads us, as physicians, to the point where it is possible to make a rational moral choice. He never tells us what to do, but he always invites us to think.

Of his hero Socrates, Roger writes:

> *He demanded of himself the full embrace of all his human capacities – rational and irrational, physical and psychological, pragmatic and idealistic.*

And that describes, precisely, the achievement of this book.

Iona Heath
September 2015

Sex and the single pronoun

English is a wonderful language, and I am privileged to have it as my birthright. But it has one blind spot, one that bedevils every author of a pedantic disposition, and that is its lack of a gender-neutral pronoun standing for 'a person of either sex'. To have to refer to a generic doctor or an anonymous patient as either 'he' or 'she' is to impose an unintended and sometimes inappropriate masculinity or femininity.

Once upon a time this was not a problem. It was sufficient for any author bothered enough to acknowledge the difficulty to dismiss it with an airy 'The masculine pronoun includes the feminine', or (more rarely) 'The female includes the male'. I am as uncomfortable with that as I am with the assumption that an atheist or agnostic, asked to tick the 'religion' box, will settle for being put down as 'Church of England'.

'He-or-she' and 'his-or-her' (or, worse, 's/he' and 'hi/her-s'), with or without the hyphens, quickly become wearisome. Too many '*one*'s and '*one*'s-es', and one begins to sound like Royalty. 'They' and 'their', while probably destined eventually to become the norm, lead to such barbarisms as 'When a doctor talks to a patient, they say to them …'

An alternative strategy would be for me to decide that my doctors were always to be male and their patients always female, or vice versa. This would antagonise at least half my readers. Another would be to divvy out the gender identities of each group either 50/50 or in proportion to the latest demographic data, whatever that is; but so laboured a gimmick just seems silly. Life, as Shirley Conran observed, is too short to stuff a mushroom.

We are between a rock and a hard place. I have to choose between the risk of offending some readers and the certainty of traumatising my own sense of linguistic nicety. Sorry, but with you, dear reader, I can plead for tolerance. You I can ask to accept that I am not intending to be sexist; and if you think I am, you can always write in and say so. But the language can't defend itself. So I would rather be protective of English syntax than of anyone's idea of political correctness.

I'm afraid I've just written my text without worrying too much about pronouns. Sometimes my doctors have come out female, and sometimes male. Sometimes my patients have come out male, and sometimes female. Occasionally one of either has become plural, and the odd 'they' has crept in. These have not been conscious choices; each individual example no doubt reflects the workings of my subconscious biases and assumptions. But, since this is a book about how a doctor's psyche contributes to the clinical process, I hope we can all can live with that.

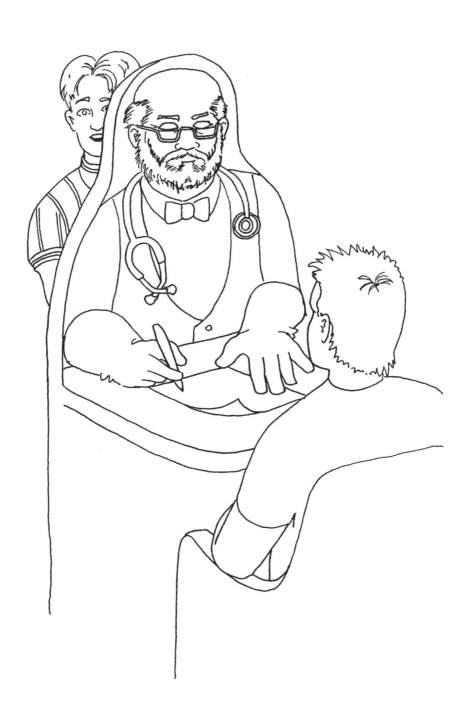

Summary

This book explores the idea that the mind of every doctor retains an untrained 'ordinary human being' part – the Inner Physician – which makes an important, although often neglected, contribution to medical practice, especially clinical generalism.

Chapter 1 ('Beginner's mind') uses the image of nested Russian dolls to explain how medicine at every level, from national institution down to the individual clinician, has at its core the doctor's own personal qualities, experience and insights.

Chapter 2 ('A backwards glance') traces the history of medicine from ancient times. Its emergence as a scientific discipline encouraged the historical split (further explored in Chapter 3, 'Inchworms and also-rans') between specialists and generalists. However, modern quantum theory has re-asserted the crucial role of the 'observer effect', i.e. that what we see depends on who we are and how we look.

Chapter 4 ('The medical gaze') suggests that, whereas the specialist looks at patients as if through a fixed-focus lens, the generalist gaze can zoom as necessary between close-up (detail) and wide-angle (context) settings, and can also be directed inwards to examine the doctor's internal awareness.

Chapter 5 ('The illness catastrophe') shows that the traditional 'medical model' is too simplistic to explain the subtleties of how people fall ill and recover, and describes a multidimensional alternative based on catastrophe theory.

Chapter 6 ('The case for big picture medicine') recapitulates some earlier ideas and concludes that it is the generalist, whose practice is informed by the Inner Physician, who is at the leading edge of contemporary medical thought.

Defining diagnosis as a search for meaning in the patient's narrative leading to 'insight on the verge of action', Chapters 7 and 8 ('What's the matter?' and 'As long as you think of it') point out shortcomings and fallacies in conventional approaches to diagnosis that rely exclusively on rational analysis.

'Crichton's switch' (Chapter 9) describes the switching-off of a doctor's human responses that is sometimes necessary to avoid being overwhelmed in fraught or shocking situations. Anecdotes from medical colleagues describe this, and also their realisation that professionalism required their Inner Physicians to be re-engaged.

Chapter 10 ('Through Johari's window') uses a well-known model to suggest that the Inner Physician represents the 'private', 'blind' and 'unknown' regions of the doctor's psyche. When these engage with their equivalents in the patient's mind, the phenomenon of emergence leads to unexpected levels of complexity in the doctor–patient relationship.

Chapter 11 ('The Greeks had a word for it') draws parallels between Socrates' 'daimonion' (his inner voice) and the Inner Physician. The Greeks were also familiar with 'phronesis', the wisdom that 'knows what to do when no one knows what to do', which is the hallmark of the modern generalist.

Chapter 12 ('In praise of innersense') reviews the impact of the Inner Physician on clinical practice, and considers how the mindset in which it best operates – awareness of the present moment and conscious control of the attention – can be developed.

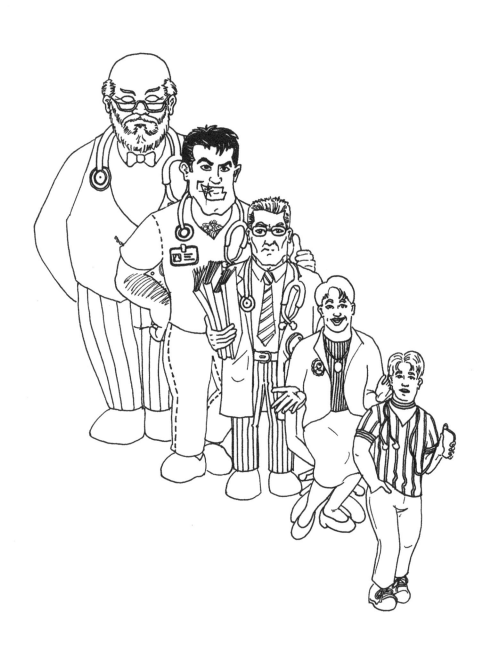

Chapter 1

Beginner's mind

> In the beginner's mind there are many possibilities: in the expert's
> mind there are few.
>
> Shunryu Suzuki (1904–1971)
> Japanese Soto Zen master

Britain has a first-class second-rate health service.

Let me explain. As second-rate systems of health care go, the British
National Health Service is first class. In its intentions, and in many of its
achievements too, the NHS is excellent – first class, in fact. Nevertheless,
the quality of the health care it delivers is – compared with what its founders
hoped for, what its clinicians aspire to, and what its consumers deserve –
sometimes second rate.

Why?

This book is intended to be an upbeat, even celebratory, enquiry into how
good medicine is practised. It is a quest for one of medicine's least explored
mysteries: how what happens in the privacy of individual doctors' own heads
– their 'Inner Physicians' – contributes to their effectiveness.

Good tales of quest often begin with a vision of distant treasure, and a
good mystery story with a puzzle or a crime. So let's begin with this puzzle.
How is it that our medical services, potentially so excellent, are so often
experienced by patients, doctors and managers alike as disappointing? In
the popular view, the NHS is something of a wounded hero, bruised and
bleeding, but much loved and somehow still standing. Yet this is a crime
without a culprit. There seems to be no assailant, no weapon, no fingerprints,
no motive. No one seems to have set out to harm the NHS, or to starve it of
nourishment or affection.

So this begs the question: where in the world can we find a first-class *first-
rate* health system? And the answer is 'nowhere'.

Practically every country – Western or Eastern, developed, undeveloped or emerging – provides health care that is either second class in conception or second rate in delivery, or both. Sometimes it's the political ideology that is at fault. There are governments that don't seem to care if some citizens are disadvantaged by geography, race or income. Others, of a more totalitarian persuasion, ignore the priorities and preferences of their populations. Then, of course, good medical care costs, and year on year it costs more and more. There are huge variations, even amongst the developed nations, in the proportion of gross domestic product devoted to health,[1] with no clear correlation between spend and benefit. All over the world, governments experiment frantically in their search for the best compromise between cost containment and electoral popularity, between public and private provision, between state subsidy and personal insurance.

The government of the USA spends a chart-topping 17-plus per cent of gross domestic product on health care, but gets only first-rate second-class health care for its investment. At its very best, the American system combines state-of-the-art hospital-based medicine with good person-centred family-orientated primary care. But not every American can afford the best, and primary care as we in Britain understand it is a luxury for the wealthy few. For the scores of millions who neither can afford the insurance premiums nor are covered by the various exemption schemes, health care of any kind, let alone the best, is a pipedream. They are second-, if not third-, class patients. What's more, the insurance-funded health maintenance organisations, their priorities financially rather than clinically determined, have skewed the concept of good medicine towards what is cost-effective and away from what is in the best interests of the individual patient. A system that so widens the health divide between the 'gets' and the 'can't-gets' can never, I would maintain, be better than second class.

---

1   Government expenditure on health care as a percentage of gross domestic product (World Health Organization data for 2013):

Country	% of GDP	Country	% of GDP
USA	17.1	Sweden	9.7
France	11.7	Australia	9.4
Switzerland	11.5	Italy	9.1
Germany	11.3	UK	9.1
Canada	10.9	Cuba	8.8
Japan	10.3	Russia	6.5
Greece	9.8	China	5.6
New Zealand	9.7	UAE	3.2

When Nye Bevan[2] established the British National Health Service in 1948, his was surely a first-class ambition: comprehensive health care for every citizen, from cradle to grave, funded out of general taxation and free at the point of delivery. But it was based on a false premise – that the amount of ill-health in the population was finite, and that the cost of treating it would therefore likewise be finite. If only the founders of the NHS had understood the medical equivalent of Parkinson's law:[3] 'Illness expands so as always to swamp the medical resources available for its relief'. But then, if they *had* understood this,[4] perhaps they wouldn't have been idealistic enough, brave enough in the aftermath of a world war, to enshrine in legislation the principle that the poorest and lowliest Briton has as much claim to succour in adversity as the wealthiest and the highest born.

So why has such a fine ambition proved only second-rate in reality? We can round up the usual suspects. The charges against them form a familiar enough litany.

For a start, we, the general public, can be held to blame. We are living longer, and we want to enjoy our lengthening decline in health and dignity. We live round-the-clock want-it-now lives in which delayed gratification is a disgrace and patience no virtue. Frailties and unpleasantnesses that previous generations might have borne with stoicism, such as sadness, worry, over-indulgence or sexual apathy, have been reclassified in our contemporary minds as health problems, and thus come within the province of the medical profession. Health care is no longer a service to be appreciated but a commodity to be shopped for and a right to be insisted upon.

Or it's the fault of our politicians and policy makers. They fail to conjure limitless resources out of an electorally tolerable tax burden. They mistake interference for improvement, and prescribe change as a panacea for every ill. They offer the illusory rhetoric of choice because it is more acceptable than the reality of rationing. They impose morale-sapping reorganisations and amateurish performance targets because they don't trust professionals to behave professionally. In fact, they don't trust the professions, full stop.

---

2   Aneurin Bevan: Minister of Health in the 1945 Labour Government led by Clement Attlee.

3   'Work expands so as to fill the time available for its completion.' Northcote Parkinson C. *Parkinson's Law: the pursuit of progress*. London: John Murray, 1958.

4   Enoch Powell, British Minister of Health 1960–3, did understand: 'There is virtually no limit to the amount of health care an individual is capable of absorbing.'

Indeed, it seems that we in the medical profession are as much part of the problem as we are of the solution. Examples of unacceptable clinical performance are too numerous to overlook. Historical squabbles and rivalries live on in the sniping between disciplines, between primary and secondary care, between the academics and the political activists, between doctors and administrators. We appear united only in the rush to feather our own nests, regardless of patients' convenience and the public purse. We are seemingly besotted with the newest technologies, the shiniest gadgets, the most expensive wonder drug. And, although we have no shortage of firm ideas about how to improve things, we can be impossibly stubborn and uncooperative for others to work with.

It is almost a defining characteristic of civilisation that it creates institutions and professions out of the universal dream of staving off disease and death. Even the most primitive communities have their shamans and witch-doctors, credited with special powers of access to the gods of affliction, who are to be invoked, obeyed and propitiated according to prescribed rituals. Yet equally universal is a sense of disappointment. And it's not just that, wriggle as we might, disease and death will inevitably catch up with us in the end. Wherever we look in the developed world we find a similar feeling that medicine aims high but, one way or another, falls short. No government, no political party, no system of administration has yet got it right. We can't even agree on who has got it least wrong. Of course, in our rational moments we understand that the 'they' who organise our lives are probably doing their best. 'They' are trying to juggle three balls: what medicine *can* do, what we *want* it to do, and what we can afford. But we look at 'them' trying as we might do at a circus juggler. We've paid our admission fee and we expect the trick to be performed, the illusion of effortless competence to be maintained. When the juggler stumbles, and the balls go flying, we feel a bit cheated, a bit foolish, and some of us want our money back.

But spare a thought for the juggler. No one likes to be a let-down, especially politicians. The reality is that modern high-tech medicine is a ravenous cuckoo in the fiscal nest, eager to gulp down far more than its fair share of resources at the expense of less assertive competitors. It is a fact of life that every individual patient wants to be the exception to the depressing statistics of disease, treatment and outcome. And it is indeed the case that the medical profession is notoriously difficult to motivate and to control. The arcane complexities of a doctor's expertise often look baffling to lay people, and can be hard to reduce to the over-simplifications in which politicians like to deal.

In June 2003, the British Prime Minister Tony Blair carried out a reshuffle of his Cabinet. John Reid,[5] who at the time had been Leader of the House of Commons for only a few months, was summoned to 10 Downing Street. The press later carried reports that Reid had looked into his leader's eyes and realised the fate that awaited him. 'Oh f*** no,' he is said to have blurted out, 'not Health!'

And yet, and yet …

* * * * *

… we must be doing something right. Almost all the doctors I have ever met count themselves blessed. They might not say as much to the Men from the Ministry, but most would continue doing the job for a fraction of the salary; it is that satisfying. The source of the satisfaction runs much deeper than the rewards of money and status. It's something more than the craftsman's pleasure in the exercise of long-honed skills – more, too, than the emotional fillip of being appreciated and trusted, although doctors are both.[6]

Searching for words to convey the nature of that deeper 'something', it's hard to avoid trite-sounding phrases such as 'making a difference', or 'doing something that matters'.

It's an everyday experience for GPs to recognise in the street the faces of people in whose lives they know at some point they made a real difference. See this noisy group of teenage lads crowding people off the pavement? 'Hello Duane,' you say to one of them. Four years ago, when his dad walked out and left him man of the house and he'd started wetting the bed again, you'd seen him a few times just to talk things over, maybe given him a hug, maybe prescribed something, and soon he didn't any longer have to bottle out of going on sleep-overs in case he embarrassed himself. 'Aw-'ight Doc?,' Duane mutters, and shoves his mates aside to let you pass. You smile to yourself. And see that middle-aged lady emerging expensively coiffed from the hairdressers? Somewhere back at the surgery you've still got the card she sent you six months earlier. 'Just to say thank you for all your help with mother,' it reads. 'It was how I know she wanted it.'

---

5   John Reid, PhD, MP, Secretary of State for Health 2003–5.

6   Ipsos MORI polls show the NHS to be the national institution that British citizens are most proud of (What the public think of the NHS, 2013). Doctors are consistently the most trusted of all professional groups (trusted by 90% of those sampled in 2013), compared with teachers (86%), judges (80%), the police (66%), journalists (22%) and politicians (16%).

All doctors, not just GPs, know the satisfaction that comes from being on hand at critical moments in patients' lives. Iain Hutchison, a leading maxillofacial surgeon, has told of how, when he was working in an Accident & Emergency (A&E) Department early in his career, 'People would come in having been in car crashes, with cuts all over their face, and I'd spend a few hours painstakingly stitching them up. And when they came in they'd feel their lives were destroyed, and just by doing a little bit of work on them … suddenly they'd feel their lives were restored again. And it was just fantastic to be able to do that, and I continue to feel immensely privileged to do what I do.'[7]

The feeling of sometimes being pivotal at a turning point in someone else's life is universally and powerfully rewarding. This is more than altruism. Altruism means doing good for its own sake. In medicine, however, doctors also do good because it makes them themselves better: not just *feel* better, but actually *become* better – more fulfilled – people. After some particularly appreciated piece of work, a doctor might modestly say, 'I was just doing my job; anyone else would have done the same.' But the patient may well see it differently: 'It's not just what you did for me; what matters is the way you did it, and the fact that it was *you*.' The patient recognises, even if the doctor may sometimes not, that the context of the human relationship within which care is given is as important as the technicalities of the care itself. And, in the doctor–patient relationship as in every other, the flow of added value is not one way. In a good piece of doctoring, the emotional rewards are reciprocal. The patient, of course, benefits from the doctor's professional experience and skill. But there is a simultaneous trade in the reverse direction, a gift from patient to doctor of what we might call 'validation', an affirmation of value, a uniquely personal endorsement not only of that experience and skill but also of the doctor's worth as a fellow human being. Individual singularities – patient's *and* doctor's – are the currency in which good medicine is transacted. The implied contract between them is that each will authenticate the humanity of the other.

Why should 'mattering' matter? Why should it be that making a difference, being the agent of relief in someone else's adversity, is such a powerful motivator, strong enough to maintain doctors' commitment despite the frustrations of real-world medicine?

---

7   Mr Iain Hutchison, Consultant Oral and Maxillofacial Surgeon, St Bartholomew's Hospital, London. Interviewed by Olivia O'Leary in *Between Ourselves*, BBC Radio 4, 24 July 2007.

Several pseudo-psychological explanations suggest themselves. One is that playing the 'good parent' to the patient's 'helpless child' bolsters the doctor's self-esteem. Or perhaps there is a more eschatological dimension. Perhaps, by embodying the role of saviour, doctors allow the fantasy to be sustained that mortals can escape their destiny and cheat death. To believe *oneself* capable of this miracle might be madness, but to credit others – doctors or divinities – with such powers of intercession allows the hope of immortality to persist while absolving oneself of responsibility when it fails to materialise.

I prefer a more biological, Darwinian, explanation. One reason for the evolutionary success of *Homo sapiens* is our capacity to extend our consciousness forwards and backwards in time, beyond the immediacy of the present moment. We have memory and imagination. We are aware not just of how things *are*, but also of how things *were* and how they *might* be. Memory allows us to learn from the past, giving us access to more information on which to base our actions. Imagination is the complementary faculty for examining the future. In our imagination, we can create as-yet nonexistent possibilities and anticipate the consequences of as-yet unperformed actions.

Being able to predict the behaviour of other people has considerable survival value for us as members of a social species. To this end, one particular facet of the imagination comes into play: namely, the ability to imagine what another person is thinking and feeling – in a word, empathy. Empathy is a social prediction tool. The better we are at empathising, the more successfully we can pick our way through the minefield of social relationships.

Psychopaths, who lack the ability to empathise, are social misfits who tend to harm others. Psychopathy is an imagination deficit disorder. By contrast, good doctors have hypertrophic imaginations. A doctor with a well-developed imagination has some sense of what it is like to be in the patient's skin, and can feel a measure of the patient's distress and worry. And when the distress is eased, and worry gives way to hope, the doctor gets a 'fix by proxy' of the patient's consolation. A portion of the relief that so matters to the patient is transformed by the power of the imagination into nourishment for the doctor's own self. Making a difference for the patient changes an already imaginative doctor for the better.

* * * * *

It can be a powerful experience to be the patient of a doctor in whom technical expertise is matched by the empathy that flows from a well-developed imagination. Most of the myriad encounters between patients and doctors are pretty humdrum: a common condition easily diagnosed and simply treated; a routine procedure uneventfully carried out; some minor adjustments made to a treatment regime. But – and it can be in an apparently straightforward consultation just as much as one where the medical stakes are high or the emotions intense – sometimes a small miracle occurs. The patient may feel unexpectedly better, unburdened, understood, out of all proportion to the apparent simplicity of whatever medical business has taken place. There may be a sense of brushing with something mysterious, of something significant happening. Perhaps just the right thing has been said, some unspoken concern given voice, some insight articulated whose life-transforming effects will play out long after the consulting room door has closed. Perhaps for the first time the patient has experienced care not as a noun but as a verb, and feels not just cared *for* but cared *about*.

'I don't generally go much on doctors,' one sometimes overhears it said, 'but mine's wonderful.' *My doctor's wonderful*: the phrase captures the preciousness of the personal bond between one patient and one doctor, and also acknowledges that some doctors somehow work greater wonders than others and are treasured for it. Medical schools and postgraduate training programmes certainly produce doctors of whom it can be said, 'My doctor's knowledgeable, or thorough, or up to date'. But 'wonderful'? We can imagine medical students leafing through their curriculum and seeing a timetable of clinical rotations, communication skills training, projects and attachments, and – particularly if they themselves have as patients experienced good doctoring – asking, 'When do we get shown how to be wonderful?'

I'll not claim for this book that it will teach anyone to be a wonderful doctor. But it *is* my belief that the factors that make some doctors admirable beyond their technical accomplishments can be identified and encouraged, and released in those who already possess them (which is most of us). I'll maintain that good doctors are as familiar with, and in command of, their own mental processes – their 'Inner Physician' – as they are with their clinical skills. Practising *adequate* medicine is a matter of aptitude and training; practising *good* medicine is additionally a matter of mindset.

This opening chapter is intended to give an overview of territory I shall explore in more detail in the rest of the book, and to prime you, the reader, to engage with various lines of thought I plan to develop. Metaphor and analogy are good ways of doing this.

You know those nests of Russian dolls, one inside another? They're called *matryoshki* ... .

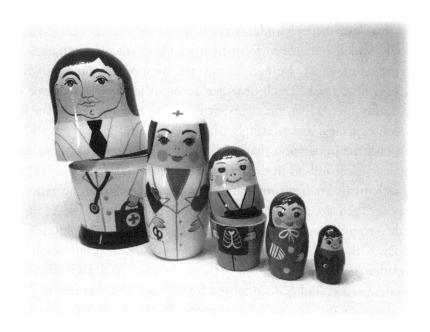

* * * * *

Medicine is like a nest of Russian *matryoshka* dolls.

Many domains of complex human endeavour are hierarchically organised: levels of functioning arranged, pyramid-wise, in order of decreasing influence from the highest pinnacle to the lowest base. An army is a good example, with its cascading chain of command linking the commander-in-chief to the lowliest grunt. This 'top-down' model is an assertive and masculine one. Those at the top are 'in charge'. They are deemed to know best; they plan strategy, issue orders and are not to be challenged from below. Such a hierarchical structure assumes and reinforces a culture of dominance and subservience. Though effective and predictable under pressure, it necessarily overrides the autonomy, and overlooks the creative potential, of individuals at all but the highest level. While an ethos of control and obedience may be appropriate in a military context, it has tended to cause problems when applied to social projects such as health care. In this area at least, doctors are notoriously reluctant to let politicians' claims to know best go unchallenged; and clinicians, while they will happily acknowledge being 'in the front line' in a battle against suffering, expect to have more influence on policy and strategy than is granted to a trench-bound squaddie.

Biology, too, has until relatively recently tried to understand life, including human life, in terms of hierarchies. Descartes started it, with his dualistic account of man's material body mysteriously governed by a non-material soul. To this day, medical students are taught how biochemical events give rise to cells, which coalesce to form tissues and organs, which make up the organ systems of which human beings are composed. Some enlightened departments take the hierarchy further, recognising that individuals come together in families, which make up societies. But many still find the fact of human consciousness as irritatingly undeniable as did Descartes, and leave students with the impression that psychology is a 'suppose we must, but it's not proper science' add-on in the medical curriculum.

The mechanistic 'man as sum of his parts' approach can lead to a disjointed and impoverished account of what it is like to be alive. The Hungarian polymath Arthur Koestler attempted to reconcile the principle of 'layered complexity' with such intangibles as emotion, art, morality, ambition, reverence and destructiveness.[8] He did it by postulating that each hierarchical level of organisation had goals imposed from above, but was free to develop its own autonomous ways to achieve them. With this 'fixed rules, flexible strategies' account, Koestler was able to model many apparent anomalies in biology and human behaviour. One consequence was that combinations of relatively simple components in a system can develop unexpected characteristics of unpredictable complexity. (A contemporary example is how a large network of computers, connected in straightforward ways, gives rise to the astonishing world-changing information system that is the internet.) This is the phenomenon of emergence, to which I shall return in Chapter 10 of this book.

But back to the Russian dolls.

Practising medicine doesn't *feel* like a hierarchical activity – not once the consulting room door has closed, and there's just you and the patient, each with the other's full attention. Becoming a doctor; hearing patients' stories and witnessing their crises; being an occasional 'maker of differences'; playing a variety of roles on a variety of stages; building a career; developing and sometimes regressing as a human being – it all *feels* like something far more three-dimensional. The image of the *matryoshka* dolls, differing in scale and detail but not in fundamental shape, seems an altogether truer metaphor.

---

8   Arthur Koestler (1905–83) was born in Budapest to a Jewish family, and studied science and psychology in Vienna. A member of the German communist party 1931–8, he fled via France to England, where he became a vehement anti-communist and anti-Nazi. He became a naturalised British citizen in 1945. Koestler worked as a journalist, novelist (e.g. *Darkness at Noon*, 1940) and philosopher of science (e.g. *The Sleepwalkers*, 1959). The ideas summarised here are from *The Ghost in the Machine*, 1967. London: Hutchinson. Reprinted Arkana, 1989.

Even if you don't have an actual set of dolls at home, you can imagine the feel of them in your hands as you open up successively smaller figures until you reach the littlest: structure within structure; innermost within inner within outermost. Each doll will stand alone, but together they form something much more intriguing. The nest is more than the sum of its parts. The fitting together is the point.

So imagine yourself curious to know how medicine ticks, and in particular how doctors tick. Allow the idea that a proper grasp calls for a simultaneous unpacking of phenomena on several levels – on *five* levels, in fact, represented by five nested Russian dolls. Each doll, each level of explanation, has its own distinctive surface features. But each is moulded to accommodate the contours of the next doll in, which it itself contains. The inner dolls impose their general shape, but not their details, on the outer.

The outermost of our five dolls is the public face of organised health care on a national scale. It's the largest doll, the most expensive-looking and the most elaborately decorated, the one designed to catch your eye as you window-shop; and it's the favourite plaything of politicians. It encompasses all the political and bureaucratic machinery it takes to service an enormous state enterprise. Policy, priorities and (horrid phrase) 'direction of travel' are set by ministers and implemented, through a pyramidal command structure, by the Department of Health, NHS England, Clinical Commissioning Groups and various service providers.[9] A measure of independent scrutiny is provided by various 'arm's length' regulatory and advisory bodies such as the General Medical Council (GMC), the Care Quality Commission, and the National Institute for Health and Care Excellence (NICE). Professional interests are represented by the medical royal colleges and the British Medical Association.

Perhaps unsurprisingly, the face of the 'organisation' doll can look hard and unsmiling. It speaks the language of politics, management and commerce. It lives in a PowerPoint world of flowcharts and surveys, spreadsheets and balance sheets. It feasts on paper. Its gaze – and we should not criticise it for this – is partly directed back over its shoulder towards the electorate. At this outermost institutional and political level, all the major players – ministers, civil servants, quangos and professional bodies – have to concern themselves

---

9   These and most similar examples are taken from the British National Health Service, and, where there are differences between the devolved UK administrations, the NHS in England. This is purely because my personal experience is chiefly of working as an English GP. Readers from other settings or at other times should, however, have no difficulty making the relevant translations to the equivalent bodies in their own countries and healthcare systems.

with what will please their constituencies. What is clinically desirable, or of limited application, may have to be subordinated to what is cost-effective and popular. On the national stage, when people speak of 'patients' they usually mean 'voters'.

It is ironic that health policy is largely determined by people who are healthy. Most legislators will have experienced illness only as a minor inconvenience or an acute emergency, or something that happens to somebody else. Their concept of what constitutes good care tends to reflect what they themselves expect in their own relatively privileged circumstances. Thus, they judge primary care by how rapidly and conveniently they can get a simple problem fixed. The quality of hospitals (a word used interchangeably with 'health care' in much political rhetoric) is measured principally by numbers of operations and length of waiting times. While these things are important, they are dangerous over-simplifications. In the painted designs on the outermost *matryoshka* there is little room for more subtle details such as the quality of medical thought or the depth of personal commitment. It is not until we open this outer doll that we see a face that is recognisably human.

* * * * *

The second in our nest of medical dolls is the medicine people think they know from film and television. It's the glamorous medicine of *Casualty*, *ER*, *Angels*, *Holby City*, even *M*A*S*H*. It's the clichéd medicine where blood flows and blue lights flash, and expensive machines go 'ping'; where we see eyes narrowed in steely resolve above a surgical mask; where the products of the pharmaceutical industry are either miracle drugs or ticking time bombs. It's headline medicine chunked into episodes and punctuated with neat resolutions. In this medical world of the popular imagination, the doctors are 'characters', who talk and act in inverted commas, marking a crucial divide between the doctor as depicted and the doctor as 'liver of an unseen life'. They are often portrayed as heroes – but heroes with an occasional endearing personality flaw, which can be redeemed as we follow them through a suitably poignant case history. Others are even more two-dimensional, and have only walk-on cameo roles: 'rude consultant', 'incompetent GP', 'over-worked junior doctor'.

Why are such hackneyed representations of medicine so widespread in vernacular culture? Perhaps the stereotyping of professionals serves a purpose in our collective semiotics – the way we create and manipulate symbols as proxies for forces in our lives that would otherwise be too difficult to understand or too powerful to control.[10] We make heroes of our fictional doctors because that is, at some level, what we want the real ones to be. Sickness and death are such formidable adversaries, and the forces of high-tech medicine such awesome weapons, that only heroes who knew what they were doing could fight and stand a chance of winning. And we give these latter-day Saint Georges their little character blemishes to reassure ourselves that they are sufficiently like the rest of us to be trusted to stay loyal and to keep us safe in their hands.

The larger-than-life, too-good-to-be-true version of medicine that the second doll represents has unfortunately imposed something of its contours onto the outermost, political, doll. If these fictions were to be believed, medicine is hypnotically popular, superhumanly powerful and unlimitedly expensive. The doctors we see on screen are either self-aggrandising demigods or adorable saints in white coats. However, combine their mass popularity with the high degree of self-confidence necessary to do their job and it's not surprising that, seen through political eyes, doctors are something of a threat. Like Gulliver in the land of Lilliput, the medical profession can seem an out-of-control giant, to be tethered and brought to heel – not with ropes, but with the tight reins of regulation. Idolatry is dangerous for the idol as well. Politicians seldom miss an opportunity to dispel any impression that the institutions of medicine are beyond criticism.

As symbolised by the outermost *matryoshka*, medicine is distorted by being scaled up to industrial proportions in order to mass-produce a commodity called 'care'. And to the second doll, 'care' is more like a story line in a soap opera, over-simplified and sentimentalised for dramatic effect.

But neither one, to my mind, is the authentic face of medicine. Beguiling though it is for doctors to play politics, and flattering though it is for our fictionalised alter egos to star so prominently in collective mythology, we should remind ourselves of one crucial premise. Historically and (I shall

---

10 The definition of what constitutes a 'profession' is controversial. However, the following rings true to me, at least as far as the traditional professions – medicine, the law, teaching and the Church – are concerned. All have as their area of expertise domains of life that are (a) crucial to the wellbeing of the individual (health, freedom, wisdom and salvation respectively), but (b) too complicated for every individual to master. We therefore subcontract to professionals, the deal being that we trust them to look after our personal vulnerabilities, and reward them accordingly, as long as they treat us 'professionally', that is, prioritising *our* interests above their own or those of the state.

It is tempting, and probably important, to ask whether a medical workforce that colluded in imposing state political and financial targets and directives on individual patients would continue to be worthy of the name 'profession'.

argue) essentially, the practice of medicine is a private and personal affair, conducted one to one behind a door closed against bureaucrats or voyeurs. To me it is axiomatic that a doctor's attention and skills are primarily focused, despite every distraction, on the unique circumstances of *this* patient, and now *this* one, and now *this*.

Recent decades have seen a stampede of innovations in health care, both technical and administrative. The ensuing impetus has been to direct the medical gaze 'outwards', towards new technologies, higher investment, greater expectations, clearer targets, more robust accountability, and tighter regulation.

But, while many of the changes have contributed laudably to the drive for higher quality, they have come at a price. In pursuit of mass efficiency, effectiveness on an individual scale has been compromised. In our hospitals, changes to consultants' contracts and training programmes seem, perversely, to be resulting in a dilution of clinical experience at senior level and to demoralising career uncertainties amongst junior doctors. In general practice, the 2004 new contract[11] that improved the management of many serious and chronic conditions has, perversely, eroded the continuity of personal care; turned out-of-hours care into a lottery; undermined doctors' pastoral and advocacy roles; and, quite possibly, by encouraging practices to recruit salaried partners to do the donkey work, sabotaged the career prospects of a generation of our brightest young doctors. The cash incentives of the new contract have introduced a government-imposed agenda into individual consultations, so that the interests of doctor and state surreptitiously compete for priority with those of the patient.

In this book I attempt a reversal of the direction of medical gaze, back towards the inner core of the individual doctor, where the humanity of medicine has its mainspring. Or perhaps a bifurcation of the gaze comes closer: good doctors can embrace the imperative to practise efficient 'public' medicine while at the same time fostering their own personal effectiveness as they strive to be the best possible help to the patients who entrust themselves to their care.

* * * * *

---

11 Key features of the contract included: financial incentives for GPs to meet supposedly evidence-based clinical and administrative targets; the right of GPs to opt out of responsibility for out-of-hours care; and the ending of patient registration with a named GP.

And so, when we come to the third *matryoshka* doll we see, for the first time in this metaphorical unpacking, the features of a clinician who works with actual patients. The face on the third doll is the face of the 'doctor as expert' – someone who knows about sickness and disease, and what can be done about them.

The doctor of the third doll is, stereotypically, the product of a traditional medical education. He – statistically it's still probable that it's a 'he', and, in a *Men are from Mars, Women are from Venus* kind of way,[12] he'll probably *think* like a 'he' – will probably have set his sights on a hospital-based career, ideally a consultant post. To this 'doctor as expert', medicine is primarily a scientific exercise – to be undertaken with respect and applied with sensitivity, of course, but at bottom a hard-nosed discipline to which the methodology and mindset of science are appropriate. He will, again typically, have gained exceptional grades in maths and sciences at school. At medical school, he will have been inducted in the 'medical model' as the rational approach to the diagnosis and management of disease. He will see illness as an indication of a biological malfunction, and accurate diagnosis as the prerequisite for evidence-based treatment. To this end, he will take pride in acquiring detailed knowledge and practical skills, and in keeping himself up to date and abreast of the latest research and technical developments. Allowing that no one doctor can any longer be expected to master the whole of medicine, or even one of its broader divisions, he will specialise and sub-specialise as his career develops. If you ask him, he will explain that, while he doesn't claim to be an expert outside his chosen field, that chosen field he knows in depth, and his advice can, as far as is mortally reasonable, be relied upon. He thinks of himself, in short, as a specialist; he provides a service called 'care'. He doesn't get much involved in politics, although he is often suspicious of management and wishes his experience at what he likes to call 'the coal-face' was better appreciated. Nor is he much concerned with medicine's public image, either the wincingly inaccurate dramas his wife watches on television or the scare stories he reads in his patients' tabloid newspapers. It is enough for him to concentrate on maintaining his skills, practising his craft, seeing

---

12 In his 1992 bestseller, John Gray used this planetary metaphor to describe his perception of how the two sexes think and communicate. 'Men offer solutions and invalidate feelings,' he wrote, 'while women offer advice and direction ... [In coping with stress, men] tend to pull away and silently think about what's bothering them, [while women] feel an instinctive need to talk about what's bothering them ... Men are motivated when they feel needed, while women are motivated when they feel cherished.'

the patients, doing – within the limits of the resources made available to him and in the best traditions of his profession – the best he can for them. He is a conduit in a white coat, siphoning aliquots of medical science from its cisterns and silos into a never-ending procession of needful souls.

It would be possible to construct an entire health service staffed, on the medical side, solely by 'third doll' doctors. Indeed, if our world were populated exclusively by robots, and if it were only our mechanical malfunctions that qualified for the attention of the medical engineers, that would be the best way to do it. And yet wouldn't there be something dispiriting, something stultifying, about such a world, if real people had to live in it? Wouldn't there be something sinister if all we had were doctors whose remorseless reliance on logic rendered them indifferent to the endearing perversities of human illogicality?

Let there be no misunderstanding: the third doll, whom I have dressed in a specialist's white coat and teased for his dry rationality, is only a metaphor. Thus caricatured, he symbolises just one aspect of medicine's multi-layered complexity. In the *real* world, real life specialists are softer, moister, rounder people. And there is nothing wrong with expertise in skilled and considerate hands.

But this doll, for whom clinical practice is a straightforward matter of applying medical science to the particular case, has a 'cat who's discovered the cream' look on his face that brings out the devilment in me. I imagine our conversation …

'Do you think,' I ask him, 'that there are any diseases that *can't* ultimately be explained by science?'

'The short answer is "no",' he replies. 'Ultimately we're all biological systems. And, ultimately, biology is just molecules, doing what molecules do, obeying the laws of physics and chemistry. Life and health depend on a set of biological variables staying within certain limits. Disease, or death, is what happens if too many of them stray from their "safe" range. As I see it, medicine is the science of coaxing wayward bits of physics and chemistry back to where they belong.' And here perhaps I frown, for the doll tells me, 'I know what you're going to say.'

'You do?'

'You're going to recite the usual list of things you think are prone to diseases *not* caused by molecules in motion – things like consciousness, emotion, thought … Well, let me tell you, the evidence shows –' (and I think he expects me to cringe before that supposedly killer phrase) '– the evidence shows that all these subjective psycho-ey things are the consequences of specific configurations of chemicals and electricity in the brain. And that puts them squarely in the frame for a scientific approach. Descartes is dead,' he continues, his eyes burning with the afterglow of the Age of Enlightenment. 'There *is* no ghost in the machine.'

'I probably don't disagree,' I say. 'But no, actually, I was going to ask you a follow-on question. Do you think there are any kinds of human hurting that doctors are not qualified to try and relieve?'

'Hurting? You mean "illness"?'

'Not just illness. Let's say "distress".'

'Well, not things like poverty, or unrequited love, obviously.'

'Why "obviously"? Isn't being poor or lovesick ultimately caused by molecules in motion?'

'Well yes, but … it's a question of scale. Some aberrations of physics and chemistry are too massive for a humble doctor to tackle.'

I let the 'humble' pass. 'So if a patient comes to you and says, "I'm ill because I can't afford proper food," or, "My heart's broken," you would say …?'

'I'd say, "As a doctor I can't help you with these matters; you need a politician, or a social worker, or just a friend." '

'And for these roles you're not qualified?'

'Not *medically* qualified, no.'

'You don't think your own personal life experience qualifies you, gives you something useful to contribute?'

'Absolutely not. Well, maybe a bit of common sense, a bit of worldly wisdom. But nothing more. In medicine, where the skilled application of science can help rectify biological aberrations, I'm a professional. That's my field of professional expertise, and it's to be kept strictly separate from my private life outside medicine. In every other field I'm an amateur, neither more nor less qualified than the next man. A good doctor is one who knows his limitations.'

A good doctor is one who *pushes against* his limitations, I'm thinking. But I don't say so. Instead I ask, 'So you wouldn't see your own personality, your own psychology, as having any bearing on your clinical effectiveness?'

My specialist makes the sound usually spelled 'pshaw!' 'Correct,' he declares. 'Boundaries, that's the thing. What goes on in here,' (and he taps his head), 'is private, nobody's concern but mine. Can't have it interfere with the business of diagnosing and treating.'

I think I hear another sound, much fainter this time, like a muffled squawk of protest. But I press on.

'So what sort of relationship should there be between doctor and patient?'

'Well, a professional one. Civil, of course. Courteous. Respectful – and that goes both ways.'

'And one where they can have feelings about each other?'

He looks horrified. Perhaps I didn't put that very well.

'Absolutely not! Highly unprofessional! That sort of thing might be acceptable in psychiatry, but I'm talking about proper doctors here. No, no, start entertaining feelings about your patients and you're up before the GMC[13] before you know what's hit you.'

I hear it again, a definite squawk, louder this time. It seems to be coming from inside the doll I'm talking to. I prise it open, and an indignant-looking smaller fourth *matryoshka* tumbles out. 'Phew,' she says, 'I thought I was going to burst.'

* * * * *

This next doll clearly has something to get off her chest, and draws a deep preparatory breath. 'As a GP, …' she begins. But I shush her with a gesture, and stand her beside the larger 'specialist', who until a moment before had been her cocoon. It is not immediately obvious that this is any kind of medical doll at all. Not for her the consultant's white coat, nor the perfection of his expensively tailored suiting. She sports – oh dear! – a cardigan.[14] Whereas he flourishes with quiet pride the tools of his trade – the stethoscope, the scalpel – she, if she has any, must be keeping them coyly concealed in, one supposes, a drawer, a cupboard, an anonymous black briefcase. Beside his self-confidently professional persona, she cuts an altogether less impressive, more timid figure.

But something rather strange is happening. I inspect the two dolls alternately, making comparisons, noting differences. And yet whenever my gaze

---

13 General Medical Council: UK statutory body with responsibilities 'to protect, promote and maintain the health and safety of the public by ensuring proper standards in the practice of medicine.' It 'maintains a register of qualified doctors; fosters good medical practice; promotes high standards of medical education; and deals … with doctors whose fitness to practise is in doubt.'

14 Some years ago, when I was Convenor of the Panel of MRCGP examiners, I invited a senior examiner for the Royal College of Surgeons to meet me at the Royal College of General Practitioners. He reported that when he had told his colleagues back at his home college where he was going, one of them had said to him, 'Oh, you're off to the College of cardigan-wearers, are you?'

flicks back to this modest-looking GP doll she seems subtly altered. I'm reminded of a butterfly fresh from its chrysalis, flexing its virgin wings as the sun warms and strengthens them. I sense beneath her unremarkable exterior an unexpected but understated complexity, in contrast to her more flamboyant companion. She has the ability, chameleon-like, to vary her appearance – and, I anticipate, her language and behaviour – according to the ever-changing circumstances of her clinical habitat. From the look on his face, I suspect number three doll is also a bit puzzled by this newcomer. With a faint pursing of the lips and a dipping of the eyebrows his expression flickers almost imperceptibly from disdain via condescension to – surely not! – fear.

Her own counterpoint of emotions plays out on the features of the GP doll as she contemplates her supposedly senior colleague. I think I may have glimpsed awe: but blink and you'd miss it. Her default position seems to be the engaging friendliness of a new puppy; but at times her eyes flash with an evangelical sparkle, and at others her teeth are bared like a Jack Russell let off the leash and locking on to a high-stepping pedigree Saluki. 'I was listening to you saying how medicine was all science and no feelings,' she tells number three doll. 'With respect, that may be true in your operating theatre, but surely medicine is an art as well as a science? General practice is, at any rate.'

'Whoa,' I say. A squabble between the *matryoshki* looks to be on the cards. Hastily, I step in with that ever-dependable gambit, 'Tell me about yourself.'

It transpires that she, like the specialist, had been good at sciences at school, though she had struggled with physics A-level and would have preferred, had the timetable allowed it, to do English alongside her chemistry and biology. Asked at her medical school interview who or what had motivated her to become a doctor, she declared Dr Tertius Lydgate in George Eliot's *Middlemarch*[15] to be her inspiration and role model. Whether the interviewers were deceived by her claim or impressed by her effrontery in advancing it she could not tell. In the event, they accepted her, and she embarked upon the 5 years of debt, cramming and belittlement that it takes the average medical school to convert a young person's vocation into a medical qualification.

Like most undergraduate curricula, that at her institution had recently undergone refurbishment. According to the brochure, the course was now 'integrated', 'problem-based' and 'learner-centred'. The students were

---

15 *Middlemarch, A Study of Provincial Life*, novel by George Eliot, published 1871–2. One narrative strand traces the career of the ardent and idealistic Dr Lydgate as he attempts to bring the benefits of the new scientific medicine to his cholera-threatened community.

'exposed to patients' from the start.[16] But through the eggshell veneer of this new educational orthodoxy (she told me) an undercoat of traditional 'teaching by humiliation' often peeped through. Some of the more conservative consultants – particularly in specialties awash with blood, high-tech gadgetry and private practice – spurred on the smarter alecks amongst the students with a vision of success in their own prestigious fields. Over the heads of the others, the prospect of 'ending up in general practice' hung as an Awful Reminder of the wages of mediocrity, much as children who don't eat their broccoli are threatened with constipation and bad skin.

The ambitions of medical students often keep pace with the specialties through which they rotate during training. Students working in Casualty, where their manual skills are useful to the junior medical staff and their enthusiasm is popular with patients, aspire for the duration of their attachment to become A&E consultants, or surgeons, or general physicians. When they move to the children's ward, where the kids are fun and would just as soon be played with as diagnosed, they want to be paediatricians. Even (though this is rarer) departments of radiology and psychiatry can prove temporarily seductive to the students passing through them.

Our GP doll – her name turns out to be Emily – Emily too had her clinical aspirations shaped by her experience of successive components of her undergraduate programme. But in her case there was a time lag. Her aspirations were out of phase. Whereas the more eager of her peers fell in love with whichever department they happened to be working in at the moment, Emily always felt she had preferred the subject she had just finished. Moving from urology to dermatology, she realised in retrospect how much satisfaction she had derived from the gratitude of the old men whose agonising urinary retention she could relieve with a simple catheter. When dermatology gave way to obstetrics, it dawned on her how mechanical were the technicalities of childbirth compared with the subtle interplay of psychology and environment manifest in diseases of the skin. Nevertheless, compared with orthopaedics, which she was due to do next, obstetrics at least brought her into contact with hope, with potential, with the extremes of anguish and joy.

Almost imperceptibly, Emily's backward glances towards the earlier stages of her training built into such a cumulative sense of disillusionment that, during her fourth year as a student, she began to question her choice of

---

16 'Exposed to patients': a revealing phrase. It makes the patients sound like a source of danger, as injurious as radiation or chicken pox. It is ironic, too, that the patients probably think of themselves as being 'exposed to students'.

career. She still passionately wanted to *be* a doctor. It was just the process of *becoming* one that disappointed her.

She understood of course that if you were to be an effective doctor you had to study, in obsessive detail and with objective detachment, how your patients' bodies worked, and what went wrong with them, and what medical science could do about it. But somehow it seemed that the more closely you examined the disease that afflicted your patient, the less store you set by the individuality of the patient who had to bear the affliction. To many of her teachers, 'the patient' looked to be an abstraction, little more than the anonymous bed-bound object of their clinical curiosity. Yet it was their individual uniquenesses and complexities that made the patients precious to their friends, lovers and relatives who trooped onto the wards at visiting time. And it was precisely those uniquenesses and complexities, Emily thought, that made them worth devoting her life to. Each patient was intriguingly different from her, and at the same time essentially the same. But medicine – at least as most of her teachers taught it – appeared to concern itself only with those anatomical, physiological and pathological ways in which human beings are pretty much all the same. Nowhere in the curriculum, it seemed, were the idiosyncrasies of their personalities and the singularities of their lives thought worthy of much attention, let alone cause for celebration or respect. It was ironic, Emily reflected, that a doctor whose purpose was to make a difference to individual lives had to be trained systematically to disregard individual differences. Whatever sense of vocation she had felt when she entered medical school was in danger of being throttled by the very educational system that was supposed to equip her with the practical skills necessary for its expression.

Once, on the obstetric delivery ward, Emily had been observing a supposedly straightforward birth. Just as labour reached its third stage, the senior house officer (SHO) had slipped out to answer his bleep, leaving matters in the hands of an inexperienced pupil midwife – and Emily. She saw the baby's head crown, then emerge. But the rest of its body failed to follow. Alarmingly rapidly, the baby's face turned navy blue, and the displays on various monitoring devices changed in ways Emily was sure they were not supposed to. One of them began to ping a warning, and the young father-to-be, wide-eyed and sweating, said, 'Oh God, what's happening?' Emily and the midwife were as if paralysed. Miraculously, the SHO returned, blasphemed, and deftly freed the baby's neck from the two turns of umbilical cord which were threatening to strangle it. 'No problem,' said the SHO; and then again, 'No problem.' But later, when the baby was safely in the arms of her smiling parents, he had looked Emily in the eye and slowly, reprovingly, shaken his head. Afterwards she had fled to the sanctuary of an on-call room, thrown herself onto the bed, and sobbed. Had anyone then asked her the reason, she would have said it was the release of tension, that she was weeping for the disaster that might have been. But, if truth be told (and now is the first time Emily has confided it), she was crying from self-pity. She was jealous of the baby, jealous of the fact of its rescue from suffocation. *What about me?*, her tears were saying; *won't someone help* me *breathe?*

The Emily-doll's eyes are moist. 'And *did* anybody?', I ask.

'Sorry about that,' she says. 'It was just a low patch. I was overtired, and that business with the baby felt like it had been a close shave. Things like that happen in medicine. You just have to get used to it. If you can't stand the heat, get out of the kitchen, and all that. And I didn't want that. Did anybody *what?*'

'Did anybody help you get through the bad patch? Help you to breathe?'

'Oh sure,' she says, more matter-of-fact now. But it is the brittle, emotions-only-just-under-control nonchalance of the widow replying to banal condolences at the post-funeral reception. 'Next was my general practice rotation, and that did the trick.'

'In what way?'

'Maybe I was lucky in the practice I went to, but I was attached to a GP who was really enthusiastic about what he did. And he knew his clinical medicine too, which came as a bit of a shock. I mean, in hospital all we ever heard about GPs was how all they saw was coughs and colds, and they couldn't diagnose anything serious, and they were always trying to get patients admitted who didn't need to come in. Particularly the registrars seemed to think general practice was where you ended up if you were an also-ran, if you were someone who fell off the hospital promotion ladder or weren't bright enough even to set foot on it. To be fair, some of the consultants would sometimes say what a difficult job it was to be a Jack of all trades, but they'd say it in a sneery kind of voice that you knew meant they were thinking, *master of none*. But the GP I was with showed me that hospital practice wasn't the only way you could be a good doctor. It was as if he could see a bigger picture than the specialists. In fact he used to say that a lot – 'the big picture'. He said if you wanted to treat patients, and not just their diseases, you had to have a wider perspective than if you were just a specialist. He said every specialty was an important piece of medicine, but it was still only one piece in a bigger picture.'

'I can see he made an impression on you. But can you summarise what you discovered about general practice that attracted you to it?'

Perhaps unsurprisingly – she is after all only a wooden doll – Emily's response, though fluent and convincing, sounds a bit mechanical. She rattles off, as if rehearsing a familiar catechism, a list of ways in which medicine as undertaken in general practice is a different enterprise from its hospital-based cousin, with its own clinical territory and working methods. In general practice she begins, ticking off this first point on her fingers, the illnesses that patients present for the doctor's attention don't always – indeed, almost never – conform to the typical profile of diseases as described in textbooks and taught in medical schools. GPs often see diseases at an early, undifferentiated stage of their evolution, before the full array of diagnostic hallmarks has had time to develop. The GP, therefore, has to find ways of living with, working in, and making decisions in spite of a fog of clinical uncertainty. What is more (second point), the ways patients in general practice present their problems are profoundly modified by their personalities and psychologies, their social and cultural milieus, and their educational, employment and financial status. Each patient brings a unique combination of emotions and worries, information and misinformation, realistic and misguided expectations, all of which have to be factored into the doctor's diagnosis and management. Moreover (and thirdly), in what Emily likes to call 'the real world' patients tend to suffer from more than one thing at once. 'Real' patients have multiple conditions and multiple therapies, which coexist and overlap and interact and quarrel, making the doctor's task one of perpetual compromise.

All this, Emily concedes, potentially applies to hospital-based medicine as well. Whereupon the third doll, the specialist, who has been listening with rising indignation, harrumphs and makes to interrupt. 'Of course it does!', he says. 'All patients are different, we know that. You GPs have no monopoly on ...'

But in hospital, Emily argues, there is a collusive fiction that individual differences, everything except the pathological process, are of limited relevance. Ideally, the patient entering hospital should – figuratively if not literally – lie still and naked on a bed while the fierce spotlight of specialism is focused on the offending part. By contrast, generalism inhabits a misty landscape in which elaborately disguised and camouflaged problems endlessly drift in complex choreography. 'High-tech medicine,' she asserts (and I don't know whom she is quoting), 'is the glorification of means above ends, of labels above narratives, of detail above context.'

I feel I should applaud. She has the grace to blush. 'It's what I like to tell my own students,' she says. 'Sorry, I know I tend to get a bit evangelical. It's just that ... remember the baby with the cord round the neck? When I was feeling suffocated and dehumanised by the way we students were being force-fed with specialty after specialty? I just knew something inside me was in serious danger as a result of the process we were being put through. But I couldn't give it a name until I did my GP attachment.'

'And then you found you could? Give it a name?'

'Yes. Emily.'

'Emily?'

'Yes. Emily the person. That's what was in danger. All the personal things that made me *me*. Me the bright one of our family, the first to be a doctor. The me who got four A grades in maths and science but didn't go on the pill until I was 22. The me who told the interview panel she wanted to be like Tertius Lydgate, and now cringes at the memory. The me who used to wince when the consultant obstetrician called the patients 'Mummy', and I had to pretend I found it charming. The me who froze when that baby nearly died. My GP placement gave me the language to put into words why scientific medicine, for all its successes, was actually incomplete and simplistic. It showed me that what kind of person you were was just as important for being a good doctor as how much you knew. You had to complement the science with your own warts-and-all humanity. But medical school didn't teach us students how to do that. On the contrary, it seemed as if the whole curriculum was geared to training it *out* of us.'

Emily pauses. Her eyes have moistened again, memories surfacing, the widow jolted back to the brink of tears by the sight of a cushion no longer crumpled on her husband's favourite chair.

'You didn't learn all that in your general practice seminars,' I gently suggest. Another pause: then …

'It so happened that the couple who'd had that baby were registered with the practice I was attached to. The GP sent me out to see them at home. He didn't know, of course. The baby was thriving and they were over the moon. They made me tea, and let me hold her, and then the father said, "Hey, you were there when she was born." I said, "Yes, I was just a student, you know, observing." And he said, "Yes, I remember. She had the cord round her neck, which was bad, apparently. And you were terrific, so calm, you didn't panic, just got the doctor back and everything was all right. We're really grateful." And do you know what I was thinking?'

'If only they knew?'

'I was thinking, *If only they knew*. When I got back to the surgery I told my tutor what a sham I'd felt, and we had a discussion about it. To this day, I find myself telling my own students and registrars the same things.

Sometimes when I'm in the consulting room, particularly with a patient who seems to expect more from me than purely medical expertise, I'll be sitting there being the cool professional, and I get a strong feeling that the professionalism is just a mask, a veneer, and that underneath I'm actually out of my depth and floundering. And with that comes a fear that I'm about to be rumbled. Someone's about to expose me as a humbug and say, 'You don't know what you're talking about. You're no more qualified than anybody else. You've no business setting yourself up as an authority.' But of course they never do. The mask stays in place. And I guess it has to. Patients take from us whatever it is they need; and they have the right to do that, even if what they take is something we don't think we have, or if what helps is something we hadn't thought would be helpful. That's a trade secret – and it's a valuable one. Knowing our *own* vulnerabilities teaches us to respect other people's. And that, I suspect, is the basis of empathy.'

I steal a glance at the 'specialist' doll, the third *matryoshka*. There is a sardonic curl to his lip; he's not taking Emily's self-exposé well. This 'we are all frail mortals' talk is not what he expects from a fellow professional. The way he sees it, he has worked and studied for many years in order to develop an expertise and to overcome his own frailties so that he may better confront those of his patients. And Emily, for all that her clinical world is a long way from the cutting edge that is his own, has been similarly trained. Or so he had assumed. Yet she seems to be claiming that, to be a good doctor, it's enough merely to have a few technical skills up the sleeve you wear your heart on. To him, this is a betrayal. The effectiveness of the medical care patients receive, he thinks, should not depend on anything so arbitrary and fickle as the mental state of the doctor who chances to treat them. *When you're hungry*, he thinks, *you're not overly concerned with the pattern on the plate. I didn't get where I am today by wearing my heart on my sleeve.* And he is, of course, correct: were he a different kind of doctor, his career would have taken a different course.

Emily has at last fallen silent. But something inside her still seems to be searching for expression, struggling to find a voice. She wishes – as we all do – to account for herself, to be understood and accepted *for* what she is and *in spite of* what she is. She is clearly a very good doctor; most of her patients and many of her colleagues will tell you so. But what it is that makes her a good – an effective – doctor is hard to pin down. Her sound clinical knowledge and skills are necessary but not sufficient. So are the soundness of her judgement, her ability to put people at their ease, and the tireless way she will argue her patients' case against the sapping inertia of NHS officialdom. Her admirers, and they are many, would describe her as compassionate, sensitive, insightful, dedicated and – as far as her ability to diagnose 'beyond the label' is concerned – instinctual. And, as we know, she can list a dozen ways in which her approach as a medical generalist differs from that of her specialist colleagues. But these attributes are the 'what' and the 'how' of her practice, not the 'why'. She has a sense that her professionalism flows from some internal wellspring, some 'inner physician' that is the source of motivation and compassion not just for her but for every good clinician – something which, could it but articulate, would have an answer to that *faux-naïf* interview question, 'Why do you want to be a doctor?'

To a doctor like Emily, 'care' is more than a commodity, more than a service; more even than a verb. Care – caring – is a response, something that arises impromptu in the face of certain human predicaments. This kind of caring may have its physical expression in the skills and routines of professional behaviour. But the process of professionalisation is only secondary. A doctor's training lays a veneer of detail over something already there, something the medical school can only take for granted in its undergraduates, an intrinsic capacity for compassion that precedes – and may indeed conflict with – the laborious business of formal education. It is as if inside every professional there is – or at least once *was* – an 'amateur within'.

* * * * *

'An amateur within': I had taken Emily to be the last of our nest of medical *matryoshki*, but this phrase prompts me to examine her more closely. And sure enough, there is a seam around her wooden waist that I had not noticed before. Cautiously I prise it apart. Emily does indeed contain a fifth and (I check) final figurine, which I gently extract. It's a fragile little thing, naïvely carved and simply decorated. It is casually dressed, and wears a wide-eyed guileless look on its youthful face. And yet it has been there all along, unsuspected, nestling inside the previous four. It has lain buried deep inside medicine at the organisational level. It has gone unrecognised, too, within the over-glamorised medicine of popular imagination. Yeti-like, it has been rarely glimpsed and is generally debunked in the 'doctor-as-applied-scientist' camp. Even Emily the generalist, the 'doctor-as-specialist-in-the-patient-as-individual', has managed to lead much of her professional life unconcerned with whatever vestiges she may be harbouring of her pre-medical self.

I propose to call this central doll – or rather, everything for which it is a metaphor – the 'Inner Physician'. It will be my contention in this book that the Inner Physician plays a crucial but under-appreciated role in how medicine is practised. The relationship of individual doctors – you and me – to our own Inner Physician forms a template shaping the whole of our professional life. Consciously or by default, we can either allow the Inner Physician to contribute to our practice of medicine or exclude it from it. That choice conditions every level of our daily work, from the loftiest of our professional values down to the minutiae of our clinical activity. At the institutional level, aspects of their Inner Physicians that most doctors have in common influence the medical profession's herd behaviour and shape its collective unconscious.

Your Inner Physician is:

- your 'amateur within'
- a psychological legacy from your pre-medical life
- the person you were before you were made into a doctor
- a subset of your thoughts, emotions, memories, motivations, attitudes, habits, principles and beliefs that you have carried into, through and beyond medical school
- a non-medical component of your present-day professional mindset
- the 'beginner's mind' you retain even as you transform yourself to 'expert' medical scientist.

To summarise and anticipate where this line of thought will lead: every one of us, including those destined to become doctors, has a private, invisible and often unexpressed inner world of thoughts, drives and feelings that shape our dealings with the outside world and the other people in it. The inner world of the neophyte medical student can seem naïve and amateurish when set against the great weight of science-based knowledge and skills that must be learned. Most medical school curricula seem to be based on the belief that the way to turn students into professionals is to train the amateurism out of them. Raw curiosity and a wide-ranging view of the human condition have to be sacrificed in favour of less flexible categorisations if human pathology is to be brought within range of medicine's therapeutic artillery. (*'There are four key principles of ethics, and five stages of bereavement. Here are the guidelines for the management of primary infertility.'*) Nevertheless, elements of the pre-training mindset of the young doctor – who probably already knows right from wrong, may have lost a loved one, and knows what it is to be worried about the future – do survive the process of professionalisation, even if in compromised or suppressed forms. This residuum, the 'amateur within the professional' is what I mean by the Inner Physician.[17]

This book will explore how doctors' Inner Physicians profoundly influence the way they practise medicine. I contend that the quality and effectiveness of what doctors do is affected by how familiar and comfortable they are with their own inner worlds, and by how far they can allow their own human uniqueness to be a factor in their clinical work.

As we shall see, doctors tend to incline towards one of two default positions. There are those – and they tend to be specialists – who believe that their personal psychology is best kept separate from their working practice. Like the third *matryoshka*, they would consider their inner worlds to be irrelevant to their clinical work, a distraction, a corrupting influence on their attempts dispassionately to bring scientific medicine to the relief of their suffering patients. There are others – and they tend to be generalists – who believe that familiarity with their own inner worlds is an advantage, adding value, power and insight to their therapeutic role. I am of this camp. They – we – are persuaded that our capacity to help over the widest possible range of human distress is enhanced in proportion to our capacity to understand and manage our most potent asset – the unique selves that we ourselves are. If this book succeeds in its task, I will bring you to the view that a vigorous and self-confident Inner Physician is not the enemy of professionalism but potentially its most valuable ally.

I have used the image of the nested *matryoshki* to convey the concept of an Inner Physician at the core of contemporary medicine. Before moving on to more substantive subjects, there is one final thought to be gleaned from the 'concentric dolls' metaphor. Each of the four outer dolls has an Inner Physician as its kernel, albeit buried at different depths. But each treats it differently.

---

17 A note on terminology. The reason for the *inner* tag will, I hope, become clearer on further reading. But why *physician*? To pre-empt the premature raising of hackles, let me explain that I mean 'physician as opposed to lawyer or layman', not 'physician as opposed to surgeon, pathologist or GP'. I could have gone with *inner doctor*, but that sounds, frankly, a bit flat and lacking in a degree of gravitas I think our profession merits. Besides, what I have to say about the inner life of doctors is less relevant to a surgeon's manual dexterity than it is to the traditional 'physicianly skills', such as diagnosis, decision-making and communication, which are the stock in trade of every practising clinician (including surgeons).

When doctors get together in groups and organisations – and particularly when they begin to engage with the machinery of state control in the form of managers, policy makers and politicians – something unfortunate happens. They start to talk in ways intended to appear remorselessly and irresistibly logical. Presumably they think that unrelenting rationality is the only properly professional approach. But it all too easily becomes the false rationality of the flat-earther, brooking no contradiction or compromise, no uncertainty or ambivalence. It is as if they were born with their minds made up. (And, to be fair, doctors' collective fluency in pseudo-rational rhetoric is easily matched by that of their managerial and political interlocutors.) Possibly it's a macho group thing. Doctors *en masse* collude in trying to look hard-nosed; anything soft and fuzzy, anything that smacks of emotion or psychology, is defined out of the equation and off the agenda. The negotiations that resulted in the 2004 GP contract[18] are a case in point. Publicly at least, discussions between representatives of the profession and the government were presented in the flinty language of cost-effectiveness and strategic planning. Only a few maverick voices such as Iona Heath[19] had the prescience to ask more thoughtful questions such as, 'Will this new contract help GPs to be the sort of doctors their patients value? Does it encourage the kind of personal service they can be proud of? Will it enhance public trust in, and appreciation of, general practice?'

Institutional medicine – doll number one – likes to keep its Inner Physician bound and gagged, and very firmly away from the action. The Inner Physician of the second doll – the fictionalised doctor of popular culture – is suppressed in a different way.

Until they actually get sick and need a real doctor, people (if they think about it at all) have clear and polarised ideas about how doctors ought to behave, and about how they imagine their inner lives to be. In popular

---

18 The contract has unquestionably improved the standard of general practice in some clinical and geographical areas. However, its consequences – possibly unintended but certainly regretted by some – include: lowering the priority of non-targeted areas of practice not susceptible to easy quantification; the erosion of one of general practice's much-vaunted virtues, continuity of care; an increase in the number of GPs employed on a salaried basis, rather than as partners, to the frustration of significant numbers of new entrants to general practice; and a significant reduction in the proportion of newly qualified doctors opting for a career in general practice, dissuaded by what they perceive as its prevailing business ethos.

19 See, for example, Heath I. The cawing of the crow ... Cassandra-like, prognosticating woe. *British Journal of General Practice* 2004; **54**: 320–1.

imagination, doctors are either heroes or (less commonly) villains – Dr Finlay or Dr Shipman.[20] Indeed, leaving aside Shipman's real-life atrocities, the imperfections of fictional doctors – such as arrogance, lasciviousness, ambition – tend to be portrayed as endearing pockmarks on an otherwise admirable character. They may contribute to a sub-plot storyline, but we don't expect our screen doctors' personal idiosyncrasies to impact on their clinical judgement. Interesting though it may be to peep into the moving parts and hear the creaks and squeaks as the doctor gears up for action, in a crisis we expect the machinery to function reliably. Given our tendency to project our need for powerful caring figures onto the medical profession, we dare not imagine them as too much like our incompetent lay selves. And so, in novels and screenplays, they are idealised to the point of implausibility. While we the audience may concede that our fictional doctors may have their Inner Physicians, and indeed may like to glimpse them from the safety of our armchairs, we don't like to credit them with any executive role in the business of doctoring. Like a small child on the arrival of a distant aunt, the imagined Inner Physician is patronised, patted on the head, and sent off to play quietly in another room.

But it is with how the third and fourth *matryoshki* – the specialist and the generalist – relate to their Inner Physicians that this book is chiefly concerned. Our specialist is rather uneasy about his. He is willing to concede the existence of his own inner life, but is nervous that it could prove disruptive if allowed to intrude into his clinical practice. Emily the generalist, on the other hand, is more at ease with hers. In principle she endorses the Delphic injunction 'Know thyself'[21] and the biblical 'Physician, heal thyself'.[22] She

---

20 *Dr Finlay's Casebook* (BBC Television 1962–71) was a series of dramas set in a pre-NHS general practice in the Scottish lowlands. The crusading energy of the young Dr Finlay was tempered with the pragmatism of his senior partner Dr Cameron, and their approach to medicine was characterised by common sense and devotion to their community.

Manchester GP Dr Harold 'Fred' Shipman (1946–2004) was unfortunately not fictitious. For reasons that have never been convincingly explained, he murdered at least 250 of his patients over a 23-year period while preserving the appearance of a devoted family doctor. An enquiry by Dame Janet Smith into the Shipman case questioned the effectiveness of the GMC as a regulatory body and led ultimately to the introduction of mandatory revalidation for medical practitioners. Four years into an indeterminate life sentence, Shipman hanged himself in Wakefield prison.

21 Γνῶθι σεαυτόν – 'gnothi seavton', 'know thyself' – was inscribed in the forecourt of the temple of Apollo at Delphi, site of the famous oracle.

22 Gospel according to Saint Luke, chapter 4, verse 23.

is not afraid to acknowledge that her own personality is an important component of her professional style, and that a little judicious self-awareness and self-disclosure can prove helpful, particularly for patients with complicated emotional problems.

Let us remember that the 'dolls' metaphor is just a metaphor. Let us be clear: the 'specialist' and 'generalist' as I have so far depicted them are stereotypes, clichés, exaggerated and parodied in order to make some general points. What really matters to real patients in the real world is how real specialists and real GPs treat them. And in this context I believe that what I am calling the Inner Physician represents something of real importance. The practice of medicine can be conducted in one of two ways – a 'generalist' way or a 'specialist' way – depending on whether or not the doctor's inner world is allowed to participate. Doctors who prefer to exclude their Inner Physician tend to think and practise in a specialist kind of way. Doctors who allow their Inner Physician a degree of involvement in the clinical process tend to think and practise in a generalist kind of way. It's a question of mindset. I am not asserting that either way is better than the other, even less that GPs are 'better' than specialists or vice versa. I do believe, however, that in the present culture of medical education generalism is under-taught, that the generalist mindset is under-appreciated, and that the generalist way of doing medicine is under-valued.

The remainder of this book is my modest attempt to redress this imbalance.

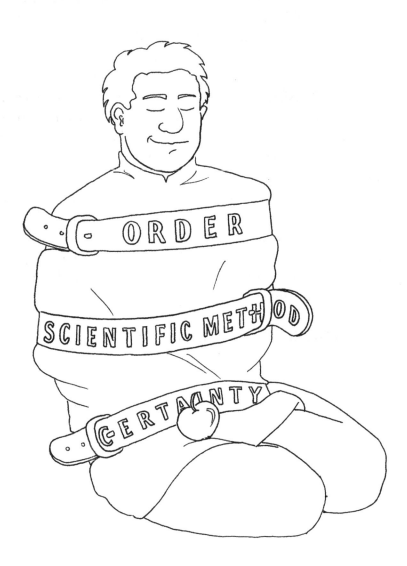

Chapter 2

A backwards glance

All science begins with astonishment, but the human being behind the instrument is much more important than the instrument itself.

Antonie van Leeuwenhoek (1632–1723)

Dutch lens-maker and microscopist

In the previous chapter I likened the current state of medical thinking to a set of nested dolls with, at its core, the private individuality of the individual doctor. This chapter will lead us towards a similar conclusion, but by a different route. By taking a historical approach and asking *How did we get to where we are?*, I shall try to set the development of medicine within the wider history of science and the scientific method. This will be a brief and selective account of medicine's contribution to the human project, and of how its prevailing ideas came to prevail. Inevitably, it will be heavy on generalities and light on detail; this is not the place for a comprehensive world history of medical science and philosophy.[23] Nevertheless, the development of medicine from its prehistoric roots to its present complexity does have important implications for the analysis I want to advance of how individual doctors mature from student via rookie to expert. History suggests that medicine has not fully caught up with the leading edge of science in understanding the importance of the 'observer effect' and other ideas culled from quantum physics. Together, this chapter and the previous one are intended to prepare us to loosen some of our assumptions about what is 'good' medicine and how 'good' doctors do what they do.

In the course of this book I shall be reflecting upon three separate medical relationships: that between different kinds of doctor (specialist and generalist);

---

23 If such a history would be of interest, I know of none finer than *The Greatest Benefit to Mankind* by the late Roy Porter (London: HarperCollins, 1997).

that between doctor and patient; and the internal relationship between a doctor's public and private selves. Each of these three is the product of the evolution of ideas and the ebb and flow of prevailing wisdom.

We know only two objective 'givens' – birth and death. But in between there are some experiences so nearly universal as to be *almost* givens, including sickness, injury, the loss of faculties. In the subjective world, the world behind our closed eyelids, there is an additional given – the inexplicable fact of consciousness. But in this world too, where 'only I know what it is to be me', we discover some further commonalities. Three are pre-eminent, in the sense that they power much of mankind's cultural development: the emotions of love, fear and – amazement. From love and fear, and particularly from the tension between them, arise many of the social institutions that unite or divide us; the systems of government that protect or enslave us; and the clashes of value and self-interest that drive our history. But *amazement?*

Amazement – the dawning realisation that things are like *this!* – must be a uniquely human experience. The infant discovering her own toes; the teenager in the maelstrom of first sexual attraction; the walker stopped in his tracks by a shaft of light in a landscape; van Leeuwenhoek examining pond water through his spherical lens and first seeing protozoa; the DNA penny dropping for Crick and Watson as they puzzled over Rosalind Franklin's X-ray diffraction plate; the Apollo 11 astronauts galumphing on the dusty surface of the moon: all are united by a sense of *Wow!* Rational and imaginative beings that we are, that exclamation is swiftly followed by questions. Following close on amazement come curiosity and reflection. Curiosity, the need to understand, impels us to ask 'Why?' and 'How?' Reflection, the 'Let me see now' response, prompts us to consider how fresh experience connects with previous.

The adventure that is science is driven by amazement. What we call 'the scientific method' is the rational organisation of curiosity and reflection. Its outcomes often take the dry forms of laws and theories, classifications, analyses and papers. But it is not the prospect of contributing to the world's accumulation of knowledge that primarily motivates the scientist: it's an innate urge to make sense of the unexplained. Newton did not sit under his apple tree, nor Darwin board the *Beagle*, intent upon formulating the laws of motion or the theory of evolution. Something unexpected

> It is their sense of amazement that makes people try to understand.
>
> Aristotle (384–22 BCE)
> Greek philosopher, pupil of Plato
> From *Metaphysics*, Book I,
> part 1 (c. 350 BCE)

happened, and they noticed it, welcomed it, allowed it to amaze them. The making of sense came later. *Wow! before How?* might be the motto of the best scientists and the best artists; and also, perhaps, of the best doctors.

Pasteur said that 'where observation is concerned, chance favours only the prepared mind'.[24] That is unduly pessimistic. Insight begins with the capacity, which we all possess, to be surprised. It is in the nature of our minds to be prepared for the unexpected. It's just that sometimes the responses of curiosity and reflection, which should come next, get trained out of us.

* * * * *

And so the history of science, including that of medicine, is the unfolding quest to explain the things that amaze us. We have to assume that it didn't take much to amaze our prehistoric ancestors. How astonishing it must have seemed that life should begin and end; that the sun should set and rise again; and that people should on some occasions survive disease and on others succumb. The passing millennia have made us blasé, and we no longer find these miracles amazing. But it is perfectly understandable that our forebears should have done, and that the explanations they came up with should have been magical ones. After all, if you have only the immediate evidence of your five senses to go on, how else are you to account for the rhythms of light and dark, of harsh and gentle seasons, other than through the agency of unseen forces of unimaginable power? How else to explain life's blessings and catastrophes, save as the acts of benign or malevolent gods, to be worshipped or placated in ways you hope they'll approve of, and given names and human-like depictions in order to encourage them to be friendly? And to whom else should you turn for support in the dangerous business of intercession, unless it be to shamans and witchdoctors empowered for the purpose, who have a foot in both worlds – the visible and the imagined – and whose rituals nevertheless make a kind of symbolic sense that may even help by driving out the demon of helplessness? (And before we get too pleased with our sophisticated selves, we should remember how many of our contemporaries continue to blame their health problems on mysterious energy imbalances and undetectable toxins, to be corrected with magical 'superfoods', by sticking pins in invisible dotted lines, or through the sacrifice of some of life's fattier pleasures!)

---

24 'Dans les champs de l'observation le hazard ne favorise que les esprits préparés.' Louis Pasteur (1822–95), French bacteriologist. Address given on the inauguration of the Faculty of Science at the University of Lille, 7 December 1854.

If we want to trace what Roy Porter calls 'the triumphal progress of medicine from ignorance through error to science',[25] we could do no better than start in the Athens of antiquity.

It is probably fair to credit the Ancient Greeks with inventing rationality, or at least with the courage to try to base an entire way of life upon it. If Greek civilisation had a single defining word, it would be λόγος – logos, which comes to us as *logic* and all the *-ologies*. The primary meaning of λόγος is the spoken word; but, together with its abstract variant λογισμός, it is used to signify all the virtues that flow from the sensible use of language by a disciplined mind: reasoning, deliberation, principle, judgement, insight. From around 900 BCE and over the next six centuries, the Greeks systematically wrested control over human affairs out of the hands of imaginary supernatural puppeteers, and brought notions of cause and effect back into the realm of the ordinary mortal's common sense. They had their gods, of course – in legions: standing room only on Mount Olympus. But gradually they came to regard this pantheon, not as the hands-on directors of events on earth, but rather as a portal giving access through myth and narrative to deep, symbolic truths about the human psyche.

As the gods grew old and impotent, the belief gained favour that the key to wisdom, health and happiness lay in harmonious relationships between man and the natural world. Take medicine, for example. Asclepius, who was probably an actual healer around 1200 BCE, was widely worshipped as a god throughout Greece in temples, such as those at Kos and Epidaurus, devoted to his name. There, the sick underwent a ritual of 'healing sleep'. They would pass what must have been a restless night in an open-air snake-infested dormitory near the temple, to be visited in their dreams by Asclepius or one of his priests, who would give advice. In the morning, the patient would depart cured, or confident of a cure. At least as therapeutic as the ritual, however, were the setting and the regime. Temples to Asclepius were situated in peaceful surroundings, with gardens and fountains, a theatre for amusement and a stadium for gentle athletics. The visitor would enjoy mineral baths, nutritious meals, moderate exercise and (snakes notwithstanding) rest and relaxation – a healing package for which folk will pay good money to this day.

Then as now, rationality did not always prevail. In the fifth century BCE the Sicilian philosopher Empedocles advanced the theory that the universe was composed of four elements – earth, air, fire and water – in varying combinations. Mainly because of its author's persuasive personality and oratory, Empedocles' model was swiftly and widely accepted. From there it was only a

---

25 *Op. cit.*, page 29.

small step to the doctrine of the four bodily 'humours' – blood, phlegm, black bile (melancholy) and yellow bile (choler) – from whose balance or imbalance health or disease resulted. The doctrine of humours, which persisted for two millennia, was well established by the time Hippocrates (*c.* 460–377 BCE) set up in practice on his home island of Kos.

Hippocrates was the first physician whose rational approach to medicine is documented. He was sure that health and disease, like every phenomenon, were susceptible to logical investigation and reasoned explanation. Writing on epilepsy, then called 'the sacred disease', he said, 'It is not any more sacred than other diseases, but has a natural cause, and its supposed divine origin is due to man's inexperience.' Lacking instruments, and barred by taboo from dissecting the human body, Hippocrates relied solely on his own powers of

---

The Hippocratic Oath

I swear, by Apollo the Physician, and Asclepius, and Hygeia, and Panaceia, and all the gods and goddesses, making them my witnesses, that to the best of my ability and judgement I will keep this oath and covenant:

To reckon him who taught me this art as dear to me as my own parents; to share my own belongings with him; if he is in need of money, to give him a share of mine; to look upon his offspring as if they were my own brothers, and to teach them this art, if they so wish, without fee; by precept, lecture and every means of instruction I will teach the art to my own sons, and those of my teachers, and to other pupils who have agreed to be bound by the laws of medicine, but to no one else.

I will apply such therapeutic measures as, to the best of my ability and judgement, I consider to be for the benefit of my patients, and to abstain from anything that is harmful or mischievous.

I will neither administer a deadly drug to anyone who asks for it, nor will I make a suggestion to this effect. Similarly, I will not give a woman a pessary to induce abortion. In purity and holiness I will live my life and practise my art.

I will not cut any person for the stone, but will leave this to be done by men who are practitioners of this work.

Whatever houses I visit I will enter for the benefit of the sick, and will abstain from every intentional act of mischief and corruption, including the seduction of any woman or man, be they free person or slave.

Whatever I may see or hear touching on people's lives, whether or not in the course of my professional service, which ought not to be made public, I will not divulge, reckoning that such matters should be kept secret.

As long as I keep this oath inviolate, may it be granted to me to enjoy life and the practice of my art, and to be respected by all men at all times. But if I transgress and break this oath, may the opposite be my fate.

observation to make a diagnosis and give a prognosis. In this latter particularly, knowing that accurately predicting the course of a disease was a sure way to build a reputation, he was spectacularly successful. Many of his clinical dicta and observations remain valid to this day.[26] In other respects, too, Hippocrates anticipated the best qualities of today's medical professionalism. His well-known oath (see box) – with the possible exception of the financial obligation of student to teacher, and his uncompromising stance on abortion and euthanasia – remains a comprehensive and up-to-date ethical creed. By all accounts, his consulting style and bedside manner were what we should today call 'patient-centred'. 'There are three factors in the practice of medicine,' he wrote, '- the disease, the patient and the physician. The physician is the servant of the science, and the patient must do what he can to fight the disease with the assistance of the physician.' And again: 'Make frequent visits,' he advised. 'Be especially careful in your examinations, and enquire into all particulars.' He continued shrewdly, 'Keep a watch also on the faults of your patients, which often make them lie about the taking of things prescribed. They will not confess to this, but blame is thrown onto the physician.'

Hippocrates personified the ideal of the learned physician, in whom science, philosophy and common sense are united and who attends the patient as a personal advocate rather than as a magician or state functionary. Given that 25 centuries have elapsed since Hippocrates' time, it is disheartening how little we have added to his understanding of medicine, beyond a massive accretion of factual detail. The history of ideas is of course beset with blind alleys and false dawns. But we might have expected the Hippocratic approach, based on the rational interpretation of clinical observation, to have advanced us further and faster than in fact turned out to be the case. What went wrong? In a word, dogma.

* * * * *

---

26 Perhaps his best known, the first in his collection of *Aphorisms*, is: 'Life is short, the art of medicine unending; opportunity is fleeting, experiment is dangerous, and judgement is difficult.' Others include: 'Desperate cases need the most desperate remedies'; 'In acute diseases, employ drugs very seldom and only at the beginning. Even then, never prescribe them until you have made a thorough examination of the patient'; 'The vomiting of blood of any kind is bad; its passage as excrement is not a good sign, nor is the passage of black stools.'

An excellent selection, including the *Aphorisms*, *Prognosis*, *Fractures* and *The Nature of Man* (a critique of the doctrine of humours), is *Hippocratic Writings* (trans. Chadwick J. London: Penguin Books, 1983).

The European locus of the ancient world's political, military and cultural influence shifted from Athens to Rome, and medicine's centre of gravity relocated with it. Hippocrates' pioneering legacy survived the move and remained the dominant tradition. The Romans' contributions to medical progress were, first (and successfully), public health measures such as running water and mains drainage, and, second (and perhaps of less benefit) – Galen. Galen (129 to *c.* 216 CE), a Greek trained in Alexandria, became the best-known and most influential amongst the physicians of Rome. His illustrious patients included the soldier and philosopher Marcus Aurelius and the emperors Commodus and Septimus Severus.

Galen's reputation rested largely on his studies in animal anatomy, largely based on the dissection and vivisection of pigs, goats and Barbary apes. He described the valves of the heart; demonstrated that the arteries carried blood, not air; identified most of the cranial nerves; and, by tying off the recurrent laryngeal nerve, showed that the brain controlled the voice. Nonetheless, as a stepping-stone in medicine's 'triumphal progress from ignorance through error to science', Galen was a disappointment.

There are two sorts of error to which scientific progress is prone. The first is to draw illogical conclusions from sound observations. The other results from applying rational thought processes to irrational beliefs. Galen was guilty of both. From his detailed anatomical studies of animals he concluded, for example, that blood formed in the liver was carried through the veins to the tissues, where it was transformed into flesh. Equally misguidedly, he uncritically applied his conclusions from animal experiments to the human organism. Dissection of the base of the calf's brain revealed a network – the *rete mirabile* – of nerves and vessels. Assuming (erroneously) that the same existed in humans, he asserted that the seepage of blood through this network resulted in the formation of 'psychic pneuma' – a subtle material, refined by the liver into something akin to a soul, that was the vehicle of conscious sensation. Galen also accepted unquestioningly the doctrine of humours, refining it so as to locate the supposed humoral imbalances within specific organs. He considered that virtually every case of human disease arose from a surfeit of one or other humour in the bloodstream. Given this irrational premise, his almost universal remedy – blood-letting to remove the excess – was a rational one: rational, but wrong.

We might perhaps forgive Galen for these errors were it not that his shortcomings as a researcher were compounded by flaws in his own character. He seems to have been a bombast and a bully. A prolific author (he wrote over 300 works, of which 150 survive), Galen's influence as a teacher owed more to his domineering personality than to his clinical acumen. For a thousand years, no one dared challenge him on matters of anatomy and physiology, even when the evidence from human dissection was plainly contradictory. Nonetheless Galen, like Hippocrates, knew the value of a good bedside manner. He understood that it was essential for a successful physician to secure a patient's trust through explanation, empathy, and responsiveness to subtle signs of anxiety. Against these virtues as a role model for subsequent generations of doctors, however, we must offset his legacy of rigidity and dogmatism. Galenic authoritarianism is a weakness still not completely expunged from the medical psyche.

Medical progress might have circumvented Galen's obstinacies and inconsistencies had his life not coincided with another momentous development in European civilisation – religion. It is hard not to see the early history of the Christian church as an intellectual road-block in the path of rational science. As the church gained in numbers and influence, it required of its adherents that they eschew the materialist ideas of the classical world and turn their gaze instead to higher things, to a world invisible and transcendental. Unlike the Greek and Roman gods, who could be affectionately indulged while mortals got on with the serious business of philosophy, the new 'one God' required faith rather than reason, and devotion rather than discussion. Granted, he also called for compassion rather than cruelty, and humility rather than pride. But what he got, in the form of his organised church on Earth, was an executive who set doctrine above evidence and obedience above curiosity. For many centuries, the response of the church to rational debate was to suffocate it with dogma and kick logic into the long grass.

Given the venom with which Rome oppressed the early Christians, this is perhaps not surprising. Tight control of your devotees and a fervent belief in a better life to come have always been strong defences against persecution, especially when administered through the hierarchical command structures of which mankind is so fond. Nevertheless, faith and dogma, whatever their merits as a basis for religious experience, do not encourage the pursuit of rationality.

* * * * *

Thus medicine, as a would-be scientific discipline, was engulfed by the dark age of medievalism, awaiting first the Renaissance and later the Enlightenment before resuming where the Hippocratic tradition had left it. During the intervening 1500 years, disease continued to be viewed as a divine test or punishment, and death as the doorway to Paradise; it was almost a blasphemy to seek to avoid either. A capacity for amazement *did* endure – was encouraged, even – but only as long as it took the form of amazement at God's creation and his unconditional love for mankind.

Ultimately, inevitably, the urge for cultural and intellectual exploration reasserted itself. During the 14th century an accommodation was reached with the ecclesiastical establishment. Art and scholarship were after all to be acceptable, provided their products were devoted to the glory of God and to reinforcing the teachings of Mother Church. The community of artists and scholars could live with that. It was like uncorking a shaken bottle of champagne. Imagination and creativity burst upon Europe and spilled into every field of endeavour. The air filled with music; poets picked up their tireless pens. The dust was blown off the old Hippocratic and Galenic texts. In order to achieve the verisimilitude God deserved, painters of the human body, Leonardo da Vinci (1452–1519) pre-eminent among them, examined it in unprecedented detail. Dissection of the dead became legitimate, and the discipline of anatomy respectable. It became once again permissible to look within the body for the causes and effects of disease. The very names of the anatomists from the medical schools of Italy, recognisable to this day, mark out the history: Vesalius, Falloppio, Eustachio.

It was in the natural sciences, however, that the spirit of the Renaissance most plainly conflicted with the teachings of the church. Galileo (1564–1642) is a case in point. Copernicus's heliocentric theory of the planetary orbits had appeared in 1543. But as long as it remained just a theory, unsupported by objective evidence, it could be dismissed by the church authorities as heretical and 'wrong by definition'. However, when Galileo, using a telescope of his own devising, made the astronomical observations that convinced him that Copernicus was right, and publicly stated as much, the Inquisition had no option but to prosecute and, by threat of torture, obtain Galileo's famously qualified recantation.[27] Galileo made many other, less controversial, discoveries in the fields of mathematics, physics and mechanics. His practice of submitting theory to the test of observation has established him as one of the founders of the experimental method.

---

27 Popular legend has it that Galileo, leaving his trial after a successful plea bargain whereby he agreed that he had been wrong to publish his belief that the Earth moved round the Sun and not the other way round, muttered under his breath, 'Eppur si muove' – 'But it *does* move.' There is, unfortunately, no documentary evidence that he made such a remark. Nor can historians confirm that his experiment of dropping weights from the Leaning Tower of Pisa ever took place. That we like nevertheless to believe these tales shows how deeply ingrained is our tendency not to let the facts get in the way of a good story.

For a long time medicine, although as keen as any other discipline to join the Renaissance party, lacked its equivalent of Galileo's telescope. Many of the agents and processes we now understand to be the physical causes of disease are invisible to the naked eye and undetectable without instruments. For lack of a microscope, medical science lagged behind the other sciences. It remained prone to Galen's error – applying rational thought processes to unsubstantiated beliefs, and thereby arriving at wrong conclusions.

The resurgent humanism of the Renaissance gave the physician a heightened sense of his own dignity as a man of learning, but was slow to deliver the empirical scientific knowledge that would have justified it. *Faute de mieux*, Renaissance doctors often talked what we now consider to be nonsense. They had nothing yet to supplant the doctrine of humours as an explanatory framework, although some of them toyed with astrology as an alternative, or performed theatrical hocus-pocus on samples of urine and stool. Their passion for venesection continued unstaunched. The physicians' rivals, the surgeons and apothecaries, had perhaps an easier time of it. At least the causes of surgical problems were usually obvious, gangrene and war injury being among the commonest, and the remedies, amputation and bone-setting, obvious as well. And the apothecaries could at least draw on a long history of practical folk wisdom when they prescribed their herbal and chemical specifics, some of which – rhubarb, coca, opium, mercury – had well-established therapeutic properties.

Then as now, some of the chattering classes saw through the medical humbug. Thus: 'I observe the physician with the same diligence as he the disease', wrote John Donne.[28] And, from John Owen:[29]

God and the doctor we alike adore
But only when in danger, not before;
The danger o'er both are alike requited,
God is forgotten, and the Doctor slighted.

* * * * *

---

28 John Donne (1572–1631), English metaphysical poet. Quotation from *Devotions upon Emergent Occasions*.

29 John Owen (*c.* 1560–1622), Welsh schoolteacher, whose command of Latin earned him the sobriquet of 'the British Martial'. His *Epigrammata* (1606), from which this quatrain is taken, was found so offensive by the Catholic Church as to be placed on its Index of Forbidden Books.

During the European Renaissance, the pursuit of reason and creativity (if offered to God) had again become respectable. Then cautiously, erratically, as the 16th century reached middle age, territories that had opened up to intellect and imagination became progressively colonised by solid information and data. Facts began to catch up where speculation had led; the Enlightenment was upon us. New intellectual virtues appeared: analytical rigour in argument; the pursuit of verifiable evidence; the testing of hypothesis through experiment. The dissemination of printed books enlarged the community of thinkers who could encourage and stimulate each other. New technologies allowed glass to be fashioned into lenses for microscopes and telescopes. An intoxicating conviction grew that consistent and intelligible principles were at work in human affairs and in the natural world. Naïve amazement was followed by its logical consequence – science. From Descartes[30] onwards, and reaching a pinnacle in Newton,[31] the scientific revolution that saw the Universe, including man, as an intricate machine was under way.

A bridge between the Renaissance and the Enlightenment was William Harvey,[32] whose discovery of the circulation of the blood, based on meticulous dissection, physiological observation and common sense, marked a tipping point in the field of medicine between error and science. According to the prevailing Galenic dogma, arterial and venous blood had quite separate functions. Galen recognised that arterial blood contained air, but thought it was sucked into the heart during diastole via the pulmonary vein, mingling with venous blood, which seeped through unseen pores in the interventricular

---

30 René Descartes (1596–1650). Born in Normandy, educated by the Jesuits, settled in Amsterdam. Descartes's early work was in algebra and geometry. After a quasi-mystical experience he set out the principles of 'natural philosophy' in his *Discours de la méthode* of 1637. Descartes expounded a dualistic model of man as a physical machine inexplicably imbued with non-material mind-stuff. His premise that everything about man can potentially be understood by science except the single axiomatic fact of consciousness – 'Cogito, ergo sum', 'I can think, therefore I exist' – anticipates by 300 years elements of Gödel's Incompleteness Theorem.

31 Sir Isaac Newton (1642–1727), English mathematician and physicist. In mathematics, he invented the infinitesimal calculus; in optics, he discovered the composition of white light. In his *Principia* of 1687, Newton set out his three laws of motion, from which, together with his work on planetary motion, followed the universal law of gravitation.

32 William Harvey (1578–1657), English physician, educated at Cambridge and Padua universities. Physician at St Bartholomew's Hospital and personal physician to King Charles I. *Exercitatio Anatomica de Motu Cordis et Sanguinis in Animalibus* (An Anatomical Exercise Concerning the Motion of the Heart and Blood in Animals) was published in 1628.

septum. Harvey, by animal experiments, showed that the volume of blood expelled from the heart during systole during the course of an hour far exceeded the total blood volume. He also demonstrated the 'one-way flow' effect of the valves in the heart and peripheral veins, and concluded – correctly but nevertheless bravely – that 'the blood in an animal body is impelled in a circle.'[33]

Other fanciful errors began to topple like stacked dominoes. Advances in chemistry finally saw off the doctrine of humours. The Italian Fracastoro, studying the spread of syphilis ('the French disease') and other epidemics, concluded that certain diseases were spread by imperceptible 'seeds' transmitted by air or by contact. The Dutchman Antonie van Leeuwenhoek reported to the Royal Society of London the first sightings of bacteria through his microscope. When the same instrument was turned onto the cellular structure of human tissues, the discipline of pathology was able to assume its proper place in the canon of medical sciences. The clinician Thomas Sydenham, 'the English Hippocrates', recalled his colleagues' attention to the importance of properly observing diseases at the bedside. In rapid succession the great theories of the biological world were proposed by the great thinkers of the age and confirmed by painstaking research: Darwin and the theory of evolution; Mendel and the gene theory of inheritance. Laënnec invented his stethoscope, Jenner his vaccination, Lister his antisepsis, Morton his ether machine. Maxwell[34] developed his theories of electromagnetism. The rest, as they say, is history.

Yet, for all that the last hundred years have transformed the technology and the techniques of medicine beyond recognition, its deep structure – the 'science' part of medical science, the commitment to reason and experiment

---

33 According to legend, Huang Ti, the 'Yellow Emperor' of China, ruled for nearly 100 years around 2600 BCE, and is credited with setting out the principles of traditional Chinese medicine in a text entitled *Huang Ti Nei Ching Su Wen – The Yellow Emperor's Classic of Internal Medicine.* More credibly, this probably consists of medical writings by various authors collated during the last two centuries before the Christian era in the name of the then despot of China, Shih Huang Ti. Whatever its provenance, the *Nei Ching*, one of the oldest medical texts in existence, contains the following:

All the blood is under control of the heart. The blood current flows continuously in a circle and never stops.

34 James Clerk Maxwell (1831–79), Scottish physicist. He unified the theoretical understanding of electricity, magnetism and inductance, and showed light to be an electromagnetic phenomenon, work which paved the way for the development of quantum theory.

guided by curiosity – has remained essentially unchanged since the time of Newton. With Newton, the outlines of the scientific method were drawn. The rest of the picture has been detail and colouring-in. More importantly, the frame that surrounds it – the system of assumptions and methodologies that demarcates science from other domains of human activity – has, at least until Einstein, remained constant.

And that word *frame* brings me reluctantly but inescapably to some discussion of paradigms.

* * * * *

---

paradigm:

'a world view underlying the theories and methodology of a particular scientific subject'

New Oxford English Dictionary (1998)

'coherent set of beliefs about cause–effect relationships within a given class of context'

www.tetradian.com/glossary

'a collection of assumptions, concepts, practices, and values that constitutes a way of viewing reality, especially for an intellectual community that shares them'

Thomas Kuhn, in *The Structure of Scientific Revolutions* (1962)

'a word too often used by those who would like to have a new idea but cannot think of one'

Mervyn King, Governor of the Bank of England

Stakeholder; *blue sky thinking*; the organisational *mission statement* of banalities in fancy dress; *choice,* that favourite excuse of the meddlesome politician: some words and figures of speech have the ability to cause disproportionate irritation, like eczema. It's not that they don't mean anything; on the contrary, the idea behind the once-striking expression is usually all too obvious. What irritates is the way some of those who use them do so with such delight you might think they'd discovered the lost gold of Montezuma. Or else – and this is more common – these originally sharp phrases have been so blunted and devalued that they now indiscriminately festoon their users' chatter like verbal bling.

The word *paradigm* is in danger of being prostituted in this way, and I am reluctant to pimp it further. But the notion of the paradigm – a coherent way of accounting for how things work – does stand for something important in the history of ideas, and we should not disparage it. One of them – the scientific paradigm – would probably claim pre-eminence, in that much of the material success of *Homo sapiens* has stemmed from it.

It is in our nature as human beings to try to understand the world we find ourselves in, such understanding being the prerequisite to exerting the control over our individual and corporate destinies that is the distinguishing feature of our species. It is said that until not many centuries ago it was possible for a single person to know everything that there *was* to know. And indeed this may have been true – not in the sense that one human brain could memorise all known facts, but rather that a dedicated polymath could achieve a working understanding of the principles of every domain of knowledge. Understanding does not depend on knowing lots of facts but on having the right conceptual framework on which they can be assembled and linked together. Paradigms are just such frameworks: agreed sets of rules and conventions about how various aspects of the world are to be understood. A paradigm defines the scope of what is to be examined, and specifies the kind of language in which questions may be asked and answers accepted. It sets the terms on which problems are deemed legitimate and explanations considered plausible.

The term *paradigm* itself has a confused history. In Greek, παράδειγμα means a *pattern* or *example*, or, interestingly, a *warning*. Grammarians adopted it to refer to a table of all the inflected forms of a Latin noun, adjective or verb. Then in 1962 this obscure little word was thrust into popular prominence by an American physicist and historian of science, Thomas Kuhn. In his book *The Structure of Scientific Revolutions*[35] Kuhn used the word *paradigm* to refer to a system of beliefs, assumptions, theories and methods generally shared by scientists at a particular period of time. Kuhn summarised the key features of a paradigm as defining:

- *what* is to be observed or studied (i.e. the territory over which it claims to hold sway)
- the kind of questions that are supposed to be asked
- the methodology whereby answers will be sought, and
- how the results of enquiry will be validated and interpreted.

---

35 Kuhn TS. *The Structure of Scientific Revolutions*. Chicago: University of Chicago Press, 1962.

On this basis we could state the traditional scientific paradigm as: The universe operates on consistent principles that can be investigated by observation and experiment, and which can be understood by logical reasoning. In Kuhn's terms, what is to be studied is how the universe operates. The essential question we ask as scientists is 'What are its consistent principles?'; and we apply the experimental method to try to discover them, using logic and rationality as the benchmark to adjudicate our results.

Typically, scientists accept the prevailing paradigm as the default position for their work, and try to extend its scope through observation and experiment. Eventually, however, their attempts at refinement may throw up insoluble problems or inexplicable data that expose the paradigm's inadequacies or contradict it altogether. There follows an intellectual crisis in which the old paradigm is supplanted by a new one with greater explanatory power. The displacement of Newtonian physics by Einsteinian relativity and quantum mechanics is one example of such a paradigm shift, prompting a rethink of the nature of reality, setting research on a radically different path, and forging previously unimaginable links between theory and observation.

Kuhn in his analysis specifically addressed that field of human activity that we call science, i.e. the attempt to discover the workings of the observable material world, the world 'out there'. What he had in mind were the so-called 'natural sciences': physics, chemistry, biology, astronomy and the earth sciences. However, Kuhn's description of paradigms and how they shift was intuitively so recognisable that other disciplines rushed to adopt and adapt his ideas within their own spheres of interest. The fuzzier sciences such as sociology, psychology, politics, economics – even painting, music and literature, even journalism – frequently drop the word *paradigm* into their discourse and feel the smugger for it. The more elderly disciplines of religion, mathematics and philosophy, on the other hand, consider themselves, I suspect, on a level above the instabilities that Kuhn describes. Religion, at least in its more dogmatic forms, relies more upon revelation than on experimental enquiry, and can dismiss as heresy any introspection that challenges its tenets. Mathematics, the pinnacle of ruthless logic, may by definition be explored but not contradicted. One and one make two: that's what 'two' *is*. And philosophy – the study of what is true and right – has avoided having to confront any Kuhnian crunch-points by endlessly procrastinating over how its postulates and conclusions are to be validated.

As Kuhn was aware, any reputable paradigm must set clear limits to its territorial ambition. In seeking to map *some* areas, it inevitably excludes others. It allows *some* questions, some methodologies, but rejects others; it can deal with some kinds of information but is flummoxed by others. In so far as any paradigm – even one with aspirations as grandiose as the scientific paradigm – deals with a subset of all possible territory and all possible information, it is necessarily incomplete. Viewed from within the paradigm itself, some territory will always remain unmapped and some observations inexplicable.

This note of caution that every conceptual framework has its blind spots – that nothing can explain everything – has received a fillip from an unexpected quarter, pure mathematics. In 1931 the Czech mathematician Kurt Gödel[36] published his *Incompleteness Theorem*, in which he proved that in any closed logical system there will always be some propositions that cannot be proved either true or false using only the system's own rules and axioms. There will always be some statements that, although true, cannot be proved to be so on the system's own terms. They might be provable by going *outside* the system and coming up with new rules and axioms, but by doing so you only create a larger system with its own unprovable statements. As Hofstadter put it in his unexpectedly successful book *Gödel, Escher, Bach*,[37] 'provability is a weaker notion than truth.'

There is always something that has to be explained from outside. Paradigms within paradigms: the image of the nested *matryoshki* dolls comes again to mind.

Paradigms, like model aeroplanes, capture some salient features at the expense of ignoring others. A plastic replica of a Boeing 747 will help us understand the shape and proportions of the real thing, but not its size, or what makes it move. If we want a sense of absolute size, a photograph of the pilot standing beside it would be better. To understand the thrust of its jet engines, we would do better to blow up a rubber balloon and let go. The question is not which is the *correct*, or even the *best*, model, but which offers the most useful representation of the particular attribute we are interested in.

---

36 Kurt Gödel (1906–78) was born in what is now the Czech Republic but took in turn Austrian citizenship, then German, and finally became an American citizen after World War II. Nicknamed *Herr Warum* ('Mister Why?') as a child, Gödel was much admired by the mathematical community, especially by Einstein. However, he never felt a part of that community, perceiving himself a perennial outsider. His 'incompleteness theorem' is a nice example of the thought reflecting its thinker. In later life Gödel developed an obsessive fear of being poisoned, which made him anorexic; at his death he weighed only 30 kilograms.

37 Hofstadter DR. *Gödel, Escher, Bach: an eternal golden braid*. New edition. New York: Basic Books, 1999.

Earlier, I summarised the scientific paradigm in these terms: The universe operates on consistent principles that can be investigated by observation and experiment, and which can be understood by logical reasoning. So all-encompassing a claim has a hubris that needs to be challenged. Several questions are begged.

- What parts of the universe, as experienced by human beings, are 'off paradigm' and, even in principle, unmappable by science?
- Is there *really* an objective world out there?
- What does *'really'* mean?
- Does rationality trump all other routes to human understanding?
- Is subjective experience – conscious awareness – something that can be understood by purely scientific methodologies; or is it rather, being itself the creator of those methodologies, ineluctably beyond their explanatory reach?

I don't presume to know the answers; but, as a doctor who thinks that there is more to human misery than science alone can relieve, I want at this stage of my book to wobble the traditional medical version of the scientific paradigm on its pedestal.

Medicine, as always, straddles several lines of demarcation between disciplines. It is at once a science, and a humanity, and art and philosophy and sociology as well. As a result it suffers from what we might call paradigm confusion.

As the history recapitulated in this chapter has reminded us, the scientific way of thinking has only relatively recently come to dominate medicine's intellectual territory. The material benefits of this conquest have been undeniably spectacular. Medical science has prevailed so successfully over irrationality and superstition that its victory sometimes looks like a whitewash. It is easy for doctors, particularly if they work in one of medicine's more high-tech provinces, to think that the scientific paradigm is the only legitimate one, or that any competition to it is the legacy of hopelessly outdated ways of thinking. This would be a mistake.

It has become fashionable to speak not of *medicine* but of *biomedicine*, as if medicine, like a detergent, also came in some alternative less potent *non-bio* forms – pseudo-medicine, possibly, or psychosocial medicine. The term *biomedicine* seemingly locates medicine wholly within the larger territory of biology, itself a province of science, over which the scientific paradigm claims sole explanatory rights. The thinking of the biomedical doctor, it suggests, should be as scientific as the thinking of the biologist. To my mind, what is being implied here is either too restricted a view of all that medicine encompasses or an over-optimistic view of what biological science is capable of explaining.

The truth of the matter is that paradigms – the ways that groups of like-minded people have of trying to get a handle on the world – are as impermanent as the human beings who embrace them. They are born, and will eventually perish. Often conceived in passion, they grow from incoherent infancy through undisciplined adolescence to eventually productive, if sedate, maturity. Along the way paradigms, like people, coexist and mix with others. They squabble and compete, interbreed and multiply, form alliances and make enemies. Their decline can be a graceful handing-over to their appointed heirs and successors; or else it can be a painful falling-away of the faculties, a time of increasing stiffness and declining comprehension leaving them creaking and grumpy, tut-tutting at the disrespect of the rising generation in its headlong headstrong pursuit of the new. Death, when it comes to man or paradigm, can be sudden and unexpected or artificially extended beyond its natural span. Both find a form of immortality in the memories and influences of those who loved them, and in the traces they lay down in the fossil record, where some future archaeologist of ideas will puzzle over them.

In a word, paradigms, like living things, evolve.

* * * * *

The biologist Daniel Dennett described Darwin's[38] theory of evolution by natural selection as 'the single best idea anyone has ever had'.[39]

The outline of Darwin's story will probably be familiar: the 22-year-old naturalist sailing for South America in 1831 aboard the *Beagle*; the qualitative studies of fossilised mammalian bones in Argentina; the quantitative observations of the differences between the finches and tortoises of the mainland and those on the Galapagos islands; the crystallising of insight on reading

---

38 Charles Darwin (1809–82), English naturalist, grandson of Erasmus Darwin and (on his mother's side) of the potter Josiah Wedgwood.

39 Daniel Dennett, American biologist and philosopher. In his book *Darwin's Dangerous Idea* (New York: Simon & Schuster, 1996) Dennett likens Darwin's idea of modification by natural selection to a 'universal acid' that spreads through every field of science and leaves them all changed in its wake.

Malthus's essay on population growth; the further decade of pre-publication anxiety, fearing the scorn and ostracism that he thought his 'anti-religious' evolutionary notions would earn him. Darwin was a martyr to sea-sickness, and spent much of his time at sea whimpering in a hammock with his eyes closed. He may have remembered, perhaps regretted, dropping out of medical school in Edinburgh after 2 years, his father's ambition for him to become a doctor drowned out by the screaming of the surgical patients. Between bouts of nausea he may have turned for distraction to the copy of Lyell's[40] *Principles of Geology* – 'the face of the Earth has changed gradually over aeons through eruptions, earthquake and erosion' – dropped into his hand by his mentor John Henslow, as the *Beagle* weighed anchor, with the injunction, 'Read this, but don't believe it.'

Natural selection is a very powerful idea. Simple, elegant and profound, it assumes little to explain much – why life is so diverse and each species so perfectly adapted to its niche. Darwin himself put it like this:

> *As many more individuals are produced than can possibly survive, there must in every case be a struggle for existence, either one individual with another of the same species, or with the individuals of distinct species, or with the physical conditions of life. … Can it, then, be thought improbable, seeing that variations useful to man have undoubtedly occurred, that other variations useful in some way to each being in the great and complex battle of life, should sometimes occur in the course of thousands of generations? If such do occur, can we doubt (remembering that many more individuals are born than can possibly survive) that individuals having any advantage, however slight, over others, would have the best chance of surviving and of procreating their kind? On the other hand, we may feel sure that any variation in the least degree injurious would be rigidly destroyed. This preservation of favourable variations and the rejection of injurious variations, I call Natural Selection.[41]*

---

40 Sir Charles Lyell (1797–1875), Scottish geologist and proponent of 'uniformitarianism' – the doctrine that natural processes observable in the recent are the same as those that operated in the past.

41 *On the Origin of* Species *by Means of Natural Selection, or the Preservation of Favoured Races in the Struggle for Life* was published in 1859. A presentation of its key ideas was made on Darwin's behalf to the Linnean Society the previous year by Lyell and the botanist–explorer Sir Joseph Hooker; Darwin himself was too distraught to attend, following the death from scarlet fever of his infant son.

Darwinian evolution has only two requirements:

- organisms must reproduce themselves, usually faithfully but occasionally with some variation, and
- environmental conditions must selectively favour the reproduction of some variant individuals rather than others.

If these are satisfied, and given enough time, all of what Darwin called 'life's grandeur' is ordained. Equally humbling is that Darwin developed his insight before Mendel worked out the laws of inheritance,[42] before we knew about genes or mutation, and before the structure of DNA was worked out.

Darwin himself was, at least publicly, no atheist. But the publication of the *Origin* accelerated one of the most profound paradigm shifts of recorded history, from supernatural to natural explanations of the universe's complexity, and signalled the terminal illness, if not the actual death, of God-as-necessary-cause. (That creationism still has explanatory power for a few otherwise rational individuals illustrates the important point that a new paradigm never completely supplants the old. Old paradigms never die; they just become quaint.)

It was not long lost on the world's thinkers that biological evolution has its cultural equivalents. Like living things, institutions and ideas also reproduce themselves more or less faithfully – institutions through tradition and the occasional revolution, ideas through teaching, word of mouth and the media. And cultural environments exercise ruthless selection over the forms of organised thought, just as does the physical environment over competing life forms. In nature it is the best adapted organisms that survive and prosper; in the realm of expressed ideas, it's the most convincing. The history of medical science sketched earlier in this chapter can be seen as a Darwinian process in which paradigms have evolved through successive mutations, selected for dominance on the basis of their ability to account for what was previously unexplained.

---

42 Gregor Mendel (1822–84), Austrian monk, botanist and 'father of genetics'. Beginning in 1856 and working in the garden of his monastery at Brünn (now Brno), Mendel studied the inheritance of the visible characteristics of garden peas, and deduced the existence of paired elementary units of heredity now known as genes. He first presented the results of his researches to the Brünn Society for the Study of Natural Science in 1865. Mendel owned, and annotated, copies of Darwin's books, but his own work was well advanced by the time the *Origin* was published.

The timescale of cultural evolution is faster by several orders of magnitude than the biological one. Global networks of written, broadcast and electronic media allow ideas old and new, established and tentative, to propagate and reproduce themselves almost instantaneously, introducing abundant varia- tions and distortions along the way. And the social environment in which they compete is largely ours to manipulate and control, as politicians and advertisers know only too well. The game of 'Chinese whispers', in which a message is passed *sotto voce* along a line of people, becoming humorously distorted in transit, is a fair analogy for the phenomenon of cultural evolu- tion. The low signal-to-noise ratio of the message whispered in the ear of each player results in imperfect transmission – mutation – of the original. The group expectation of being amused has the effect that each participant will selectively 'hear', and pass on, a version with the potential for further degradation and better adapted to the party environment.

Complicated entities, such as living creatures or entire systems of thought, are not the only things that undergo evolution. Simpler ones do too, as long as they can replicate with variation in a discriminating environment. In the biological realm, genes do it, their sporadic mutations helping or hindering their host's competitiveness in life and love. And the cognitive sphere, too, has something equivalent to the gene: the *meme*. What genes are to the living world, memes are to the world of ideas. Genes are made of DNA; memes are made of thought.

As Kuhn gave us *paradigm*, the word *meme* is the gift of the biologist Richard Dawkins.[43] A meme is a chunk of cultural information, a piece of thought, copied from person to person by any means of communication at human disposal – speech, image, print or internet; by deed, example or systematic teaching; via the arts graphic and narrative, representational and symbolic. And memes undergo evolution. Every channel of communication introduces an element of distortion: what the transmitter intends to transmit is never quite what the recipient understands. If some versions of the meme prove more robust in the prevailing cultural environment, the conditions for social evolution on Darwinian lines are met.[44]

---

43 C. Richard Dawkins (born 1941). English evolutionary biologist and evangelical atheist. The concept of the meme is elaborated in his book *The Selfish Gene* (Oxford: Oxford University Press, 1976).

44 Or as someone for whom the word *paradigm* holds no terrors might put it: 'Successive *step changes* lead to *pushing the envelope*, resulting, on an un-*level playing field*, in *mission creep*.'

At its simplest, a meme might be just an idea or a phrase. Or memes can be more complex – beliefs, opinions, assumptions and slogans, such as 'justice', 'truth', 'consumer choice', 'freedom and democracy!' Much of everyday life consists of passing on memes to each other – reading a newspaper, following a recipe, setting an example to the children. Most memes are benign and trivial – the latest television catch phrase, or the height of this year's hemline. But others can be exploitative, even sinister – cults, prejudices, irrational '-isms' such as racism, imperialism or anti-Semitism. The most powerful and enduring forces in human history – the great religions and philosophies, communism, capitalism and everything in between – all function as memes. Many of these components of our intellectual and social life are so familiar that we take them for granted, and credit them with a legitimacy they don't deserve. Rigidity of thought is perhaps the cruellest form of imprisonment; if we are to avoid it, we need to recognise even our most cherished beliefs and assumptions for what they are – temporary configurations of thought caught up in an evolutionary process, in which some may flourish and others wither but where none has the right to go unquestioned.

* * * * *

After this cautionary diversion into the evolutionary nature of knowledge and the impermanence of received wisdom, I want to return, admiration tempered with a dash of irreverence, to the scientific paradigm and medicine's place within it.

I suspect that the version of the scientific paradigm that exists in the minds of most non-scientists (and of many scientists too, if you catch them off guard) is essentially little different from Isaac Newton's. As the 20th century dawned, the workings of the universe that science revealed seemed to have a comforting familiarity. The worlds of the very large and the very small, it appeared, were not much different from our own everyday one. The galaxies ran like giant clockwork. Atoms behaved like tiny billiard balls. Some things were certain: time ran steadily forwards at 60 seconds to the minute, and a yard was a yard. There were laws and regularities. Things were reassuringly explicable. Events had antecedent causes that could be identified, and consequences that could be predicted. There seemed no mystery that might not yield to systematic rational enquiry. The man on the Clapham omnibus, even if he hadn't personally cracked the nature of reality, thought he might know a man who had. Some even went so far as to propose that God himself be relieved of his 'design and build' responsibilities.

Then in 1905 a giant intellectual meteor crashed into Planet Smug, in the form of Albert Einstein.[45] The son of a German Jewish featherbed salesman, the young Einstein had fled the military draft and taken Swiss nationality, becoming, despite an evident talent for physics and mathematics, a humble clerk in the Bern patent office. There, bored, he daydreamed about what would happen if you tried to race a light beam. In 1905 – an *annus mirabilis* during which he published four papers in the prestigious journal *Annalen der Physik* – the 25-year-old Einstein set out his conclusions. $E = mc^2$: substance is actually energy, enormously concentrated. *The special theory of relativity*: there is only one absolute – the speed of light in a vacuum. Everything else is relative. Things we think of as separate, such as space and time, are actually inseparable. What to us seems obvious common sense is just how things happen to look from where we happen to be.

Einstein's ideas seemed to catalyse an entire generation of theoretical scientists to break the shackles of conventional thought. Within 30 years, classical physics, and the notion it embodies of what 'good science' consists of, had imploded.

On 24 October 1927, a conference of the world's greatest theoretical physicists, including nine future Nobel prize winners, met at the Metropole Hotel in Brussels. They emerged a week later with the key features of quantum theory – which has been called 'the most successful set of ideas ever devised by human beings', explaining all of chemistry and most of physics – in place. The oldest contributor was Max Planck, who in 1900 had shown that electromagnetic radiation came in discrete chunks of finite size that he called *quanta*. Einstein himself was there, still puzzling over why light sometimes behaved as a wave phenomenon and at others as a stream of particles. Another participant, Louis de Broglie, thought he knew the answer – *wave–particle duality*. Everything (said de Broglie) – electrons, matter, energy – is both wave *and* particle. *Which* it behaves as depends, as Heisenberg (of whom more shortly) agreed, on how the observer carries out the process of observation.

Someone else at the Metropole that momentous week was 'the great Dane', the physicist Niels Bohr. Taking as his starting point Rutherford's 1908 'planetary' model of the atom, in which negatively charged electrons orbited a positive nucleus containing most of the atom's mass, Bohr had postulated that electrons were arranged in a small number of stable 'shells', from which

---

45 Albert Einstein (1879–1955), German-born theoretical physicist. Winner of the 1921 Nobel Prize for physics and of the 1999 *Time* magazine 'Person of the century' award.

only the arrival or discharge of a quantum of energy could budge them. Exactly *where* an electron was to be found could never be determined, even in principle. The most it was possible to know was the relative probability of its being in *this* location or *that*. Einstein hated Bohr's probabilistic notions, prompting him famously to expostulate that 'God does not play dice with the universe!'

God may or may not play dice; but, as Werner Heisenberg, another Brussels participant, appreciated, he plays a mean game of poker. You can never know the contents of his hand with complete certainty.

Heisenberg's often-quoted *uncertainty principle* applies, in his original formulation, to moving particles on an atomic or subatomic scale. To have a complete understanding of the properties of such a particle, an observer would need, at a given instant in time, to know both its precise location, i.e. its spatial coordinates relative to some fixed reference point, and, simultaneously, its momentum, i.e. the product of its mass and velocity. According to the uncertainty principle, it is impossible for the observer to establish both the position of the particle *and* its momentum with complete accuracy. The act of measuring either one of these independent variables changes the other. The more you know about the one, the less you know about the other. Even the single photon of light needed to 'see' where the particle is disturbs its momentum irretrievably. And if you measure how fast it's going, to some extent you stop it in its tracks.

Heisenberg's uncertainty principle – that something cannot be measured without changing it – is, like Darwin's theory of evolution, one of those ideas that, although conceived within a narrow field of enquiry, nevertheless apply more generally in other contexts. Information cannot be obtained without loss of truthfulness. This is the case not just in the eerie world of quantum mechanics but also in the mundane one of daily life. Pushing a meat thermometer into the joint as it roasts to see if it's done cools the meat slightly and fractionally prolongs the cooking time. Your electricity bill is always higher than it should be, by the price of the power it takes to spin the disc that turns the dials in the meter.

A concept allied to the uncertainty principle is the *observer effect*. Observing a system alters its properties at the instant the observation is made. But it doesn't stop there. It follows that, if you change the starting conditions, you change what happens next. Once an observer is involved, both process and outcome deviate from what would otherwise have been the case. As generations of young GPs in training have long protested, video-recording their consultations makes them consult differently (though whether for better or worse is a matter of conjecture: how, the uncertainty principle reminds us to ask, could anyone ever tell?)

Unlike thermometers, electricity meters and video cameras, human observers are not simply the passive recorders of information. People tend to see what they want to see or expect to see, and to interpret what they see in the light of their own previous experiences. This has both advantages and disadvantages. On the down side, where the closest possible approximation to objective truth is what's wanted, the unpredictable variability of the observer is a corrupting source of bias or inaccuracy. It's for this reason that scientists rate double-blind trials (where who did what to what is not revealed until the experiment is over) more highly than single-blind ones, or more than mere anecdote. The 'contaminating' effect of the scientist/observer's mindset is something to be factored out by the way the experiment is designed. On the other hand there are situations, when what is sought is not facts but insight, where the observer effect makes a positive contribution. In a novel, it is the author's 'take' on the events described that holds the reader's interest. In a counselling setting, the counsellor's ability to filter and interpret the client's narrative is the whole point. There is evidence from the Rogerian school of non-directive counselling that qualities in the counsellor such as empathy and staying non-judgemental are at least as important for success as the therapeutic models and strategies invoked.[46] The personal idiosyncrasies of the observer/novelist/therapist allow the emergence of a different, non-scientific but sometimes more valuable, kind of truth.

At first sight it would seem that, where scientific truth is being pursued, the observer effect should be designed out of the process of enquiry, and that, where a more humanistic kind of truth is wanted, the observer effect can be acknowledged and encouraged. This sounds an attractive compromise. In a medical setting, it would allow the science-orientated cardiac surgeon and the person-orientated psychotherapist to operate with equal self-respect. Neither need denigrate the other. But this compromise, however beguiling, is not possible. Heisenberg cautions us that any attempt to factor out the observer effect is futile. It can't be done. There is no such thing as the detached observer. If you make an observation, you become part of the system and you

---

46 Counselling also provides another, beneficial, example of the Heisenbergian principle that things are altered when you try to describe them. The therapist's 'Tell me about it' not only elicits an account of a client's problem but also begins to change the emotional response to it.

change it. If you are unwilling to have any effect on what you are observing, there are limits to what you can find out.

This question – *What is the effect of the doctor-as-observer?* – will be one of this book's main preoccupations. For now, let us just suspect that the conventional view of medicine as 'Newtonian science applied to human pathology' may probably be due for a radical update if it is to stay under the scientific paradigm's new umbrella.

* * * * *

Of all the ideas spawned by the new physics, Heisenberg's uncertainty principle is perhaps one of the easiest to get the gist of. Other notions that fell out of the post-Einstein *Intellekt-Fest* are a good deal more bizarre. Many of them are, at least to a lay mind like mine, counter-intuitive – which is to say that they seem to run counter to what in everyday experience passes for common sense. Some are so dizzying that they have been given names that emphasise their phantasmagorical nature. For example:

- *Quarks.*[47] Quarks are one of two fundamental subatomic particles, the other being the lepton. They apparently come in six *flavours*, and have properties like *charm* and *strangeness*.
- *Superposition.* If (at least in the quantum world) a system could be in any one of several possible configurations, it actually exists in all of them simultaneously – until the instant an observer looks to see which one is the case. This paradox led Erwin Schrödinger to propose his famous 'cat' thought experiment.
- *Schrödinger's cat.* A live cat is placed in a sealed box containing a small quantity of radioactive material, sufficient to decay, on average, at the rate of one atom an hour. The box also contains a Geiger counter so connected that, if an atom decays, a hammer is released that breaks a flagon of cyanide, killing the cat. After one hour, an atomic decay is just as likely as not to have occurred, and the cat is just as likely as not to be dead. On

---

47   The name *quark* was invented in 1963 by Murray Gell-Mann, who thought it was a nonsense syllable with a nice sound. In physics, it rhymes with *squawk* or *dork*, not to be confused with the line 'Three quarks for Muster Mark' in James Joyce's *Finnegan's Wake*, where, though equally incomprehensible, the word rhymes with *dark*. The various flavours of quark, combined in threes, make up neutrons and protons.

the hour, superposition has the cat just as much alive as dead – until the box is opened, whereupon it becomes wholly one or the other.[48]

- *Non-local reality.*[49] It is possible for a pair of electrons to be in what is called a singlet state, in which one spins 'up' and the other 'down', the spins cancelling each other out. Now separate them, and send them off so far apart that, according to the locality principle, the behaviour of one should be unable to affect the other. Superposition says that, until someone determines which one is 'up' and which 'down', they both exist in a hybrid 'both-up-*and*-down' state. OK; so now measure the spin of one of them, and discover it to be, say, 'down'. Instantly, in order to preserve the singlet state, the other loses its 'down' option and collapses to the complementary 'up' state. Somehow the two have remained caus-ally linked even over limitless distances. Something – communication?, influence? – seems to have taken place between them at infinite speed, in apparent contravention of Einstein's axiom that absolutely nothing can travel faster than light, not even information.

Intriguing though these mysteries are, we might think them so far removed from everyday science, let alone everyday life, that they could perhaps be left for the quantum *cognoscenti* alone to worry about. But that would be to underestimate the full impact of the new physics as it rippled out into the wider scientific community, changing for ever the ways scientists, pure and applied, in disciplines both strict and fuzzy, set about their thinking. In particular, the quantum revolution forced a rethink of how cause and effect operate.

Before Einstein, causality was generally assumed to be 'linear', of the form:

$$A \rightarrow B \rightarrow C$$

---

48 Schrödinger intended his thought experiment to be a *reductio ad absurdum* disproving what he considered the foolish concept of superposition. However, to his chagrin, the fallacy, if there is one, has not been identified by quantum theorists; and in fact some evidence from experiments on electron interference suggest that the 'all at once until you look' effect is real (though, on the cat scale, very small!).

49 According to the *locality principle*, enunciated by Einstein, an object is influenced directly only by its immediate surroundings; widely separated objects can't influence each other. Unfortunately for Einstein, experiments by John Clauser at Berkeley in 1978 and in 1982 by Alain Aspect in Paris, using photons, have confirmed that interaction *can* take place instantaneously and is not diminished by distance.

where state B has only one cause, namely condition A, and only one consequence, state C. Each state is determined by its predecessor in accordance with the immutable (and therefore in theory completely predictable) laws of nature. Post-Einstein, accommodation had to be made for non-linear causality, whereby events might have multiple or remote causes, and consequences predictable only in terms of probabilities, and where the process of observing and measuring had inescapable effects on the system being observed.

Many fields of study found these ideas to be unexpectedly liberating. They freed up ways of thinking about complicated phenomena that had hitherto seemed beyond rational analysis, such as how cancers and weather systems form, or how economies and human beings behave. Reductionism – trying to understand the whole by studying the properties of its smallest parts – was no longer the only option. New intellectual toolkits such as systems theory, complexity theory, fuzzy logic and chaos theory were developed, and usefully applied in fields as diverse as computing, financial modelling, neurophysiology and population dynamics. Reductionism met its antithesis in the phenomenon of *emergence*, when complex systems exhibit properties that could not have been predicted by studying their components.[50]

> The opposite of a fact is falsehood, but the opposite of one profound truth may very well be another profound truth.
>
> Niels Bohr (1885–1962)
> Danish physicist

Some philosopher–scientists were struck by apparent homologies between the world views propounded by the new physics and by ancient Eastern philosophical traditions such as Taoism and Zen Buddhism. Among the first was Fritjof Capra, whose 1975 book *The Tao of Physics*,[51]

---

50 Emergent phenomena include:
  - the information-handling capacity of a computer chip essentially built up from millions of interconnected transistors
  - the effects on human culture and society of the internet, the world wide web of linked computers
  - conscious awareness, which (according to the best available understanding) emerges from a big enough collection of brain cells, synapses and neuro-endocrine chemicals, and which (as we have only our own consciousness with which to study it) is probably incomprehensible even in principle.

  Emergence as a phenomenon in general practice will be further considered in Chapter 10.

51 Capra F. *The Tao of Physics*, 3rd edn. New York: Flamingo, 1992.

while showing some signs that its author was slightly intoxicated with his own delight, nevertheless suggested that the methods and conclusions of science and mysticism are not so irreconcilable as might be supposed. Both acknowledge that some forms of understanding are to be arrived at by suspending conventional rational analysis. The concept of interrelatedness is common to both: 'Everything touches everything,' as the Argentinian writer Jorge Luis Borges put it. Heisenberg's uncertainty principle closely mirrors the Buddhist insight that what we take for separateness between things is more a creation of the human consciousness that observes them than a feature of ultimate reality.

There is no need for us to get too heavy, or to force the scientific and esoteric traditions into a loveless marriage. It's enough that this brief excursion into the quantum world should caution those of us brought up with an essentially Newtonian version of the scientific paradigm, as Shakespeare's Hamlet did his sceptical reductionist friend, that:

> Natural science does not simply describe and explain nature; it is part of the interplay between nature and ourselves ... What we observe is not nature itself, but nature exposed to our method of questioning.
>
> Werner Heisenberg (1901–76)
> German physicist and
> philosopher

There are more things in heaven and earth, Horatio, Than are dreamt of in your philosophy.

* * * * *

I hope it will be apparent from this chapter that, in the course of its evolution, the scientific paradigm – how we try to make sense of the world 'out there' – has, over the course of the last 25 centuries, made a kind of 'spiral excursion' through successive phases of cultural evolution. It has come back to a position close to where it started, but has advanced in the process. Primitive explanations of the natural world were, in hindsight, magic stories, created by unsophisticated minds without the benefit of technology. With the advent of suitable gadgetry, naïve ignorance yielded to rational evidence-based explanation. The scientist was pure explorer, pure map-maker; driven by logic and curiosity, but, as far as the territory was concerned, pure sight-seer. Finally, come the quantum era, the scientific paradigm has returned to a position where we have to put inverted commas around 'what we know'.

'Reality' is a hybrid concept of the objective and the subjective, any view of how things *are* being necessarily distorted by the lens of the human observer. In a sense, the latest version of the scientific paradigm is once again a magic one, our understanding of the world out there being shaped by factors we cannot completely explain. But now it's a different kind of magic, this time performed by sophisticated minds conscious that a proportion of what they would have us believe is actually just smoke and mirrors, and that what we see is in fact shaped and coloured by the internal filters of the viewer. We have returned not to the origin, but to its projection on a more mature plane – which is why the trajectory of our intellectual excursion is a spiral and not a circle.

It's inevitable, in a condensed account such as this, that the history of science, including medical science, will appear a smoothed-off affair. Viewed from afar, it may seem that older versions of the scientific paradigm always yield gracefully to the newer one when the evidence requires it, and that yesterday's ageing minds are only too grateful to defer to the insights of today's bright young ones. If only. Unfortunately, progress neither in natural science nor in medicine is ever a seamless jolt-free 'onwards and upwards' business. Viewed from close up, it is all too apparent that there are false starts, blind alleys, voices ahead of their time, seed that falls on stony ground.

For example: the same idea may arise simultaneously but independently in more than one place.[52] Or a discovery, inopportunely timed, may sink into temporary oblivion, only to be rediscovered later by someone else who gets the credit.[53] We may fail to see an answer staring us in the face because no one has clearly framed the question.[54] Some promising ideas can be left marooned when the paradigm that spawned them moves on, even if they still

---

52 In the USA of the 1840s, Crawford Long, Gardner Colton, Horace Wells and Charles Jackson would all challenge William Morton's claim to be the discoverer of inhalational anaesthesia.

53 In 1872 – long before Fleming's 1928 'discovery' of penicillin – Joseph Lister established that a growth of *Penicillium glaucum* would kill bacteria in liquid culture, and, in a letter to his brother, proposed using a *Penicillium* extract to 'observe, should a suitable case present, if the growth of the organisms be inhibited in the human tissues'. Such an experiment was actually carried out in 1895 by Tiberio in Naples, and in 1897 by a French army doctor named Duchesne.

54 Antonie van Leeuwenhoek, peering down his microscope in 1676, saw 'tiny animals', which we now know were bacteria. By that time, germ theories of disease had already been proposed. But, because no one had speculated what germs might look like, or where they might be found, he failed to make the connection.

have something of value to contribute.[55] Conversely, some obsolete ideas – memes left over from an outmoded paradigm – can persist as 'living fossils' long after the accumulating weight of evidence ought to have rendered them unsustainable. Medicine is particularly prone to anachronisms of this kind. The continuing popularity of tonsillectomy is one example. Another – more insidious, and one that I propose to challenge in this book – is the widely presumed superiority in medicine of the specialist over the generalist.

If we were all good scientists, theory and practice would develop in sync with fresh validated evidence as it comes in and is promulgated through the profession. But that's not how things happen. It always seems to take more than just facts to change beliefs and behaviour. Why? Why can't human systems adapt swiftly and ungrudgingly to changes in their informational environment? Why is it so often the case that, in a parody of Newton's third law of motion, 'to every proposed action there is a larger and hostile reaction'? Partly, I suppose, it's a matter of inertia and friction. The forces of change have to achieve a critical magnitude before a tipping point is reached. Pour sand into a pile, and it's quite some time before one extra grain will cause the heap to topple. There is also what psychologists call the 'figure/ground effect'. New knowledge that in hindsight we can tell was important didn't seem important at the time; it didn't sufficiently stand out against the background. We are not good at recognising beginnings. And of course there is vested interest. The new always makes a victim of the old. The prospect of change, however enticing, is always a threat to someone's security, status, reputation or self-confidence. If it is our innate sense of amazement that drives us to explore the world and our place in it, it is the complexities of our own psychology that lead us to mistrust what we discover.

It's that observer effect again, muscling in on the process of rational analysis. But we are stuck with it. Having to factor in the observer effect is what

---

55 A good example is the placebo effect, which has made something of a 'spiral excursion' of its own. In medicine's pre-scientific era, every doctor had a favourite inert nostrum that, plus or minus the therapeutic impact of the doctor's personality, was often beneficial. But, as therapeutics became more potent, the placebo effect was largely dismissed, or, worse, denounced as trickery. While conceding its power – the placebo effect still has to be controlled for in clinical trials, and any benefits of so-called 'complementary' medicine are usually attributed to it – orthodox medicine turned its back on what it considered a deceitful sham.

More recently, however, the placebo effect seems set for a come-back. The issue of the *British Medical Journal* of 3 May 2008 contains several articles and editorials establishing its effectiveness in irritable bowel syndrome, and extolling the therapeutic power of a good doctor–patient relationship: something that will bring a smile and 'I told you so' to the lips of many an 'old-fashioned' clinician.

toppled classical Newtonian physics into the ultimately liberating insights of the quantum age. The mind of the participating observer is not to be filleted out of the process of investigation. And as it is in physics, so should it not be in medicine?

> [We shall hope to] discover the kind of question that it makes sense to ask and the kind of answer we can expect to get; we shall hope to discover something about the nature and the degree of the certainty that is attainable. And we shall hope to end up with more knowledge, more wisdom and a clearer understanding.
>
> But if the ardent seeker after truth is not content with that, if he is only interested in answers that are right or wrong, if he wants final conclusive certainty he must go elsewhere – to the study, for example, of pure mathematics. As he does so he will be shutting with a clang the door that leads to the world of 'it all depends'. And this will be a pity for it is the world in which we live.[56]
>
> E.R. Emmet (1909–80)
> Schoolmaster at Winchester College

Medicine, too, is embarked upon a spiral excursion of its own. Any benefits that accrued to patients during medicine's pre-scientific age came more from the qualities of the doctor-as-person than from the misguided justifications he offered for his therapies. Then, come the glory days of rational science, it was the doctor-as-scientist who claimed his place at the top table, leaving the doctor-as-person to slink shamefacedly away from the feast of innovation on which his white-coated alter ego greedily gorged. But, if medicine's excursion were to follow that of the physical sciences, we should expect it to move into its own version of the quantum age, where classic models of illness and disease have to be tempered with concepts of uncertainty, emergence and non-linear causality, and where a doctor's human properties are seen not as an obstacle to clinical effectiveness but as a source of insight complementary to his intellect. The personality of the practising clinician is not to be filleted out of the clinical process.

Such a rediscovery of the observer effect in medicine is far from complete. By most doctors and by many of their patients (though a smaller proportion) the doctor-as-person is still cast as the embarrassing, impotent poor relation of the doctor-as-scientist. But I want to offer a diagnosis of why modern

---

56 Emmet ER. *Learning to Philosophise*. London: Longmans, Green & Co., 1964.

medicine, for all its technological triumphs, nevertheless disappoints on some deep level. And that diagnosis is that we have not yet successfully reunited the two. Ambivalence about whether and how to deal with the observer effect runs like a fault line through medical practice. One result of this ambivalence is the schism that has grown up – and sadly to some extent persists – between specialists and GPs. The next chapter will remind us just how wide that schism can be. Then I want to reframe it in less confrontational terms, namely, as a difference in perspective on how medicine is to be practised, and an example of a false duality to be reconciled by a shift in our thinking.

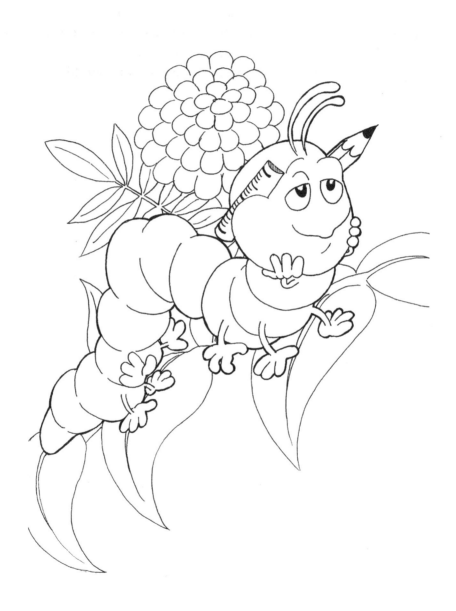

Chapter 3

Inchworms and also-rans

The specialist knows more and more about less and less and finally knows everything about nothing.

Konrad Lorenz (1903–89)

Austrian zoologist

A generalist is someone who knows less and less about more and more and finally knows nothing about anything.

Anon.

From *The 'Quote ... Unquote' Newsletter*, 1997, vol. 6, no. 1, p. 5

If ever you want to hear teeth grinding like the gears on a Chieftain tank, say to a GP at a party, 'Oh, you're a doctor are you? Are you a specialist, or just a GP?' It's the *just* that does it. I don't know a good reply. 'I specialise in general practice' sounds a bit clever. 'There's nothing *just* about being a GP' sounds, and is, a bit belligerent. The party conversation takes on a more acerbic edge if the questioner is also medical, and a consultant to boot.

'What's your field? Or are you just a GP?' (Thinks: *A GP, if the cardigan is anything to go by.*)

'Family practice, actually.' (Thinks: *A gynaecologist, if the bow tie is anything to go by.*) 'And yourself? Are you a generalist, or just a partialist?'[57]

'Actually, I'm a plousiatrist.[58] (*The pager in his pocket goes off.*) 'Sorry, you'll have to excuse me – bit of an emergency.'

'One of your private patients taken a turn for the poorer?'

And they part, two terriers kept from each other's throat by the thin leashes of decorum.

---

57 I am indebted to Professor David Haslam for this quip.

58 One who specialises in diseases of the wealthy; from the Greek πλούσιος – *rich*.

My father, who smoked 30 a day for most of his life, had enormous regard for the vascular surgeons who operated first on his ruptured cerebral aneurysm and later, unsuccessfully, on the one in his abdominal aorta. He took great pride in my decision to become a doctor, but rather less in my opting for general practice. I, on the other hand, had encountered hospital consultants only as bosses and not as saviours, and I had greater regard for my own childhood GP, Dr Heap. Ben Heap had a voice like fine sandpaper on balsa wood, and a kindness that was as warm in the touch of his hands as his stethoscope was cold. One hot summer, when I was 12, I fell ill with high fever and delirium after visiting a swimming pool that was implicated in an outbreak of poliomyelitis. I have only a hazy recollection of his twice-daily visits, but my mother always reckoned that Dr Heap saved my life. Half a century later, reason tells me that a surer way of saving my life might have been to admit me to hospital. But whether his decision to keep me at home, and the admiration for him that flowed from that decision and which shaped my subsequent choice of career, was ultimately of more value in the great scheme of things, I have no way of knowing.

* * * * *

A longstanding and almost universal fault line runs through the heart of the medical profession, dividing doctors into two camps – generalists and specialists. The commonest and most egregious manifestation of this divide is that between general practitioners[59] and consultants. Lesser examples can be found in tensions between, on the one hand, general physicians or surgeons and, on the other, their colleagues working in the more rarified sub-specialties.

If the distinction served no purpose other than to differentiate doctors who work in the community from those based in hospital, or to indicate whether a

---

59 A note on nomenclature: unless otherwise stated, I am using the terms *general practitioner* (GP), *family doctor*, *family physician* and *primary care doctor* as interchangeable synonyms for what is essentially the same role, i.e. a doctor based in the community and providing an initial point of contact for patients regardless of their presenting clinical problem. Different countries have their own preferences on terminology. The term *primary care* implies the infrastructure and clinical teams in which family doctors work, and is to be distinguished from *secondary care*, which is provided by specialists, largely hospital based, and often accessed only after some filtration process in primary care. *Tertiary care* refers to the concentration, on grounds of cost and efficiency, of ultra-specialised clinicians and resources into a small number of centres drawing patients needing particular expertise from secondary care.

particular doctor is a patient's primary or secondary point of contact with the medical services, or whether the doctor's range of clinical activity is relatively broad or narrow, then all might be well. But the generalist–specialist divide goes much deeper than just a description of their different roles. For many people, both medical and lay, to speak of the difference between generalists and specialists is also to make assumptions about the relative calibres of their professional skills, and to make value-judgements about their relative worth. The popular perception is often that specialists are superior to generalists: superior in status, in expertise, in usefulness, and in power and influence. To become a hospital specialist is commonly thought to be a nobler – the ultimate – ambition for a young doctor; and this expectation continues all too often to be reinforced during medical students' undergraduate years by the hospital specialists who still undertake most of their teaching. General practice, the subtext still goes, is where the also-rans end up.

Perhaps I'm being over-sensitive. In the UK at least, as health services feel themselves more and more stretched and beleaguered, relationships between consultants and GPs have never been more cordial than they are now. Amongst the medical royal colleges and other professional bodies there is no lack of mutual respect between the two main arms of the profession. Nor is there much disharmony when it behoves doctors to appear united against a common, often political, threat. But the historic belief that 'specialists are better than generalists' dies hard. It remains an acceptable snobbery at dinner parties. Government ministers almost invariably use the word *hospitals* as shorthand when referring to the National Health Service, as in 'Our top priorities are schools and hospitals.' Yet, in Britain, primary care employs about 50% of the medical workforce and deals with about 90% of patient demand, but receives only about 10% of NHS resources. And such knowledge as I have of international health care systems leads me to think that, particularly in countries where patients are free to refer themselves directly to the hospital services, the status gradient between community-based generalists and hospital-based specialists is as steep as ever.

I lament these inequities. *Well* (you might think), *you would, wouldn't you, being a GP*. But the cause for lamentation is not jealousy or injured vanity; it is that the status gap between generalists and specialists indicates a widespread failure of insight into how they each go about their business, a failure that distorts and weakens the contribution of both.

If this book succeeds in its ambition, the perceived superiority of the specialist will be seen in hindsight to be, like the Newtonian view of physics, an understandable but unfortunate anachronism. The belief that specialists are better than generalists is, by the previous chapter's lights, an out-of-date meme stranded in a shifting paradigm. If patients are to benefit as they deserve from the vocation and commitment that make people become doctors, this particular meme needs to be booted into the long grass of history. In this chapter I shall try to give it a good kick, beginning by looking at some of the ugly stereotypes and assumptions that, graffiti-like, disfigure the popular imagination.

* * * * *

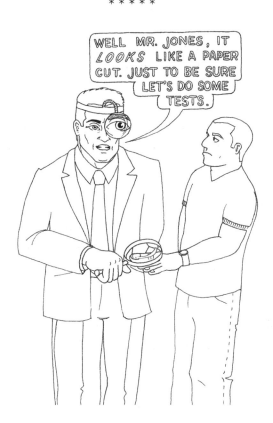

One thing that irks the layman about specialists is our ambivalence towards them; we need their expertise, but hate needing it. John Owen's *God and the doctor we alike adore …* has already been quoted. Ambrose Bierce in *The Devil's Dictionary*[60] expressed similar sentiments:

> **Physician**, *n. One upon whom we set our hopes when ill and our dogs when well.*

---

60 Ambrose Bierce (1842–1914), American journalist and satirist.

A specialist is a person who fears the other subjects.
> Martin H. Fischer (1879–1962)
> German-born physician

We're not sure whether or not to admire the narrow range of the specialist's skills.

A specialist is someone who does everything else worse.
> Ruggiero Ricci (1918–2012)
> Italian American concert
> violinist

No man can be a pure specialist without being in the strict sense an idiot.
> George Bernard Shaw
> (1856–1950)
> Irish playwright

Nor are we convinced that it's a good thing to know quite so much about anything.

Do not be bullied out of your common sense by the specialist; two to one he is a pedant.
> Oliver Wendell Holmes
> (1809–1904)
> American physician and poet

One thing is generally agreed: you can't understand what specialists tell you:

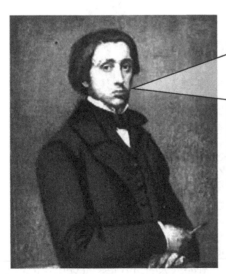

What a charming thing is the conversation of specialists! One understands absolutely nothing, and it's charming.

Edgar Degas (1834–1917)
French painter and sculptor

The criticisms commonly levelled at specialists have rather a naughty feel to them. They remind me of how at school, during a lesson from the strictest disciplinarian on the staff, the class clown would attempt to keep despondency at bay by pulling faces at the teacher when his back was turned, disrespect being the best antidote to fear. The public tends to hold specialists in awe, and sniping at them under the cover of wit tends to be as much as it feels it can get away with. GPs, on the other hand, are more ordinary, more 'like us', and as such can be affectionately teased:

> *General practice is a system of care provided by dinosaurs and guarded by dragons.*
>
> Anon.

However, the 'specialists are cleverer than GPs' meme is firmly entrenched in vernacular culture:

> *A general practitioner can no more become a specialist than an old shoe can become a dancing slipper. Both have developed habits which are immutable.*
> Frank Kittredge Paddock (1841–1901)

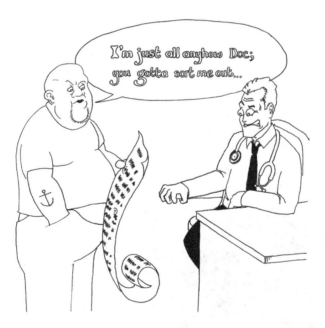

Another common concern about GPs is that they don't keep their knowledge up to date. This is not a new charge; Osler, no less, levelled it a century ago:

> *For the general practitioner a well-used library is one of the few correctives of the premature senility which is so apt to take him.*
> William Osler (1849–1919)
> Canadian physician

In medicine's pre-scientific era, when to do no harm but with a good bed-side manner was all that could be hoped for in a doctor, this may not have mattered too much. However:

The good old 'family doc' was a wonderfully affable, understanding man, who replaced his lack of knowledge with human kindness and human warmth. When medicine encompassed a broad, but not a colossal, quantity of knowledge, the old-fashioned general practitioner could practice with some degree of success. But let's face it: he has no reason to exist in this modern age.

Jerome J. Rubin (1963)

Unfortunately, stereotypes like these are alive and flourishing, even within the medical profession. I recently had the opportunity to invite an audience of newly qualified doctors, as yet uncommitted to particular career paths, to brainstorm[61] the images and assumptions they had about GPs and specialists. This they did with worrying enthusiasm. Fifteen minutes later the flipcharts looked like this:

Specialists	GPs
■ *Suits, expensive cars* ■ *High prestige* ■ *Tunnel vision* ■ *Arrogant, think they're the best* ■ *Run late, no time, always in a hurry* ■ *Can never get to see them* ■ *Poor communication, don't listen, can't explain* ■ *Work harder, more academic* ■ *Their exams are harder* ■ *Jealous of GPs' lifestyle* ■ *Always do private practice*	■ *Cardigans, sandals, leather elbow patches, tree-huggers* ■ *Dumb, lazy, pen-pushers* ■ *Failed consultants, hospital drop-outs* ■ *Not good enough to specialise* ■ *Not good clinically, miss diagnoses, refer inappropriately* ■ *Easy option, lots of time off, golf* ■ *Over-paid* ■ *'Lovely man, my doctor'* ■ *'Known me since I was a baby'*

* * * * *

---

61 Apparently, the term 'brainstorm' is now politically incorrect, being deemed insensitive to people with epilepsy. According to more than one medical royal college, I should have asked them to 'thought-shower'.

Beneath the levity of what I have so far written lie some serious matters. Charges against both arms of the medical profession can be laid, and by each a defence can be mustered.

Generalists can be arraigned on charges of soppiness and sloppiness. It can be alleged that the breadth of their clinical responsibilities compromises their competence so far that they become ineffectual or, at worst, dangerous. The defence would argue that this need not be the case; and, furthermore, that over-attention to the physical substrate of ill-health militates against appreciating the mental, social and cultural contexts in which real people experience illness. Counsel for the prosecution would counter that such considerations are an irrelevant luxury with which professional bio-scientists need not overly concern themselves.

Specialists, on the other hand, stand accused of anatomising patients so minutely that the sense of the patient as a unique and complex individual is lost. Patients, it will be put to them, are more than the sum of their biological parts. There is more to illness than organic pathology, and more to recovery than a mechanic can achieve. Moreover, counsel will continue, thinking of patients as automata is dehumanising for the doctor, in whom, for lack of practice, human sensitivities can wither. Nonsense, retorts the defence; humanity and science are not incompatible, and the best specialists successfully combine the two.

There are, of course, elements of truth in both sets of charges and in both defence arguments. And, indeed, as more and more medical schools acquire flourishing departments of primary care that contribute increasingly to the undergraduate curriculum, we can hope that future generations of doctors will be less prejudiced than their predecessors. Nevertheless, as the young doctors' flipcharts showed, the veneer of mutual respect between specialists and generalists can sometimes still be thin. I am reminded of H.L. Mencken's[62] observation that 'we must respect the other fellow's religion, but only in the sense and to the extent that we respect his theory that his wife is beautiful and his children smart'.

How is it that specialist–generalist tensions, so unproductive and demeaning, have become so entrenched? Part of the answer is to be found in history – in the rise of the classical scientific paradigm described in the last chapter.

---

62 Henry Louis Mencken (1880–1956), American journalist, essayist, satirist and social commentator. Known as 'the sage of Baltimore', Mencken had something of Oscar Wilde's wit and the temperament of a Doberman Pinscher.

The mechanistic approach to medicine, and the specialisms it spawned, brought great practical rewards and fuelled mounting public expectations. One corollary, however, was that areas of human suffering that were too subjective or too complicated to yield readily to the scientific method were marginalised and – like the mind in Cartesian mind–body dualism – defined as beyond rational understanding. In the UK and the USA the old-fashioned family doctor, for whom the subjective and the complicated held few terrors, was left gaping as 20th century medicine threw itself into the arms of science. The more his patients clamoured for scientific medicine, the more patently he, a small-scale operator, could not compete with the mighty hospital, bulging with specialists, to provide it.

Mencken was sharply critical of 'folksy' values. In an essay published in 1956 he wrote:[63]

> *Very little of the extraordinary progress of medicine during the past century is to be credited to the family doctor, though he is still the official hero of the craft ... He is, at best, a humble artisan, not an artist or scientist. The man [we] should really fight for is the research man, [whose] greatest value lies less in enriching medicine with new ideas than in exposing and destroying the old ideas that family doctors cherish.*

In a further delicious dose of vitriol,[64] Mencken is sceptical about the value of the personal doctor–patient relationship, and scathing about the danger he thinks it can pose to clinical competence:

> *The current sentimentalizing of the old-time family doctor is, like any other sentimentality, mainly buncombe ... The idea that the doctor should be a family friend flows out of the prevailing delusion that most illnesses are largely psychic. This nonsense has been preached so long that many otherwise intelligent people, including even doctors, believe it. It is very seldom true.*

> *The best doctor is not one who has had years of experience with the actual patient before him, but one who has had years of experience with multitudes of other patients ... The best the family doctor can do is ... to send them to*

---

63 *Minority Report: H.L. Mencken's Notebooks*, section 41. Baltimore, MD: Johns Hopkins University Press, 1997.

64 *Op. cit.*, section 115.

this or that special clinic. Now and again he falls into error, but it is hardly important, for the specialists quickly recognize it and rectify it.

The chief area of errors is the abdominal region, where symptoms are often obscure and those of quite different diseases are deceptively similar. But in this region as in others, the specialist has enormous advantages over the family doctor – indeed, his advantages are so gigantic that the family doctor's work could be dismissed as trivial if doing it badly were not so dangerous. All the errors that lead to burst appendixes are made by family doctors ... who are supposed to know the patient inside out.

Oh dear; truth is always so vulnerable to a journalist's expertly wielded invective. *The delusion that most illnesses are largely psychic*: with the factually inaccurate 'most' and 'largely' and those scorn-laden words 'delusion' and 'psychic', Mencken dismisses even the possibility that idiosyncrasies of mind as well as of body could have a role in how disease manifests in an individual patient. Why should he wish to do that? Could it have been to impress the influential medical specialists he numbered among his close friends in Baltimore, including the 'Big Four' founding fathers of Johns Hopkins Hospital and Medical School – Sir William Osler, William Halsted, William Welch and Howard Kelly.

Mencken was a man of notoriously fixed opinions, boasting that 'converting me to anything is probably a psychological impossibility'. It's a shame that he didn't recall a story carried in *The American Mercury* of April 1926, a magazine he himself edited, concerning Mellzo McCoy, a 12-year-old boy from Colquitt County, Georgia, who developed symptoms suggestive of acute appendicitis. The lad's father took him to a local physician – not a specialist, mark you – who discovered that the problem stemmed from Mellzo's having eaten the family Bible, all bar its covers and two pages on which the family records were kept. I'll wager that young McCoy, had he fallen instead into the hands of a surgeon, would have undergone an immediate but unnecessary laparotomy.

Domestic politics during the middle years of the 20th century hastened the decline in the prestige of the family doctor in both the USA and the UK. In the USA, referral by a family doctor was neither required nor expected in order to access the services of a specialist. Patients seldom saw much reason to obtain (and pay for) a generalist opinion, relying instead on their own diagnostic skills to decide whom they needed to see. Even only moderately well-off families would expect to retain their own obstetrician/gynaecologist, paediatrician, dermatologist, surgeon, even psychiatrist – with predictable consequences for over-investigation, missed diagnosis and unnecessary treatment. It is only recently that American research[65] has shown how much suffering and money would have been saved had generalist primary care not been squeezed out of the system. Too late: the primary care physician acting as the patient's advocate and providing cost-effective one-stop care is now an endangered species in the USA.

In the UK, events took a different course. The National Insurance Act of 1911 and the advent of the NHS in 1948 gave every citizen the right to his or her 'own' named doctor, with whom the personal relationship so despised by Mencken could be established. Unlike their American counterparts, however, British GPs forfeited the right to attend their patients in hospital, retaining instead the 'gate-keeper' role whereby their signature on a referral was required for all non-emergency admissions. To be sure, specialists' reliance on GPs for their stream of private referrals encouraged a degree of civility, and the now-defunct practice of joint GP–specialist consultations in the patient's home fostered mutual respect between local colleagues. But GPs, denied access not only to the wards but also to the clinically and intellectually challenging atmosphere of the hospital, found themselves excluded from the very environment where they might have been able to hone and update their knowledge of the scientific foundations of their practice.

To a patient – sick, frightened or in pain – to be admitted to hospital is to enter a world that might have been designed to induce deference. They speak an alien language there, work to unknown rules. On every side machines blink and hum, laying bare the workings of our inmost parts. Tubes and syringes infuse, it seems, life itself. Periodic miracles occur, often out of sight and by unknown hands. At ease amid the maelstrom, the senior doctors parade, fluent and powerful, their mastery awe inspiring in proportion to their patients' bewilderment. Even if *we* know, and *they* gladly concede, that these specialists are ordinary fallible mortals like the rest of us, it is inevitable that expertise delivered in such a setting will impress us more profoundly

---

65 Notably by Professor Barbara Starfield of Johns Hopkins University School of Medicine. In innumerable papers over several decades, Starfield has amassed evidence for the greater beneficial impact of primary care than of secondary care on a wide array of health outcomes. For example: Starfield B. Is primary care essential? *Lancet* 1994; **344**: 1129–33.

She summarises the international evidence in a chapter entitled 'The effectiveness of primary health care' in: Lakhani M (ed.). *A Celebration of General Practice*. Oxford: Radcliffe Medical Press, 2003.

than the same degree of expertise demonstrated in familiar surroundings by someone we know and who dresses and speaks much like *we* do. Despite a hundred years of criticism of the medical profession's vainglory; despite challenges to its hubris by commentators from Bernard Shaw to Ivan Illich to the latest Secretary of State; despite the welcome shift in public attitude from deference to scepticism – doctors are still accorded high status. But the status of the specialist has proved more resistant to the forces of social erosion than that of the generalist. The pedestal on which the GP stands never *was* as high as the specialist's.

For the first two decades of the NHS it was possible – indeed, it was the norm – for doctors entering general practice to do so without any further education beyond their 12 months' medical and surgical pre-registration house jobs. Although by the 1950s some visionaries were actively canvassing a system of postgraduate training for general practice, and allowing that some family doctors were clinicians of the highest calibre, it has to be conceded that general practice harboured a significant proportion of doctors who practised to poor standards and had little interest in improving them. It is hardly surprising that the impression grew amongst their colleagues in the highly competitive world of hospital medicine that GPs were the also-rans in the race for professional advancement. As so often in medical politics, issues of principle and value were boiled down to squabbling over money. In 1958 the Royal Commission on Doctors' and Dentists' Pay, chaired by Sir Harry Pilkington, heard evidence from the then President of the Royal College of Physicians, Lord Moran.[66] The following exchange took place:

> The Chairman: It has been put to us by a good many people that the two branches of the profession, general practitioners and consultants, are not senior or junior to one another, but they are level. Do you agree with that?

> Lord Moran: I say emphatically 'No!' Could anything be more absurd? I was Dean at St Mary's Hospital Medical School for 25 years, and all the people of outstanding merit, with few exceptions, aimed to get on the staff. It was a ladder off which they fell. How can you say that the people who fall off the ladder are the same as those who do not? ... I do

---

66 Moran was Sir Winston Churchill's personal physician, and at the time the most influential doctor in the country. His was the principal 'mouth' that Aneurin Bevan famously 'stuffed with gold' in 1947 in order, by allowing consultants to continue private practice, to buy their grudging cooperation with the NHS.

not think you will find a single Dean of any medical school who will give contrary evidence.

Lord Moran subsequently attempted to retract, explaining that he had merely sought to improve the financial lot of junior hospital doctors, who spent long years in training on low salaries. But his talk of a 'ladder' had touched a nerve. GPs – or at least those who were proud of the under-recognised achievements of family medicine and who appreciated its potential as an essential counterpoise to the hospital services – were galvanised into action. The College of General Practitioners, which had been founded in 1952 despite fierce opposition from the Royal College of Physicians, realised that only a sustained drive to establish the defining hallmarks of good general practice, and to guarantee appropriate training in its core skills for all new GPs, would salvage the reputation and future of the discipline. On both counts it was spectacularly successful. John Horder, who later became President of the RCGP, wrote in its Journal:

> *Specialists expect to remain under part-time training until they are from 33 to 40 years old. Is it surprising that some of them have feelings of superiority – and some of us feelings of inferiority – when our own training is so much shorter? Unless this differential is altered what right have we to expect much change in the other differential?*[67]

Under Horder's chairmanship, the College's Vocational Training Working Party presented evidence in 1966 to the Royal Commission on Medical Education that persuaded them that general practice was a distinct discipline within medicine, requiring its own system of formal postgraduate training. In 1972 the (by then Royal) College published *The Future General Practitioner*,[68] a seminal book cataloguing the key skills and attributes required for general practice, and providing a template for systems of vocational training in the UK and worldwide. The 1960s and 1970s must have been an exhilarating time, which saw general practice rescued from the rocks of disdain and reinvigorated with academic respectability. Subsequent decades have seen

---

67 Horder JP. Training for general practice. *Journal of the College of General Practitioners* 1964; **7**: 303–4.

68 Working Party of the Royal College of General Practitioners. *The Future General Practitioner: learning and teaching.* London: RCGP, 1972. The working party consisted of John Horder (chairman), Patrick Byrne, Paul Freeling, Conrad Harris, Donald Irvine and Marshall Marinker.

the accumulation of a substantial body of literature articulating the unique scientific, humanistic and philosophical features of generalism – a corpus to which I hope this book will be allowed to contribute.

* * * * *

Summarising in order to look forward: medicine has always been a hybrid of the rational and the intuitive, of science and the humanities. As the scientific paradigm grew in confidence, the unitary concept of medicine as the compassionate face of reason was threatened. A variety of historical, social and political factors conspired to divide doctors into specialists, who did 'proper' science in hospitals, and a lower order of generalists, who dabbled in sociology, philanthropy and an amateurish kind of medicine in the community. The status gradient that ranks specialists above generalists exists to this day, perpetuated in popular culture and, amongst doctors, in attitudes inculcated at medical school. In recent decades the gulf has to some extent been bridged, and the stereotypes challenged, by a public backlash against the dehumanising effects of scientism and by generalists' belated attempts to explain that what they do isn't as easy as it looks. But the specialist–generalist divide nevertheless persists.

Does this matter? Yes, it does. Internal discord, even if it were only light-hearted, disfigures a profession and undermines public trust. And this at a time when public and political opinion is suspicious of the very concept of professions, which are sometimes portrayed as elitist, self-serving and exploitative. Medical professionalism has recently been described as 'everything it takes to maintain doctors' trustworthiness in the eyes of patients'.[69] On this basis, sniping between specialists and generalists – if it implies that one type of doctor is 'better', or does more valuable work, than the other – is unprofessional. It is as if two people, one of whom has gone blind and the other deaf, fall into argument over whether painting or music is the superior art form. *When there are two midwives* (a Persian proverb goes), *the baby's head is crooked.* And yet neither faction has quite managed to dampen the smouldering rivalry between them. Tension between specialists and generalists will not be resolved by agreeing to differ; co-existence would suggest that patients,

---

69 Royal College of Physicians. *Doctors in society: medical professionalism in a changing world.* London: RCP, 2005. The report of a working party of the Royal College of Physicians of London. This excellent analysis offers the following short definition (considerably expanded in the text): *Medical professionalism signifies a set of values, behaviours and relationships that underpins the trust the public has in doctors.*

their illnesses and problems change in some mysterious way as soon as they cross a hospital threshold. Nor is there any want of fundamental goodwill on either side; each camp contains many excellent, rounded, clinically competent and patient-serving doctors who, intellectually at least, understand the others' approach.

> In order properly to understand the big picture, you should fear becoming mentally clouded and obsessed with one small section of truth.
>
> Xun Zi
> Chinese Confucian philosopher
> c. 300–230 BCE

In some ways medicine now finds itself in a situation similar to that of classical physics in 1905. The Newtonian model of physics and the specialist model of medicine are both based on what we might call 'the mechanistic assumption' – that the natural world and the human body are machines that behave in predictable ways when you do things to them. Both brought tangible benefits on a scale undreamed of in the long centuries before the advent of formalised science. But Einstein and the rest of the quantum gang showed that there were limits to what the mechanistic assumption could account for. They asked questions that classical science could not answer, even in principle. They pointed out phenomena that conventional analysis could not begin to explain. They reached conclusions that left the Newtonians bewildered and helpless: logic is not always linear; causality is complex and multi-dimensional; things can behave as if they are more than one thing at once; what you see depends upon where you stand; what you find depends upon how you search and upon who you are.

The generalist tradition in medicine has very similar things to say about the limits to the specialist model. The generalist knows that the body might well function as a machine, but its owner hates being treated as one. Patients can be rational and irrational at the same time. They suffer from several problems at once, which interact in complex and unpredictable ways. They ask unscientific questions such as *Why me? What does all this mean?* The generalist knows that the course of an illness can be profoundly affected by the patient's psychology, and by that of the doctor, and by the relationship between them.

Although classical and quantum physics were at first uneasy bedfellows, and the gulf between them probably seemed wider at the time than that between specialist and generalist doctors has ever been, the world picture that eventually sprang from their union was bigger and more vigorous than before. It wasn't that Newtonian physics was shown to be *wrong*, or that quantum physics replaced it. For many purposes, even putting men on the moon, Newton worked fine. Rather, each was enhanced by accommodating the insights of the other. We now have a bigger picture of physics, in which the Newtonian and the Einsteinian both sit comfortably. The gaze of the 'big picture physicist' can, if necessary, shift away from the everyday to the world of the infinitesimally small or the astronomically large. He can 'think classical' or 'think quantum' as the situation calls for, without internal contradiction.

I believe medicine is now called upon to make a similar synthesis between its specialist and generalist traditions. It is time for us to sketch out medicine's 'big picture'.

In 'big picture medicine', specialist practice and generalist practice are not 'either-ors'. Nor are they the prerogative of doctors who work in a particular setting or who see patients with a particular class of problem. Specialism and generalism are matters of mindset, ways of doing your medicine, distinguished not in terms of *who does what where*, but of how you think about your practice. The 'big picture doctor' can also 'think specialist' or 'think generalist' as the situation calls for, without internal contradiction. The two cultures should be integrated not at the organisational level but internally, within the skills repertoire of the individual clinician.

Every patient needs understanding, solace and remediation in some unique combination. Deciding what form of each, and in what proportion, is the challenge facing every doctor – specialist or generalist – every time a patient consults. The specialist mindset has most to offer in the field of remediation, working out what biological or technical intervention will most benefit the 'body-as-machine'. The generalist mindset comes into its own for ensuring that the patient is properly understood and comforted. One of my personal heroes, John Heron, has described a professional as 'someone with a wide range of options, and who can move cleanly and elegantly amongst them.'[70] Cleanly and elegantly: isn't that how a good doctor should aim to draw on the best of both specialist and generalist ways of working?

> One of the perennial curses of thought is the making separate of what is only distinguishable.
>
> L.A. Reid (1895–1986)
> Professor of the Philosophy of Education
> University of London

---

70 John Heron, personal communication, *c.* 1980 and 2007. Heron, born 1928, is a humanistic psychologist. He founded the Human Potential Research Project at Surrey University in 1970, and was later Assistant Director of the British Postgraduate Medical Federation until 1985, working extensively with hospital doctors and GPs interested in personal development. He developed Six-Category Intervention Analysis as a framework for communication in a therapeutic setting.

Practising 'big picture medicine' is as much a question of achieving a flexibility of mindset as it is of acquiring specific skills. The next chapter will flesh out some of the details. But I want to close *this* chapter by attempting to convey something of the experience of being in the 'big picture' mindset. Metaphor may prove a more successful vehicle than explanation. Bear with me ... .

* * * * *

The caterpillars of moths of the family Geometridae ('earth-measurers') are commonly known as 'inchworms' or 'loopers'. About 2.5 centimetres (one inch) long, they have six true legs at the front of their bodies and four pro-legs at the back; but, unlike most other caterpillars, they lack pro-legs in the middle. They move by grabbing hold with their front legs, then arching the body so that the rear end is drawn forward. They then grip with the back legs, let go with the front, and reach forward for a new attachment, giving the impression that they are measuring off the journey inch by inch.

In Charles Vidor's 1952 film *Hans Christian Andersen*, with songs by Frank Loesser, Danny Kaye plays the eponymous Danish story-teller. There is a scene in which children are learning arithmetic in a classroom. Mournfully they sing over and over:[71]

> *Two and two are four*
> *Four and four are eight*
> *Eight and eight are sixteen*
> *Sixteen and sixteen are thirty-two.*

Andersen, listening just outside, gazes at an inchworm crawling on the flowers, and sings:

> *Inchworm, inchworm,*
> *Measuring the marigold,*
> *You and your arithmetic*
> *You'll probably go far.*
> *Inchworm, inchworm,*
> *Measuring the marigold,*
> *Seems to me you'd stop and see*
> *How beautiful they are.*

---

71 A track of Danny Kaye singing *Inchworm* can be downloaded from: http://beemp3.com/download.php?file=1245463&song=Inchworm.

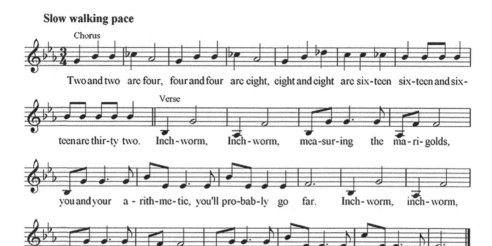

Slow walking pace

The Inchworm
Words and Music by Frank Loesser
© Copyright 1951 and 1952 (Renewed 1979 and 1980) Frank Music Corporation
MPL Communications Limited
All Rights Reserved. International Copyright Secured.
Used by permission of Music Sales Limited.

Put yourself inside the skin of the various players in this wistful little scene.

First the inchworm, absorbed – contentedly, as far as we can tell – in looping his way across the face of a marigold. He doesn't question the value of botanical mensuration, nor his role as a specialist in it. He is just doing what inchworms do. If you've got any marigolds needing measuring, he's your man.

But we sense from the children's doleful refrain, as they recite their numbers, that they *do* have doubts. Is arithmetic, they seem to be wondering, a fit thing to be doing on a summer's afternoon, when the whole of nature lies effulgent just beyond the classroom door? If later on they become medical students, they will experience many such moments of inescapable pointlessness – better get used to it. But we can sympathise with their resignation.

Andersen – free, mature, blessed with imagination – can respect the thoroughness of the inchworm's activity. He can also see it in a wider context: one where *what* the creature is measuring also has immeasurable qualities that, could it but notice them, would give it pause and open its eyes to the mystery and loveliness of its surroundings. (The musically trained reader may note how the rising sixth to the submediant on the first syllable of 'beautiful' implies a plagal cadence, with its noble or religious associations.) What

Andersen cannot know at first hand, however, is just how satisfying an inchworm finds its marigold measuring. All he can say, from his generalist perspective, is that if *he* were the inchworm, he would take stock now and then to allow the beauty of the flowers to register.

But imagine what it would be like to be the kind of inchworm that could respond to what Andersen is saying – an inchworm with a sense of aesthetics; an inchworm with 'big picture awareness'; an inchworm able to switch cleanly and elegantly between measurement and wonderment.

And imagine what it can be like, as a doctor, to take pride in the technicalities of your work and at the same time to have a sense of the richness of the context in which you operate – to be able to stop and see how beautiful, and mysterious, and intriguing and unique are the patients who put their trust in you.

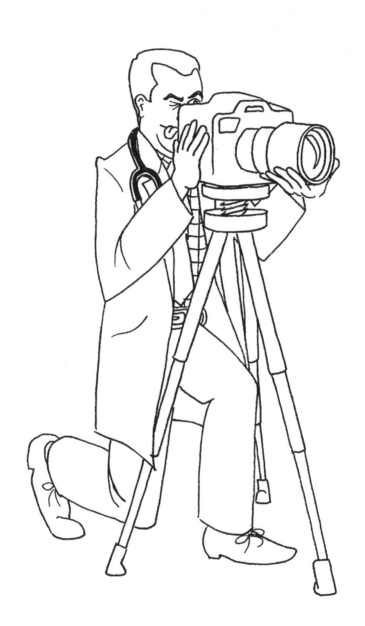

Chapter 4

The medical gaze

The businessman who assumes that this life is everything, and the mystic who asserts that it is nothing, fail to hit the truth. No; truth, being alive, was not halfway between anything. It was to be only found by continuous excursions into either realm.

E.M. Forster (1879–1970)

English novelist

From *Howards End* (1910)

The previous chapter explored the traditional divide between specialists and generalists, and proposed that the important differences between them are neither the types of patients and diseases they deal with, nor whether they work inside or outside hospitals. The distinction, I suggested, is more a cognitive one – a matter of what goes on in their heads, a question of how they each think about the work they do. There are distinctively specialist and generalist ways of thinking about what medicine is and how it is to be practised. An individual doctor might use one way more than the other in his everyday setting, or might have a preferred style that emphasises one rather than the other. But we are dealing with a continuum, a spectrum, a range. The most effective clinician, I believe, is one who can draw upon skills from across the whole range, sometimes practising in a more generalist way and at others in a more specialist way, moving cleanly and elegantly throughout the range as the patient's needs dictate.

In this chapter I want to enquire more closely into what differentiates the generalist from the specialist way of doing medicine. I shall develop the idea that the distinctions are largely perceptual – by which I mean how the doctor selects which features of the clinical situation are to be taken notice of, and the quality of the attention that is to be paid to them.

Neurophysiologists tell us that perception is a more complicated process than just afferent sensory messages reaching consciousness. Our sense organs are subject to a degree of efferent control by the cerebral cortex and limbic system; what we perceive is modified by past experience, distorted to fit with what we expect, and conditioned by our emotional and hormonal state. What a doctor *sees*, and therefore subsequently *does*, is modulated by what kind of person that doctor already *is*.

I need a phrase for how an individual doctor views and interprets the job and the patient, some words to mean *how things look and sound through the doctor's personal eyes and ears*. 'Perceptual set' sounds a bit psycho-babbly. *The medical gaze* would be a good term. *Gaze*, being both noun and verb, narrows the gap between seeing and doing. *Gazing* is how mothers look at their infants, something that lovers do, or travellers when they chance upon a fine view. A *gaze* is less cursory than a glance, more confident than a peek, less aggressive than a stare. A *medical gaze* sounds a promising thing for a doctor to confer upon a patient as a prelude to fruitful action.

Unfortunately, the phrase *medical gaze* has already been used by the French philosopher Michel Foucault,[72] or at least by his translator. In his 1963 book *The Birth of the Clinic* Foucault wrote, pejoratively, of *le regard médical* as the often dehumanising way doctors paid attention only to the physical body, and ignored the patient's sense of being a unique self. To Foucault, the medical gaze was an instrument of corporate subjugation and control; it was how doctors as a group looked upon patients merely as biological phenomena in which they the doctors, and only they, were the experts. Foucault, of course, can only have based his analysis on the doctors he himself encountered in France over 50 years ago, and so we should not assume that he intended to disparage every doctor for ever more. The concept of a medical gaze should be essentially a neutral one – at least until it is embodied in the particular behaviour of a particular doctor – and I should like to reclaim it for my own use here. The turning of a doctor's medical gaze towards a patient, viewing that patient, as it were, through a lens, is the first stage in their interaction.

Some doctors – they tend to be specialists – do their medical gazing through a lens of fixed focal length. They have only one pre-set field of view, giving only one perspective and taking in only a fixed amount of the patient's

---

72 Michel Foucault (1926–84), French philosopher, historian and sociologist, best known for his critical studies of social institutions such as medicine, psychiatry (*Madness and Civilisation*, 1961) and the prison system (*Discipline and Punish: the birth of the prison*, 1975). He was particularly interested in how knowledge and power are related.

background and setting. They look at every patient in the same way that they always do, notice only what they always notice, and interpret what they see in much the same way every time. The fixed-focus lens of the specialist is often a close-up lens, picking out fine detail at the expense of context. Doctors with a fixed close-up gaze tend to work in the clinical specialties such as surgery, cardiology or dermatology, where attention to detail is at a premium. Other specialist colleagues, such as those working in public health or epidemiology, may be fitted with a fixed wide-angle lens, through which their clinical work appears in panoramic view uncluttered by too much detail of individual patients.

At all events, the doctor with a fixed gaze, whether close-up or wide-angle, is potentially restricted, even trapped, by it. So, more importantly, are his patients. He can be a sorry figure: the harassed dermatologist, for example, whose overstretched clinics seem full of patients inexplicably reluctant to put steroid cream on their eczema but evangelical enough when it comes to faddy diets or unlicensed herbal remedies. Both he and they are imprisoned by an inflexible medical gaze.

In contrast, the defining quality of the generalist medical gaze is its adjustability. The lens of the generalist is a zoom lens, capable of adjusting its field of view from close-up to wide-angle and everything in between. Moreover, as a further refinement, the generalist's zoom lens is mounted on a swivel, so that it can be pointed away from you the doctor, towards your patient – or, should you wish, directed back towards yourself. In its most sophisticated form, the medical gaze has these two degrees of freedom – 'field of view' and 'direction of point'.

If you view the patient with a fixed close-up gaze, what you see is detail: the organs, the cells, the molecules; the anatomy, the physiology, the chemistry; the fine structure of normality or abnormality. If you swop the close-up lens for a wide-angle one, you see not detail but context. You see generalisations, populations, distributions; roles, relationships. As well as biology you see psychology, biography, sociology, economics. But if you gaze upon your patient through the generalist's adjustable zoom lens and move it around throughout its range, you see the interplay, the connectedness of all these dimensions. You see complexity; you sense meanings and significances. You see the beauty of the marigold as well as its measurements. And sometimes you see the unfolding of time. Rather than a static picture, you see a narrative: strands of causality emerging from the past into a present crisis and heading off into a future of consequences; a story that in due course will be recollected and recounted to an audience not yet gathered.

How we look and what we see have powerful effects on how we think and act. The fixed-focus gaze of the specialist views patients predominantly in close-up and dwells chiefly on their components. If you focus mainly on the detail of a clinical problem, and if what fascinates you is its micro-structure, you will find yourself thinking that detail is paramount and practising in a way that concentrates on detail. You will tend to interpret what you discover, and to frame the problem that is to be solved, in terms that call for a solution at your favourite level of detail. Here, by way of example, is a case history illustrating the specialist gaze in action.

> A 27-year-old woman attends the Accident and Emergency department at 11 p.m. complaining of 'palpitations', and is seen by the registrar in cardiology. She says that her heart races and thumps for up to an hour at a time, several times a week for the last 3 months. On arrival, her pulse is regular, 80 beats per minute. She has no symptoms in between attacks. She has no significant past or family history, and is on no medication. She came off the oral contraceptive pill 3 months ago, as she and her husband are trying for another baby. There are no abnormalities on examination. Routine blood tests and resting ECG are normal. The registrar arranges thyroid function tests, chest X-ray and ambulatory heart monitoring, all of which, when she is reviewed in the outpatient clinic, are normal. The registrar makes a provisional diagnosis of atrioventricular nodal re-entrant supra-ventricular tachycardia, and proposes a therapeutic trial of a beta-blocking drug. The consultant cardiologist agrees, but suggests that she should be further investigated as a possible case of Wolff–Parkinson–White syndrome, potentially treatable with radio frequency ablation via catheter. The patient fails to attend her follow-up appointment.

I don't mean to imply that the specialist gaze is insensitive, or obsessive, or blind to beauty. Seeing things in close-up brings its own kind of delight. On 7 September 1674 Antonie von Leeuwenhoek, the inventor of the micro-scope, wrote the following letter to Henry Oldenburg, Secretary of The Royal Society. It powerfully conveys how discovering the complexities of the natural world can excite the amazement of the explorer/scientist:

> *About two hours distant from this Town there lies an inland lake, called the Berkelse Mere, whose bottom in many places is very marshy, or boggy. Its water in winter is very clear, but at the beginning or in the middle of summer it becomes whitish, and there are than little green clouds floating through it*

... Passing just lately over this lake, at a time, when the wind blew pretty hard, and seeing the water as above described, I took up a little of it in a glass phial; and examining this water next day, I found floating therein divers earthy particles, and some green streaks, spirally wound serpent-wise, and orderly arranged[73] *... Among these there were, besides, very many little animalcules, whereof some were roundish, while others, a bit bigger, consisted of an oval.*[74] *On these last I saw two little legs near the head, and two little fins at the hindmost end of the body.*[75] *These animalcules had divers colours, some being whitish and transparent; others with green and very glittering little scales; others again were green in the middle, and before and behind white; others yet were ashen grey. And the motion of most of these animalcules in the water was so swift, and so various, upwards, downwards, and round about, that 'twas wonderful to see.*

Leeuwenhoek's was what we might call 'the awe of the close-up'. There is another kind – 'wide-angle awe' – that comes from glimpsing the immensity of things. Astronauts, whom one might expect to be among the hardest nosed of scientists, have often been profoundly moved by what they see from their privileged vantage points. Yuri Gagarin, the Russian cosmonaut, who on 12 April 1961 became the first human being to orbit the Earth, wrote on his return:

What beauty! I saw clouds and their shadows on the distant dear Earth ... When I watched the horizon, I saw the abrupt, contrasting transition from the Earth's light-coloured surface to the absolutely black sky. I enjoyed the rich colour spectrum of the Earth. It is surrounded by a light blue aureole that gradually darkens, becoming turquoise, dark blue, violet, and finally coal black.

Within 9 years of Gagarin's flight, Neil Armstrong walked on the Moon.[76] But 'what was most significant about the lunar voyage,' wrote the political journalist Norman Cousins, 'was not that men set foot on the Moon but that they set eye on the Earth'. As Apollo 11 left Earth's orbit, Armstrong said,

---

73　This is the first known description of the green alga *Spirogyra*.

74　Almost certainly protozoa.

75　Probably rotifers.

76　During the 1969 Apollo 11 mission, its lunar module, *Eagle*, touched down on the Sea of Tranquility. On 20 July mission commander Neil Armstrong took mankind's first extra-terrestrial step.

It suddenly struck me that that tiny pea, pretty and blue, was the Earth. I put up my thumb and shut one eye, and my thumb blotted out the planet Earth. I didn't feel like a giant. I felt very, very small.

Likewise Edgar Mitchell, lunar module pilot on Apollo 14:

Suddenly, from behind the rim of the Moon, in long, slow-motion moments of immense majesty, there emerges a sparkling blue and white jewel, a light, delicate sky-blue sphere laced with slowly swirling veils of white, rising gradually like a small pearl in a thick sea of black mystery. It takes more than a moment to fully realise this is Earth ... home.

And James B. Irwin, during Apollo 15:

As we got further and further away, the Earth shrank to the size of a marble, the most beautiful you can imagine. That beautiful, warm, living object looked so fragile, so delicate, that if you touched it with a finger it would crumble and fall apart. Seeing this has to change a man.

Finally, Loren Acton, a Lockheed research scientist who flew on Spacelab 2 in August 1978:

Looking outward to the blackness of space, sprinkled with the glory of a universe of lights, I saw majesty – but no welcome. Below was a welcoming planet. There, contained in the thin, moving, incredibly fragile shell of the biosphere is everything that is dear to you, all the human drama and comedy. That's where life is; that's where all the good stuff is.

That tiny pea; a pearl in a sea of black mystery; I saw majesty, but no welcome: the very language gives the lie to conspiracy theorists who claim that the Moon landings were a hoax. Here are some of the most rational and analytical of people finding, in the very places to which the triumph of science has transported them, that the language of science is eclipsed, and that, for fuller truthfulness, they must also invoke metaphor and poetry. They truly are 'inchworms with big picture awareness'. Committed scientists though they are, when the astronauts' field of view is so dramatically widened, other aspects of their awareness are drawn irresistibly into the frame. Their gaze takes in sights and associations that demand to be understood in other, non-scientific, paradigms. Again, their language is a pointer. For the Russian

Gagarin to speak of 'beauty' rather than of Mother Russia's technological triumph was at the time an act of considerable bravery. When Armstrong blots out the Earth with his thumb and feels, paradoxically, 'very, very small', he is not talking of optics and parallax, but rather facing his own isolation and helplessness. Mitchell, seeing 'a pearl in a thick sea of black mystery', confesses he cannot analyse what it is that makes Earth precious, other than that is where he belongs. Irwin's fantasy that everything dear to him could crumble at a finger's touch seems to express a universal sense of human frailty and mortality. In Acton's hymn to life we can hear his longing for acceptance, for love and laughter – better (he implies) to be fragile and alive than majestic but indifferent.

What the astronauts were experiencing (admittedly more intensely than do most doctors during a busy clinic) was 'the generalist gaze'. What really got to them was the way their perspective kept shifting between the vast and the personal: Armstrong's juxtaposition of planet and thumb; Mitchell's realisation that the 'small pearl in a thick sea of black mystery' was also home.

In medicine too – as the generalist widens and varies the gaze with which the patient's presenting problem is examined – domains beyond the purely physical come into the frame and are incorporated into an increasingly comprehensive understanding. The specialist's systematic approach to diagnosis and treatment, based on expertise in pathology and therapeutics, remains highly relevant. But, as the doctor zooms back and forth between detail and context, those details that fill the specialist field of view come to occupy a diminishing fraction of the expanding clinical panorama. Other, contextual, considerations come into the picture: the story the patient tells; the meaning they attribute to what troubles them; the effect of their illness on the people and things that matter to them; their web of social roles and personal relationships; their inner life of fears and hopes, plans and motives, values and beliefs.

Here is another case history.

Giuseppina Thompson is an Italian-born woman of 27, married for 5 years to Gerry, a sheet metal worker. They have one child aged 3, Marko, who was born with moderate cerebral palsy after a difficult forceps delivery. Caring for Marko is hard work for Giuseppina, who feels that she is not a good mother for him; indeed, she partly blames herself for his handicap. Gerry is keen to have a second child. He hopes the next one would be 'a proper kid, one I could play football with.' Three months ago, after a furious row, Gerry threw away Giuseppina's contraceptive pills and ordered her not to get any more. The next time he tried to have sex, Giuseppina had some kind of 'attack', in which her heart raced and pounded so much that they had to stop. The same thing now seems to happen whenever they begin to make love, which is not very often. Giuseppina tells Gerry that she wants another baby just as much as *he* does, but it wouldn't be safe for her to get pregnant, not while she's suffering from these palpitations.

The GP whom Giuseppina consulted examined her and said her heart was normal. She told her she thought her symptoms were a 'kind of replacement form of contraception', and referred her to a counsellor. When Giuseppina tried to explain this to Gerry he said, 'So there's nothing wrong you?', and became angry. However, the next time they attempted intercourse Giuseppina's palpitations were so intense, and she became so breathless, that he thought she was having a heart attack, and called an ambulance, which took her to the A&E Department. Because it was 11 p.m. and there was no one else to look after Marko, Gerry did not go with his wife to the hospital.

The patient in this case history is the same as in the earlier one, but her story is told in a way that makes her arrival in the hospital A&E department more understandable. We can also begin to imagine why, faced with more alarming investigations, Giuseppina defaults from follow-up by the cardiologist. This second description, emphasising background and context, reads more like an episode in a television soap opera. On the other hand, it arguably provides a better answer – or range of possible answers – to the question *What is going on here?*

Imagine how Giuseppina and her story might have appeared to the wider angle gaze of her own GP. As Giuseppina walks nervously into your consulting room, much of what scriptwriters call her 'back story' is already familiar to you. You recall prescribing contraception for her when she was a newly-wed, brought from Naples to the UK by Gerry after a holiday romance. You remember her pregnancy as a period of happiness, shattered by Marko's traumatic birth and the diagnosis of his cerebral palsy. Your records chart Giuseppina's post-natal depression, the intensive involvement of your health visitor, frequent attendances with minor physical illnesses, the unexplained bruising on her wrist on one occasion … . As she describes her 'palpitations' in still-hesitant English, you think the account of her symptoms doesn't seem medically consistent. You notice how tears well up in her eyes when you ask her how things are at home, and how she shakes her head as she tells you, 'I cannot have more baby!' She gives you no reason to suspect thyroid disease, she doesn't look anaemic, her pulse is regular, and the ECG done by your practice nurse looks quite normal. You are alert to the danger of 'somatisation' – when unexpressed anxiety takes the form of physical symptoms, which then become the focus of misplaced medical attention and thereby entrenched. You decide not to suggest a cardiology referral; you consider this would be a fruitless diversion away from the real problem. So you try to explain to Giuseppina that, because she has not been able to tell Gerry how scared she is of another pregnancy, her body has developed symptoms that protect her from it. You refer her to your practice counsellor, hoping the counsellor can improve the communication between husband and wife, who are both so unhappy in their different ways.

Here are two approaches to Giuseppina's complaint, each highly professional by its own lights. The cardiologists zoomed in on her heart as the organ in trouble, and investigated the details of its electrophysiology and microanatomy. Their diagnosis, and the course of action they proposed, were pitched at this 'micro' level. The GP, on the other hand, took a wide-angle view. She tried to see Giuseppina's symptoms as part of a larger picture. She concentrated more on where and when they occurred, on their timing in relation to other events in Giuseppina's life, and on the effects they were having upon her and those close to her. Her proposed solution – counselling – was intended to change the context that evoked the symptom, rather than its physical manifestation.

All have done their best. But the best of none of them is good enough. None of Giuseppina's doctors has served her as well as she needs. The cardiologists (if she ever goes back to see them) will find no underlying biological abnormality. To them, her case will be 'inappropriate' and they will feel they have nothing to offer her. The GP – irked that the hospital has become involved, and unsurprised that all the tests have so far been negative – will nod sagely to herself and think *I could have told you that.* And yet her action plan, too, failed to do full justice to the situation. She was not able to sufficiently contain Giuseppina's or Gerry's mounting anxiety, resulting in their precipitate arrival at the hospital late one evening.

Giuseppina has fallen between two stools. Her GP, taking the wide-angle view and seeing her symptoms in their various contexts, saw how they might spring from her complex family and social circumstances. But Giuseppina did not feel confident enough that the possibility of physical disease had been taken ruled out, and turned to the hospital for reassurance. Later, she fled the specialists because she could sense that their close-up organ-centred approach was not going to resolve the wider ramifications of her problem. She is the victim, twice over, of fixed medical gaze. What the gaze of both GP and specialist lacked was 'adjustability'. Had the GP been able to complement her contextual approach with elements of a specialist perspective, perhaps by arranging some further investigations, she might have bolstered Giuseppina's trust in her to the point that it could withstand the late-night panic that took her to the hospital. Had the hospital doctors enquired a little more into the background of Giuseppina's symptoms, as well as the symptoms themselves, they might perhaps have held back from some of their investigations, perhaps have encouraged her to attend with Gerry as well, perhaps have seen whether explanation and reassurance might be treatment enough.

Inevitably, there is a trade-off between detail and context. Going exclusively after detail can make you context-blind. Become too preoccupied with context, on the other hand, and you risk overlooking crucial details, as Mencken so trenchantly reminded us in the previous chapter. Adjustability is key. To re-work the line of Forster quoted as this chapter's epigraph: 'the generalist gaze is not halfway between close-up detail and wide-angle context. It is to be found by continuous excursions into either realm.'

* * * * *

My visual metaphor for this chapter is a zoom lens mounted on a swivel, giving the medical gaze two degrees of freedom – 'adjustability' of the field of view and 'direction of point'. I want now to turn to the second of these.

Throughout our consideration of the field of view, the assumption has been that the medical gaze is always directed outwards, on to the patient. It might zoom in, specialist-wise, on the patient as a biological system, or pull back in a more generalist way to take in the patient's psychological, social and cultural contexts. But nothing as it were 'behind the lens', no glimpse of the observer/doctor, ever comes into the picture. However, with the additional degree of freedom conferred by a swivelled mounting comes just this possibility.

The astronauts knew about 'swivel', their gaze taking in their own inner responses as well as the marvels they were witnessing through the windows of their spacecraft. Neil Armstrong could feel himself no longer a giant but 'very, very small'; confronted with the vastness of space, Loren Acton became aware of his own need to know where he belonged. 'Swivel' adds a further capability to the doctor's gaze, allowing it to be directed not just externally

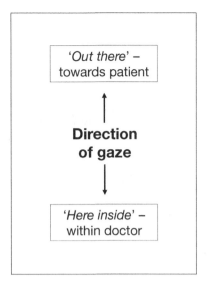

Figure 4.1 'Swivelled gaze'.

towards the patient in *her* world but also internally, towards the doctor's own private inner world. The doctor's attention can encompass what is going on *here inside* as well as what is *out there* (see Figure 4.1). And *here inside* is the realm of the Inner Physician, the doctor-as-person.

As a rule, the specialist gaze is not swivel mounted; it remains resolutely outward facing. It is almost axiomatic to the specialist mindset that medicine is conducted *out there*, where objectivity rules, and that the doctor-as-person is too subjective to be allowed to figure in the picture. It is, moreover, also possible to practise a kind of generalist medicine in which the gaze is kept pointing steadily outwards. Clinical decisions often need to be made as dispassionately as possible, without the doctor's own idiosyncrasies muddying the water. But not always. On occasion, patients are better served if their doctor can supplement the technical accuracy of what he knows with the human richness of what he thinks and feels.

If ever I have a heart attack, I want the doctor who attends me to be fully au fait with the latest guidelines on managing my cardiac pathology, yet at the same time alert to all those aspects of my life that may have contributed to it and which could be affected by it.[77] A doctor like that, detail *and* context aware, will on that day suit me just fine, and I shall count myself lucky if

---

77 Be careful what you imagine! Shortly after first writing this passage, I did have a small myocardial infarction. I was lucky both in my cardiac pathology and in my consultant.

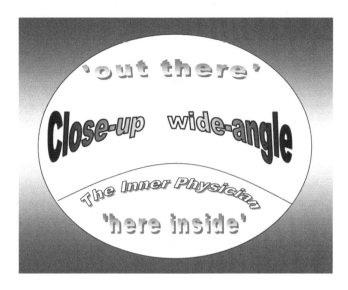

Figure 4.2 'Big picture' medical gaze.

such a one is on duty. But if I survive, I shall hope for a doctor who is all that and more besides. I should like someone who understands what unexpected illness and the proximity of death can do to a person; someone who can empathise with how the experience might have affected me; someone who may even be personally glad I was still around. Such a doctor, whose medical gaze can encompass the biggest possible picture, is likely to be one at ease within his or her own mind; someone whose life experience as well as medical know-how is at my service; someone whose self-awareness is developed to the point that empathy cannot but flow from it.

I am trying to describe what seems to me to be a comprehensive 'big picture' medical gaze, of which the more familiar specialist and generalist gazes are both subsets. Figure 4.2 is a graphical representation of what I have in mind.

Conventionally, the territory surveyed by the doctor's gaze is limited to the external world, the world beyond his own skin, the tangible world as explored by science, the public world where the patient lives and suffers in accordance with the established laws of physics and biology and the fuzzier laws of human relationships. This territory 'out there' can be viewed either in close-up or in wide-angle, specialists tending to favour the former and generalists the latter. Each has its advantages and its shortcomings. Each leads to medical interpretations and interventions on its own scale. Nimble-minded clinicians, however, can adjust their field of view as required, and pursue detail and context with equal facility.

This account of the conventional medical gaze (represented by the upper portion of Figure 4.2) is analogous to the classical Newtonian view of the natural order that obtained before 1905. And it contains fallacies analogous to the ones that Einstein and the quantum theorists identified in physics. The new paradigm in physics has made us accept as valid a good many notions which, when first articulated, seemed counter-intuitive.

1 There is only one absolute – the speed of light in a vacuum; how everything else looks depends on where we happen to be looking from.
2 Even fundamental particles such as quarks can come in varieties with different flavour, charm and strangeness.
3 Time is a separate dimension in its own right.
4 There is always an inescapable element of uncertainty in what we take for 'knowledge' that cannot be resolved, no matter how hard we try.
5 Events sometimes have to be described in terms of probabilities rather than certainties.
6 Causality is not always linear or local; events remote in time and space can have unpredictable effects on what happens now.
7 It is possible to be in more than one state of being at the same time – until someone checks to see.

Each of these updates to the classical scientific paradigm corresponds to a way in which the modern generalist medical gaze has developed and extended the conventional, specialist, version.

1 Everything doctors deal with – disease, illness, health, cure, consolation and especially death – can be understood and managed in more ways than the purely scientific.
2 Individual patients differ from one another, not only physically but also in their functioning, thinking and behaviour. Individual variations are clinically significant.
3 To the patient, an illness is not a one-off event but an episode in a longer and continuing story.
4 Even the most comprehensive medical diagnosis or prognosis is riddled with uncertainty, which has to be managed in its own right.
5 Rational systematic analysis is not the only way of making a diagnosis. Sometimes shortcuts or 'educated guesses' are all that is practicable.
6 The causes of medical problems are usually more complex, and their effects more far ranging, than can be neatly pinned down.

7   The act of consulting a doctor constrains the patient into a limited role and closes off other options. For example, a person with undiagnosed symptomless hypertension is, rather like Schrödinger's cat, both well and ill at the same time – until, that is, someone checks the blood pressure.

However, this list is incomplete. It does not incorporate what was probably the most important message of the new scientific paradigm – the significance of the observer effect. The new physics teaches us that there is no such thing as an uninvolved and detached observer. The observer is part of the system observed; the nature of the observer determines what is perceived; and the act of observing inevitably changes the system.

Mainstream medical thought has been reluctant to take the observer effect on board. Our medical schools continue to concentrate on training the doctor-as-scientist, in the mistaken belief that only the medically trained parts of a doctor are what matter when it comes to dealing with patients. Medical students are taught that the doctor-as-person, with idiosyncratic thought processes and undisciplined reactions, is as little welcome in the consulting room as the embarrassing cousin at a family gathering. But, whether or not patients know it, it is always a doctor's totality with whom they consult – doctor-as-person as well as doctor-as-scientist. The observer effect cannot be kept out of medicine any more than it can out of physics. A 'big picture' medical gaze includes the gazer.

If you are a practising doctor, you will know that, all the time you are consulting with a patient in the world 'out there', much is going on in the privacy of your own head. Thoughts come and go, some medical, some not. Small 'currents of emotion ebb and flow. Assumptions and prejudices surface. Feelings arise towards the patient, positive and negative. Remarks are being silently rehearsed, strategies planned, possible actions considered. Daydreams briefly seduce your attention. Unexpected ideas spring up from the unconscious.

Conventional wisdom is that we should do our best to suppress this internal noise as a distraction with no contribution to make to the clinical process. But we simply can't: it's there. The Inner Physician is present in the consulting room whether we like it or not, whether the patient realises it or not. The lesson of the new physics, and a key feature of modern generalism, is that we cannot, need not, *should* not try to factor it out. The observer/doctor's stream of conscious awareness *here inside* is integral to building up a comprehensive understanding of the clinical world *out there*. The lower sector of Figure 4.2 is intended to depict how a 'big picture' medical gaze, incorporating the observer effect, points inwards as well as outwards.

There are practical and clinically important consequences to broadening the medical gaze in this way. Acknowledging the doctor-as-participant-observer has implications for how empathy and insight can be fostered, for making therapeutic use of the doctor–patient relationship, and for maintaining the doctor's own well-being. Later chapters in this book will expand on these. For now, let me suggest that E.M. Forster, in this chapter's opening epigraph, was over-simplifying things when he proposed that the search for truth required continuous excursions into two realms. In medicine at least, there are three. In the realm of detail, where the doctor's gaze is in close-up mode, the search is for the right level of explanatory detail to manage the patient's problem as effectively as science will allow. In the realm of context, the doctor, with gaze zoomed to wide-angle, will be exploring its connections and ramifications as widely as is necessary to make the patient feel properly understood. Excursions into the third, inner, realm are marked by the doctor periodically wondering *What do I notice going on within myself?* The true generalist, mindful of John Heron's dictum, will allow his or her attention to dance 'cleanly and elegantly' in and out of all three realms.

What if Giuseppina's GP had from time to time turned her gaze inwards as well as outwards, and allowed her Inner Physician to make its contribution? Again, imagine yourself in the doctor's chair as Giuseppina enters your consulting room. What is your immediate reaction on seeing her? Are you pleased to see someone whom you admire for her fortitude? If so, maybe telling her so, later in the consultation, might bolster her self-esteem. Do you, your own parents perhaps no longer nearby, have an insight into the loneliness of this young émigrée? If so, words of comfort will probably hover within easier reach of your tongue. Or does your heart sink at the burden Giuseppina looks like becoming? Perhaps, in that case, you have an inkling of what Gerry might be feeling. Do you find yourself surreptitiously looking at Giuseppina's wrists, wondering if there are any fresh bruises? As she tells you how angry her husband gets when her palpitations compel him to break off their love-making, does your own heart begin to race in its own little display of somatisation? Do you feel frustrated at Giuseppina's ambiguous English when she says, 'I cannot have more baby'? Might you possibly be picking up *her* ambivalence too? Or Gerry's? Do you notice how she recoils slightly as you advance your 'palpitations as unconscious contraception' theory? Perhaps she is showing you that her fears of physical illness have not been completely allayed, and you might need to reinforce your judgement with some credible investigations. You notice that your wall clock shows the consultation has already lasted 18 minutes. Impatience makes you rush your explanation, neglecting to make sure Giuseppina has understood it and will be able to relay its gist to her husband. And what is it that makes you pass her over to a counsellor? Is it *really* that you have neither the time nor the skills to help her yourself? Or could referring her carry a covert message of rejection: *you need cherishing, but not by me*?

And so on. Back at the hospital, the specialists have probably summarised Giuseppina's case quite succinctly in the clinical notes:

C/O 'palpitations' 3/12. O/E – NAD. Ix including Holter negative.
Δ – ?PAT, ??W-P-W.
Rx – trial of β-blocker. Review, ?for ablation.

Does this do her justice? Has the close-up gaze produced the right, the most helpful, picture? Will it result in what to Giuseppina feels like care?

On the other hand, isn't there a danger that the generalist's 'big picture' gaze will lose sight of the medical essentials on a limitless canvas of possibilities? How big does a big picture have to get before it becomes too big to be manageable?

There is no crisp answer to this – certainly not from the mouth of science, anyway. Selecting the best view, highlighting the most telling features, putting a well-proportioned frame around it – this is perhaps what people mean when they speak of medicine also as an art.

* * * * *

I want to conclude this chapter, as I did the previous one with the *Inchworm* song, by attempting to convey something of the felt experience of being a participant observer in 'big picture mode', making continuous excursions into three realms – the realms of detail, context and inner awareness. For me, the poem *Judging Distances*, written in 1943 by Henry Reed,[78] succeeds in doing this crisply, elegantly and movingly.

Reed's sequence *Lessons of the War*, from which this is taken, juxtaposes the bullish voice of a sergeant, instructing a squad of new recruits in basic

---

78 Henry Reed (1914–86) started his career as a teacher and journalist. In 1941 he was conscripted into the Royal Army Ordnance Corps, but was invalided out the following year after a serious bout of pneumonia. He was later seconded to the Government Code and Cipher School at Bletchley, where Alan Turing (the 'father of the computer' and the breaker of the Germans' 'Enigma' code) also worked. Reed's best-known poem is *Naming of Parts* (1942), a companion to *Judging Distances*. The extract from *Judging Distances* is reproduced with the kind permission of the Royal Literary Fund.

military procedures, with the inner responses of one of his listeners. In
Judging Distances, we first hear the voice of the weapons-training sergeant as
he attempts to teach the recruits, in the style of the official military manual,
how to report the location and range of a potential target. Then we share
the private thoughts (shown in italics) of one of the recruits as his attention
wanders on to other more civilised and peaceful matters.

Not only how far away, but the way that you say it
Is very important. Perhaps you may never get
The knack of judging a distance, but at least you know
How to report on a landscape: the central sector,
5   The right of arc and that, which we had last Tuesday,
And at least you know

That maps are of time, not place, so far as the army
Happens to be concerned – the reason being,
Is one which need not delay us. Again, you know
10 There are three kinds of tree, three only, the fir and the poplar,
And those which have bushy tops to; and lastly
That things only seem to be things.

A barn is not called a barn, to put it more plainly,
Or a field in the distance, where sheep may be safely grazing.
15 You must never be over-sure. You must say, when reporting:
At five o'clock in the central sector is a dozen
Of what appear to be animals; whatever you do,
Don't call the bleeders *sheep*.

I am sure that's quite clear; and suppose, for the sake of example,
20 The one at the end, asleep, endeavours to tell us
What he sees over there to the west, and how far away,
After first having come to attention. *There to the west,*
On the fields of summer the sun and the shadows bestow
Vestments of purple and gold.

25 *The still white dwellings are like a mirage in the heat,*
And under the swaying elms a man and a woman
Lie gently together. Which is, perhaps, only to say
That there is a row of houses to the left of arc,

And that under some poplars a pair of what appear to be humans
30 *Appear to be loving.*

Well that, for an answer, is what we might rightly call
Moderately satisfactory only, the reason being,
Is that two things have been omitted, and those are important.
The human beings, now: in what direction are they,
35 And how far away, would you say? And do not forget
There may be dead ground in between.

There may be dead ground in between; and I may not have got
The knack of judging a distance; I will only venture
A guess that perhaps between me and the apparent lovers
40 *(Who, incidentally, appear by now to have finished)*
At seven o'clock from the houses, is roughly a distance
Of about one year and a half.

The sergeant is a specialist in his field. His close-up gaze picks out only those features of the landscape that are relevant to his task, i.e. firing guns at it. He is concerned only with an object's direction and distance. For his purposes, it's enough to recognise just three sorts of tree. The sergeant is a cautious man, averse to speculation, reluctant to label a building a barn, or an animal a sheep, until he can be sure. He knows (*line 2*) that few of his students will ever attain his level of mastery, and quite enjoys teasing them for their ignorance (*lines 8–9*). His bullying tone of voice, when in the fourth verse he picks on one of the recruits, will be familiar to anyone who has been a student on an old-fashioned consultant's teaching ward round.

The recruit whose awareness we enter at the end of this verse has not yet been brainwashed into the Army's restricted way of seeing. His wide-angle gaze takes in what the sergeant sees, and more besides. He sees the beauty of the landscape, how the setting sun dresses the fields in 'vestments of purple and gold'. He knows the proper name – elms – for the trees under which a man and woman are making oblivious love in a war zone, brought there by who knows what chains of circumstance. However, he has the presence of mind to report in the sergeant's own preferred language (*lines 28–30*), earning grudging approval in return (*verse 6*).

The final stanza is what does it for me. The recruit's gaze turns inwards, and he becomes 'the self observing the self'. He is still monitoring the world *out there* in sergeant-land, and refreshing his own wider interpretation of it (*line 40*). But with that final frame-breaking phrase, '*a distance of about one year and a half*', his individuality will not be denied any longer: it must be 18 months since he himself had such carefree sex. The young man's wistfulness comes rushing up to overwhelm him, and us. The image is turned to narrative, and the narrative gives the image meaning.

Please now read *Judging Distances* again.

When I first heard it read aloud – at the age of 11 by my form teacher, who did the voices brilliantly – I thought this poem was (though the word had not then become fashionable) 'awesome'. I still think that, in the sense that it has the power to convey a kind of awe. Unlike Leeuwenhoek's 'close-up awe' or Yuri Gagarin's 'wide-angle awe', what Reed has captured is 'big picture awe', the awe one feels when awareness dawns of the interconnectedness of things on every scale. Elsewhere in *Howards End* E.M. Forster famously wrote, 'Only connect the prose and the passion, and both will be exalted.' Again, he was two-thirds right. It takes the gaze of a third party, that of the participant observer, to make the connection. And the opportunity to make it is there every time a patient comes into a consulting room and says, 'Hello doctor, I've come about …'

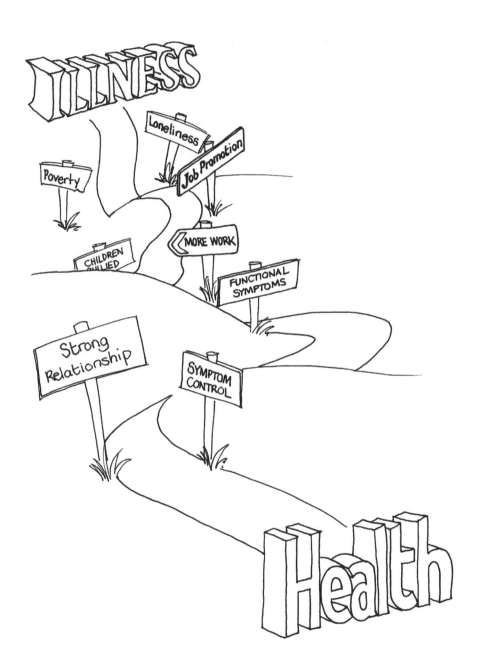

Chapter 5

The illness catastrophe

… sun destroys
The interest of what's happening in the shade

Philip Larkin (1922–85)

English poet

From *The Whitsun Weddings*

Once upon a time, people consulted doctors when they fell ill, in the hope that medical attention would get them better.

The Arcadian simplicity of this arrangement has been somewhat compromised in recent years. A touching faith in the effectiveness of preventative medicine now prompts people to consult while they still feel well.[79] In the UK, at least, a battery of government-imposed targets allows the state, rather than patients or even doctors, to define what is meant by 'better'. And the pharmaceutical industry's insidious profit-driven mission creep increasingly encourages people whose physiology or behaviour is towards the edge of a normal distribution to think of themselves as 'ill'.[80]

Nevertheless, at the heart of what doctors do are some assumptions about how people come to fall ill, and what it takes to get them better. In essence, the clinical process consists of asking, 'What has gone wrong, and how

---

79 Or, as the likes of Bernard Shaw and Ivan Illich would have it, a conspiracy by the medical profession to disempower and enslave a gullible public.

80 Examples include: 'social phobia' (formerly known as shyness, now 'treatable' with the antidepressant moclobemide); male pattern baldness (for which finasteride has been promoted); 'female sexual arousal disorder' (prompting a search for the elusive 'pink Viagra'); 'pre-hypertension' (in which systolic blood pressure is between 120 and 139 mm Hg and diastolic between 80 and 89 mm Hg – a definition encompassing 31% of adult Americans). See Moynihan R, Heath I, Henry D. Selling sickness: the pharmaceutical industry and disease mongering. *British Medical Journal* 2002; **324**: 886–91.

can it be put right?' What differentiates the specialist from the generalist approach to medicine is the number of dimensions in which those questions are answered.

As we shall see in this chapter, specialists, viewing their patients through a zoom lens set to close-up, tend to see illness and recovery in only two dimensions. They link health and illness almost exclusively to the absence or presence respectively of biological abnormality. To the generalist, however, the lens of whose medical gaze can be turned to a wide-angle setting, the processes of becoming ill and getting better are multidimensional affairs.

Doctors who, like the third Russian doll from Chapter 1, confine their view of medicine to the rational application of biomedical science base their understanding of illness and recovery on the *medical model*. As taught to countless generations of medical students, the medical model is a method of problem-solving based on the traditional scientific paradigm. Follow these steps meticulously and in the prescribed order (the label on the tin claims), and the most stubborn medical problem will yield to logic and science.

Whether explicitly or by implication, doctors in training have been so intensively and unquestioningly exposed to the medical model that most take it for granted, believing that it represents the only right way for a doctor to think. And indeed, it remains a sound analytical tool that every generalist falls back on when stumped for a clinical answer. Nevertheless, the medical model is not a 'one size fits all' approach. Its apparent rigour conceals some important fallacies, assumptions and over-simplifications that make it not so universally applicable as its enthusiasts like to believe. You could think of the medical model – shedder of much light though it can be – as the 'sun' in the lines by Larkin that are this chapter's epigraph, destroying 'the interest of what's happening in the shade'.

* * * * *

The conventional medical model (Figure 5.1) begins with a view about what health and disease consist of, and then prescribes a strategy for how the doctor should set about dealing with a sick patient. According to the medical model, disease is what happens when some biological parameter strays too far from normal, producing symptoms that the sufferer presents to the doctor. To identify the wayward bit of biology, the doctor first takes a detailed history, beginning by asking what the patient is – unfortunate phrase in our consumerist times! – complaining of. Interrogation is followed by a systematic and preferably complete physical examination, backed up by whatever special

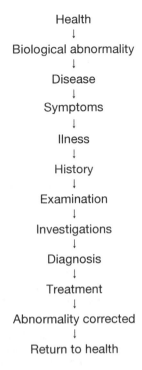

Health
↓
Biological abnormality
↓
Disease
↓
Symptoms
↓
Ilness
↓
History
↓
Examination
↓
Investigations
↓
Diagnosis
↓
Treatment
↓
Abnormality corrected
↓
Return to health

Figure 5.1 The medical model.

tests and investigations will resolve uncertainties in the doctor's mind. From the array of facts and findings thus gathered the doctor arrives at a diagnosis – ideally the identification of that singular biological abnormality that has caused the trouble. The doctor's expertise will suggest one or more treatment options which, followed through, will restore the errant biology to as close to the status quo as possible, and the patient to health.

As an example, let's take a straightforward clinical example – a case of duodenal ulcer. The patient is a businessman aged 45 – let's call him David Wren – who generally thinks of himself as being in good health.

Biological abnormality	*Helicobacter pylori* bacteria colonise the stomach's lining mucosa, and begin to multiply.
Disease	The bacteria stimulate gastric acid secretion. Erosion and ulceration of the duodenum result.
Symptoms	The patient begins to develop pain high in the abdomen, initially relieved by food and commercial antacids. Recently he has been woken by the pain.
Illness	His symptoms begin to affect his concentration at work, and his wife is concerned at his consumption of antacids. She shows him a magazine article about stomach cancer which he cannot get out of his mind, so he arranges to consult a doctor.

History	Asked what the problem is, he begins, 'I've been getting stomach pains for the last few months. I'm sure it's just indigestion, but, you know, my wife thought …' The doctor establishes no significant past or family history. There has been no weight loss and no use of aspirin-like drugs. The patient drinks 28 units of alcohol a week and smokes 15 cigarettes a day.
Examination	There is slight poorly-localised tenderness in the epigastrium. Apart from moderate obesity, no other abnormalities, including masses or hepatomegaly, are present.
Investigations	Full blood count, liver function tests and serum amylase are normal. Anti-*Helicobacter* antibodies are present at high titre. Endoscopy shows duodenal inflammation and erosion. Biopsies of antral and duodenal mucosa show no evidence of malignancy, but a CLO test for urease is positive.
Diagnosis	The differential diagnosis includes: simple dyspepsia; peptic ulceration; gastric carcinoma; gastro-oesophageal reflux disease; pancreatitis. Dyspepsia alone is insufficient to explain the history and investigation findings, which also tend to exclude reflux and pancreatitis. Carcinoma has not been positively excluded, but a diagnosis of duodenal ulceration is fully consistent with the clinical findings and investigations.
Treatment	A week-long course of twice-daily doses of the antibiotics amoxicillin 1 g and clarithromycin 500 mg, combined with the ulcer-healing agent lansoprazole 30 mg, is prescribed.
Abnormality corrected	This treatment regime eradicates *H. pylori* in up to 87% of cases.
Return to health	Following successful eradication, 95% of patients, including this one, experience full relief of symptoms.

Shorn of these case-specific details, the process of medical thinking would seem to boil down to this:

1   when presented with a problem
2   gather detail about it until
3   you're sure what the fundamental problem is
4   then think what could be done about it
5   decide what would be best, then …
6   do it.

What common sense that sounds. How neat. Yet, as someone said, 'There is always an easy solution to every human problem – neat, plausible, and wrong.'[81] Well, in this case not *wrong*, perhaps; this particular patient, after all, was cured. But, as a general template for how to tackle medical problems,

---

81   H.L. Mencken (1880–1956). From his essay *The Divine Afflatus* (1917).

the medical model is too over-simplified and incomplete to be used in all situations. Let's unpack its various stages and see how some of its thinking stands up to scrutiny, beginning with the stage of 'something going wrong'.

* * * * *

Medicine concerns itself with people whose health is endangered and with helping them to retain or regain their own personal version of it. And so the medical profession's remit depends on how *health* is defined. Immediately we are up to our necks in moral philosophy.

In 1946 the World Health Organization took a wide view, and defined health as follows: 'Health is a state of complete physical, mental and social wellbeing, and not merely the absence of disease or infirmity.'[82] Bear in mind that this definition was conceived in the immediate aftermath of world war, and perhaps reflects its authors' longing for peace and contentment as much as for the relief of suffering. And, indeed, few would deny that there is more to health than merely not being ill. But broadening the concept of health until every tiniest spasm of psychological or social discontent is deemed unhealthy would, if taken seriously, place intolerable responsibilities on the health professions and would medicalise everyday life into an Orwellian nightmare.

Complete physical, mental and social wellbeing sounds more like a description of perfect happiness than of health. Health and happiness are not the same thing. Sigmund Freud, suffering from advanced cancer of the jaw and after obeying his doctor's orders to give up his beloved cigars, wrote, 'I am now healthier than I was, but not happier.' Moreover, it is possible to be in poor physical shape yet still maintain a sense of well-being. Conversely, some people are wont to seek medical treatment for imperfections most of us manage to take in our stride, such as facial wrinkles or male pattern baldness. There are serious dangers in confusing health and happiness. The individual search for happiness is never-ending, but we cannot afford, either financially or morally, to legitimise a similarly open-ended demand for health services. To make happiness the business of doctors would be to spread their ambitions so widely and so thin as to render them effectively impotent. Some doctors with highly developed social awareness, seeing how much of their patients' illness stemmed from poverty and social disadvantage, have indeed

---

82 Preamble to the Constitution of the World Health Organization as adopted by the International Health Conference, New York, 19–22 June 1946, and signed by representatives of 61 states on 22 July 1946. It has not been amended since.

embraced political activism as a therapeutic option.[83] But, for practical purposes, the conventional medical model is content to define both health and disease mainly in terms of the functional integrity of the physical body.

The classical scientific method that underpins high-tech medicine was founded on careful observation and accurate measurement. Clinical scientists soon discovered that normal healthy functioning depended on *homeostasis* – on critical biological variables resisting perturbation and staying within a limited range of tolerance. The 19th century French physiologist Claude Bernard captured the principle in his dictum, 'The stability of the *milieu intérieur*' (by which he meant the body's internal environment) 'is the condition of free and independent life'. Health – at least in its narrow corporeal sense – requires a host of anatomical structures, physiological mechanisms and biochemical processes to stay in the 'normal' state to which evolution has brought them, plus or minus not very much. Disease is what happens if they don't. Granted, some parameters are more critical than others, or less tolerant of variation: femurs only work properly if they stay in 1 ± 0 pieces, while the blood glucose level can fluctuate 25% either side of normal without too much ill effect. Others – height, for example, or sleep–wake cycles – are distributed on such wide-based bell-shaped curves, and are sufficiently forgiving of individual differences, for it to be a matter of semantics whether we talk of the extremes of the range as being 'abnormal' or just 'atypical'.

When I was studying pathology as an undergraduate, I was taught to classify diseases in two ways. The first was in accordance with the nature of the abnormality causing the damage. Faced with an unexplained symptom or physical sign, we learned to rattle off long lists of the various categories of aetiological process that could in theory be responsible: congenital or genetic; infection (viral, bacterial, fungal or parasitic); inflammatory, allergic, autoimmune or degenerative; metabolic or hormonal; trauma; tumours, benign or malignant; and, finally, to ensure that no pathologist was ever at a loss for words, idiopathic – 'of cause unknown but not unlabelled'. The second system of classification, favoured by textbooks multi-authored by consortia of specialists, was by organ system affected: diseases of the ear, nose or throat; of the skin; of the locomotor, cardiovascular, digestive or reproductive systems. The diagnostic question we ought constantly to be asking ourselves, these classifications implied, was, 'What kind of damage has been sustained by which bodily system?'

---

83 One such was David Widgery (1947–92), a socialist GP working in London's East End. An account of his life and influence is to be found in *Confronting an Ill Society*, by Patrick Hutt (Oxford: Radcliffe Publishing, 2005).

What we were *not* taught was to think about diseases in terms of how they affected patients. That would have been useful. It would have helped in the early stages of a medical career to learn some mental strategies for trying to make sense of symptoms that, for example, hit you suddenly, or that come and go unpredictably, or make you feel tired all the time, or are worse when you run, or make you just feel awful. This after all is the kind of language patients use when presenting their complaints, and that the doctor has to interpret and translate into the language and thought processes of science. If the classification of disease by aetiology and organ system had been triangulated by the more generalist notion of 'classification by impact', it might have speeded up our acquisition of clinical acumen quite significantly. As it was, however, we were left with the impression that diseases were discrete entities that could each be located in their own separate box on a two-dimensional grid, with *'pathological process'* along one axis and *'organ system'* along the other, each disease corresponding to a particular type of failure of a particular bodily component. Disease, according to the medical model, consists of the body's reaction to a parts failure.

The medical model is a big fan of Occam's razor, according to which the explanation of any phenomenon should make as few assumptions as possible. The simplest explanation, says Occam,[84] is the best. So the medical model of disease, as well as preferring its causative agents to be singular and classifiable, likes to think of the disease process as a straightforward linear sequence of cause and effect. Think back to David Wren, our businessman with the duodenal ulcer. It is not normal to have *H. pylori* organisms in one's stomach. But they can get there. And multiply. If they do, the body reacts by secreting excessive amounts of hydrochloric acid. The acid erodes the duodenal mucosa. A leads to B, and C follows, resulting in D. Abolish A, and B, C and D fall back into line.

The medical model also likes to restrict its attention to a narrow time span. It can readily understand how bacterial growth might quickly affect gastric acid secretion, leading within days to acid burns of the duodenum. But it feels much less happy tracing the chain of causality back into the more remote past. The further back you go in time looking for causes, the medical model reckons, the less likely you are to find anything you can *do* anything about. So what, if Mr Wren is drinking more heavily because a year ago he was promoted beyond his capabilities? So what, if he started smoking at the age of 14 because his mates thought it was cool? Historical factors like these,

---

84 William of Ockham, 14th-century English logician and Franciscan friar.

to the medical model's close-up gaze, are of passing biographical interest only, and not relevant to the therapeutic goals of eradicating the *Helicobacter* and reversing the erosive changes in his gut. It would be good if he cut back on his alcohol intake and stopped smoking. But mainly he needs to take the tablets.

Unfortunately, some patterns of human distress simply refuse to fall in with the medical model's preference for a 'single identifiable recent cause'. They decline to submit themselves to Occam's razor. Among these are the so-called 'functional' illnesses, where, despite an evident impairment of function, no underlying biological abnormality can be found.[85] An analogy might be of a car in perfect mechanical order being driven on the clutch at 30 miles an hour in first gear. Hearing the scream of tortured metal and seeing the erratic kangaroo hops, you might assume there was something wrong with the vehicle, but no mechanic, examining it under calm conditions, will find anything wrong. Medically unexplained 'diseases' currently include chronic fatigue syndrome, irritable bowel disease, abdominal migraine, urethral syndrome, tension headache, food allergy, persistent low back pain, fibromyalgia, attention deficit–hyperactivity disorder (ADHD), post-traumatic stress disorder, and a variety of psychosomatic and non-organic psychological conditions such as anxiety states and panic attacks. These are medicine's Cinderella conditions. The lack of clear physical correlates can make them pariahs in the snobbish world of clinical orthodoxy. But they, and numerous conditions like them, remind us that the question *What causes disease?* doesn't always allow a crisp, unitary and physical answer.

* * * * *

Usually one of my favourite books, the *Oxford English Dictionary* is disappointingly unclear about the difference between *disease* and *illness*. It starts promisingly enough. *Disease*, it says, is 'a disorder of structure or function … especially one that produces specific signs or symptoms.' But then it goes wobbly, defining *illness* simply as 'a disease or period of sickness', as in 'he died after a long illness' or 'I've never missed a day's work through illness.' Well (I want to ask), which is it? Is illness just a synonym for disease, an episode of disordered function? Or is it something less definable and more

---

85 In order to leave no hostages to fortune, I should perhaps add *or have yet been found.* The conditions listed have been *associated with* numerous physical agents, e.g. virus infection, nutritional deficits, food additives, enzyme deficiencies, genetic traits. But no unequivocally *causal* relationships have been demonstrated.

subjective, the sort of thing that makes some people but not others call in sick and stop off work?

We must make a distinction between a biological abnormality that jeopardises normal functioning and the effects of that abnormality on the person who is host to it. The first – disease – is what goes wrong; the other – illness – is what it does to you. Disease is an event in the third person, an *it* that happens to a *him or her* and which a pathologist can objectively observe and investigate scientifically. Illness, on the other hand, is a felt experience, an event in the first person, something that happens to *me*. Disease is a fact to be analysed and categorised; illness is a narrative to be told and understood. Through the microscope, in the laboratory or on the operating table, two people suffering from the same disease can look pretty much the same. But talk to them, and the stories they each tell of their illness will be as unique as the rest of their lives.

In the medical model, the way objective disease converts to subjective illness – the process of 'becoming ill' – is straightforward. The onset of a disease is often quite insidious, and may go unnoticed by its host. Bacteria invade; cells start to divide over-exuberantly; deposits of fat begin to form in the walls of a coronary artery. Then at some stage a point is reached when the disease process reaches conscious awareness in the form of a symptom – a pain, a lump, a fever. At first, if the pathology is not too catastrophic, symptoms might be dismissed as insignificant: random fluctuations within an overall state of well-being. But, if they persist or worsen, another threshold is crossed and the disease host, now a patient, tips over into a state of illness. 'Becoming ill', in the medical model, is a sequence of developing some objective pathology, feeling a variety of subjective symptoms, and reacting to them. The *reaction* phase includes behavioural responses. There is a social role – a set of illness behaviours – that someone becoming ill is expected to carry out. A kind of social contract is implied. Entering the sick role entitles the patient to time out from their usual responsibilities, to practical, emotional and financial support, and to access the whole range of health care. In exchange, the ill person is expected to want (and try) to get better, to cooperate with treatment, and to resume normal social functioning upon recovery.

The medical model happily acknowledges illness behaviour such as self-medicating, or staying off work, or consulting a doctor. But people have psychological reactions to symptoms as well as behavioural ones. When we fall ill, the inside of our head becomes a noisy place. Unpleasant physical feelings clamour for attention. A turmoil of thoughts crowds out our usual daily preoccupations. The intellect puzzles over what is happening, trying to explain it. Emotions range from frustration to anxiety and pulses of dread. The imagination cartwheels into scary territory populated with 'what if's. We are not sure whether we want sympathy or distraction, company or solitude. We become 'not ourselves'.

Internal noise like this is inevitably present when a patient consults a doctor, and is likely to spill over into the telling of the story, particularly its early stages. We can imagine David Wren, asked about the onset of his symptoms, saying something like, 'It must have been Tuesday, because I'd had to miss lunch, we were that busy. Anyway, I felt this – not what you'd call a pain, exactly ...' Unfortunately, to a doctor schooled in the traditional medical model, prolix details of a patient's individual experience of becoming ill seldom provide much illumination; rather, they seem to be a distraction, obscuring a clear view of the revelatory symptoms and signs that point towards a diagnosis. As we have seen, the medical model likes its diseases to have compact diagnostic labels. And anecdotal accounts of illness that glory in individual variation frustrate the labelling process. 'Yes yes,' Mr Wren's gastroenterologist might interrupt. 'Point to where the pain was. Was it sharp or dull?'

At this point, there's going to be a little excursion into graphs and topology. Please bear with me and do not panic. My own maths stopped at O-level, so I couldn't make it hard even if I wanted to. The intention here is to give you a visual way of getting your imagination round some of the odd ways people behave when they become unwell.

Figure 5.2 shows how the conventional medical model relates *disease* and *illness*, and the process of becoming ill. The horizontal axis represents the objective range of biological normality and abnormality. The origin O is the

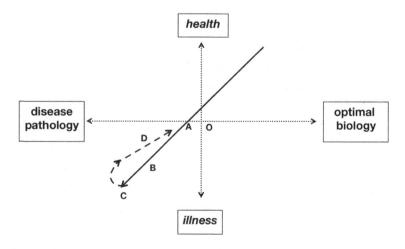

Figure 5.2 The relationship between 'disease' and 'illness'.

point where biological parameters have deviated sufficiently from optimal to threaten effective functioning: to its left is worsening disease. The vertical axis is the subjective spectrum between health (in its widest 'total well-being' sense) and illness, the origin representing the point where realisation dawns that all is not well. The oblique line charts the patient's descent from health into illness. Its displacement slightly above the origin, rather than through it, shows that the patient's usual 'resting' condition is to feel generally well. The line intersects the disease axis at A, with O–A representing the small amount of 'sub-clinical' pathology that can be tolerated without triggering the experience of being ill.

As I have drawn the diagram, the upper right-hand quadrant suggests that the closer our biological variables come to their 'normal' values, the greater our sense of well-being. This is arguable. *Super-normal equals super-healthy* may be a slogan that sells vitamins and nutritional supplements. It may also be a belief underlying much of the language of alternative medicine, with its talk of 'energy imbalances' and 'detoxifying regimes'. But the orthodox medical model need not, and does not, much bother itself with degrees of well-being. The medical model is chiefly concerned with the left-hand half of this diagram, and with its bottom left quadrant in particular.[86] Here the oblique line suggests a direct link between the severity of pathology and the degree of illness it produces. I have shown it as a straight line relationship, with illness directly proportional to the extent of abnormality, which is an over-simplification of the medical model's position. Nevertheless – as B on the line depicts – the model does make a general assumption that 'the worse the disease, the worse you feel'. The converse principle is perhaps more important. Underpinning the medical model's concept of therapeutics is the belief that *the patient gets better if, and only if, the disease regresses*. C on the graph is the point where treatment begins, reversing the biological abnormalities and bringing about the recovery phase shown as D.

For reasons that will shortly become clear, I want to redraw Figure 5.2, adding the notion of events unfolding over time, and converting a two-dimensional graph to a model in three dimensions (Figure 5.3).

---

86 The upper left-hand quadrant, where subjective health is experienced despite the presence of objective pathology, is the realm of 'symptomless disease'. Orthodox medicine and the pharmaceutical industry have their colonialising eyes on this territory, where 'symptomless hypertension', 'pre-diabetes' and genomic screening offer mouth-watering opportunities.

   The bottom right-hand quadrant, on the other hand, where people feel ill despite being biologically healthy, is where hypochondriasis and somatisation are to be found. Conventional medicine has little time for such conundra.

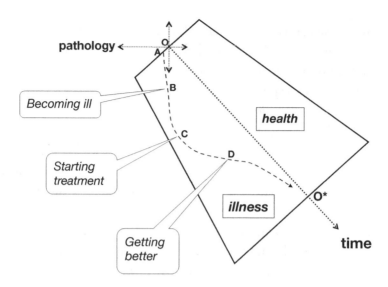

Figure 5.3 Illness and recovery over time.

See the main part of this figure, the trapezoid shape, as a tilted rectangular sheet coming out of the page towards you. The time line O–O* is also coming out of the page, towards you. Figure 5.3 shows the same information as 5.2, but developing over time. If you were to put your eye at O*, end-on to the inclined plane, and look backwards along the time axis towards O, what you would see is Figure 5.2. The point of this re-drawing is to show health and illness not as one-dimensional measurements but as surfaces over which one can range as time unfolds. This will be important as we now look at some of the weaknesses and anomalies in the medical model's concept of how people become ill.

* * * * *

There are several aspects of how people in real life move between states of health and illness that the conventional medical model finds it difficult to account for.

- People feel and act 'ill' for many reasons besides organic disease, or even in the absence of it. Well-off or privileged people get ill less often than poor or socially disadvantaged people, and they behave differently when they do. Having confiding relationships within a stable and supportive family lessens the impact of disease, while loneliness and anxiety tend to magnify it. People's beliefs and value systems are also relevant. Someone who believes in 'fresh air, regular exercise and a balanced diet' will deal with illness very differently from another who reckons that 'there is a pill for every ill'.

- Switching from a state of well-being to one of illness is, from a subjective point of view, often a relatively sudden event, as the phrase falling ill suggests. Disease pathology tends to be steadily progressive, but the felt experience of realising that one is unwell seems to strike more abruptly, as if some kind of tipping point is suddenly reached. The reverse process – feeling well again – can similarly feel like a more sudden transition than can be correlated with the gradual restoration of normal physical functioning.

- As well as health ↔ illness transitions often being sudden events, they do not always correlate in time with changes in the degree of physical pathology. Doctors sometimes see patients who present so early in the evolution of their illness that no objective signs of disease can be found, and who make a bid for the sick role on what seems at the time like flimsy grounds. In other patients, by contrast, their illness behaviour lags well behind the advance of their disease. They present late, make light of their symptoms, and endeavour to continue their normal lives in the face of obvious incapacity. It is as if some people are disproportionately attracted to a state of either health or illness, and can show an unusual eagerness or reluctance to switch from one to the other.

- It is not always clear which comes first – objective disease or subjective illness. In the medical model, disease causes, and therefore precedes, the appearance of symptoms and illness. But to the patient it is usually the other way round. People get ill before they know they have disease. What the patient *knows* at first hand is the felt experience of illness and symptoms. To the patient, disease is an abstract concept, a post hoc explanation supplied by the doctor. As the humorist said, 'Illness is what you have on the way to the doctor's surgery. Disease is what you have on the way back home.'

So – as a description of how health, pathology and illness are interrelated, and of how people behave when they fall ill and recover – Figure 5.3 won't do. For a 'big picture' view, we need a more comprehensive model, one that can help us to understand:

- the multi-factorial nature of health and illness
- the suddenness of the transitions between them

- the non-linear causal relationship between pathology and illness, and
- the non-synchronous timing of pathology and illness behaviour.

To find such a model we can draw on a branch of mathematics called catastrophe theory.[87]

Much basic mathematics has to do with understanding change, and – at the level I learned it at school – predictable, smooth change. The equations of elementary algebra allow us to know, if we alter x, exactly what y will do. Increase the force on an object and it accelerates, predictably and smoothly. What's more, it never does anything *other* than accelerate predictably and smoothly. Classical Newtonian science models a world where continuous incremental changes in one variable produce steady continuous changes in another. Adjust the rheostat, and the light gets steadily brighter or dimmer. And, according to the medical model, as the pathology gets steadily worse, so does the illness. Gradually reverse the biological abnormality, and the patient is progressively restored to health.

But in many real-world systems, change is an abrupt and unpredictable event. Steady small changes in one variable produce either no effect or a sudden large one. Heat ice steadily, and at some point it suddenly melts. Tectonic plates inch slowly over each other until, unexpectedly, an earthquake is unleashed. Gradually reduce the uptake of measles vaccination and, out of the blue, an epidemic is upon us. David Wren's wife sees him chew just one more indigestion tablet, and – '*No buts!*' – the doctor's appointment is made.

Catastrophe theory is the branch of mathematics concerned with 'discontinuous' phenomena like these, where small changes in circumstances produce sudden large changes in behaviour.[88] The behaviour we are con-

---

87 Let me again reassure the reader who is no mathematician and say, *It's OK, neither am I.* To the mathematically sophisticated reader, let me say, *Sorry if I have misunderstood.* To both, I would add that I have included this section, mathematically shaky though it may be, in order to try and convey a sense that the complex ways people behave when they are ill do have some underlying coherence and comprehensibility.

88 'Catastrophe' derives from the Greek καταστοφή, meaning 'a sudden reversal'. In this context it does not carry the connotation of 'disaster'. Catastrophe theory, developed by the French topologist René Thom, is generally considered a branch of geometry because the variables and resultant behaviours are usefully depicted as curved surfaces.

For a readable lay guide, see Woodcock A, Davis M. *Catastrophe Theory.* London: Penguin Books, 1991 (new edition).

cerned with here – how people move between health and illness in response to changes in biological variables – can be modelled, I hope helpfully, by one particular catastrophe know as the *cusp catastrophe*. Here's how to visualise it.

Figure 5.4 is a simplified version of the previous diagram, to be seen in three dimensions as a tilted flat plane coming out of the page towards you.

Now imagine the plane to be made of stretchy flexible material, and put a pleat in it, so that the upper *health* part of the surface overrides the lower *illness* part (Figure 5.5).

We now have a three-dimensional surface on which to locate *health* and *illness* and to trace the patient's transitions between them (Figure 5.6).

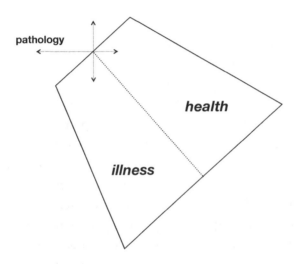

Figure 5.4 A two-dimensional plane surface.

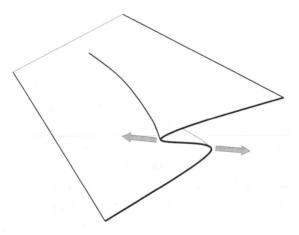

Figure 5.5 Putting a pleat in the plane.

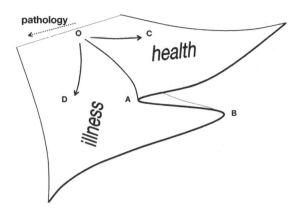

Figure 5.6 'Health' and 'illness' surfaces.

Imagine yourself standing on this surface at point O, the apex or 'cusp' of the pleat, facing forwards 'out of the page'. To your left, and inclining gradually uphill, is the surface representing *health*. Looking to your right, you see the *illness* surface sloping downhill and away from you. From O, you could, if you were healthy, walk in the direction OC, up onto the *health* plane; the healthier you were, the further you could go. Alternatively, if some pathology was at work impelling you right-wards, you might go down the OD track; the sicker you got, the further out onto the *illness* plane you would go.

Back onto the *health* surface. You're at point C, facing forwards 'out of the page'. Now look to your right. Gently curving away from you is the edge of the overhang OA. Walk towards it and look over. Beneath you is a sheer drop down onto the *illness* plane; the further you have come out onto the *health* plane, the further you have to go to reach the cliff edge, and the greater is the drop. If you start off well, that edge OA is where disease has to pull you to before you abruptly – catastrophically – fall into illness.

Let's now imagine that you're ill. You've had a degree of disease pathology that has brought you, let's say, to point D on the *illness* plane. And you'd like to get better, i.e. to make the reverse transition back onto the *health* plane. Stand at D, again facing 'out of the page'. To your left and above you, out of reach, is the overhang of the *health* plane, OA. On your level, further to your left, is the curving horizon OB, marking the limit of the *illness* plane's corresponding '*under*hang': it is partly concealed in Figure 5.6. Your route back onto the upper *health* surface requires you to get to a point somewhere along OB and then – miraculously, gravity operates upwards at this point – you 'jump' back up into health. The pleat in the *health–illness* surface means that restoring your abnormal pathology completely to normal is not sufficient to bring you to a tipping point along OB; there is still a way to go health-wards before you reach the edge of the illness plane and make the transition back to the felt experience of being well again.

Let's track what happens to David Wren, the dyspeptic businessman, as he moves over the three-dimensional surface of the cusp catastrophe (Figure 5.7).

When we meet him at point (1) on the *health* plane, David feels pretty well, although he is slightly ashamed of his sedentary lifestyle. He decides to start jogging three times a week and to cut back on his alcohol intake. As a result he feels – and indeed *is* – healthier; he advances further, to point (2). There is no way of knowing when the *H. pylori* first became established in his gut. But from now on its pathological effects, at first imperceptible, draw him a little further towards the *illness* plane. At (2) David begins to feel the first twinge of what he takes to be simple indigestion. At first this does not worry him; he still continues to think of himself as a basically fit man, who just happens to have an occasional touch of indigestion. But by the time he has slipped back to point (3) he cannot pretend all is as it should be. At (3) he buys his first packet of antacid tablets. And between (3) and (4) they seem to be working. He feels better; at point (4) he is nearly as far out on the *health* plane as he was before his symptoms first appeared. Then, at (4), he begins to be woken by epigastric pains. He still does not regard himself as ill; it's just that the tablets aren't suiting him, and he resolves to try a different brand. At point (5), however, Mrs Wren notices how much antacid her husband is con-suming, and alarm bells ring. Her concerns, and the booking of a doctor's

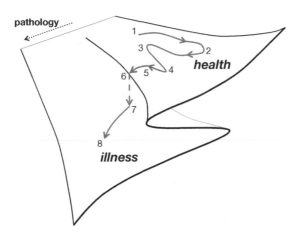

Figure 5.7 Falling ill.

appointment, propel him, by the time he enters the consulting room, to the brink of the overhang (6), where *health* plunges into *illness*.

In the space of a 10-minute consultation – the drop from (6) to (7) in Figure 5.7 – David Wren experiences the 'catastrophe' of falling ill. Until this encounter with the doctor he was 'a well person suffering from indigestion'; now he has become a 'patient', an ill person with a disease, who hitherto had been kidding himself. A Rubicon has been crossed, and he has mixed feelings about it. There is relief, in that what to him had been mysterious will prove, to the expert, no mystery. But there is also a feeling that the ground is slipping from under him, and he is no longer fully in command of events. He has exchanged his narrative for a label, and with the label comes a measure of helplessness. His subsequent course on the *illness* plane, to point (8) and beyond, will be steered by others: with his consent and cooperation, of course, but by others nonetheless. That the doctor will take professional pride in seeing him safely through this episode is of course a comfort. That he should *need* such assistance is a blow to his invulnerability that will take some getting used to.

Let's now briefly show how David Wren negotiates the reverse 'catastrophe' and moves from illness back to health. We'll fast-forward his clinical journey, skipping the technicalities of investigation and diagnosis, and pick him up [Figure 5.8, point (1)] as he begins his triple therapy.

As the drugs do their work and the pathological processes in his digestive tract are reversed, David's position on the catastrophe surface moves back in the direction of *health*. When the last *Helicobacter* succumbs and his duodenal mucosa is again normal, he has reached point (2), level with the origin

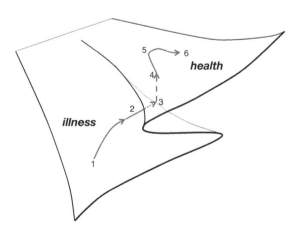

Figure 5.8 Getting better.

representing the absence of significant pathology. Seen through a specialist's close-up gaze, he is now disease-free – cured. But although no detectable biological abnormality remains, he doesn't actually *feel* cured. He is still down on the illness plane. He is, in that ambiguous idiom that is uniquely English, better but not *better*. Psychologically he still has the distance from (2) to (3) to travel before he reaches the illness horizon and can make the upwards leap to regain the *health* surface at point (4). As he does so, something subtle happens inside him – unconscious at first but soon registering as a conscious shift in self-perception. Before the leap, poised at point (3), he was 'an unwell person who is getting better'. After it, at point (4), he is suddenly back to being 'a healthy person who was recently ill'. He is at first a little unsure, half-expecting a relapse. Probably he still carries a packet of antacid tablets in his pocket 'just in case' (5). But before long, as he remains symptom free and resumes his previous lifestyle, and he is pretty much back to where he was before the *Helicobacter* struck (6).

* * * * *

Reading through the last section of this chapter as dispassionately as I can, I can imagine the reader wondering *Why bother with all this pseudo-mathematical modelling stuff?* My response would be that making conceptual models of complex phenomena is how we turn bewilderment into understanding. The cusp catastrophe model helps us appreciate that the subjective experience of flipping between well-being and illness is complicated but not mysterious, puzzling but not unfathomable. It offers an insight into aspects of illness behaviour that, as we saw earlier, the narrow medical model struggles to explain. Specifically, it clarifies:

- why the experiences of falling ill and getting better often feel, subjectively, to be sudden events, in contrast to the often gradual onset or reversal of disease pathology
- why reversing a pathological process or returning some errant physiology to its normal range may not be enough to restore a patient's sense of well-being
- why sick people can feel much worse, or much better, than the extent of their organic pathology might suggest.

A model such as this, which can represent and illuminate the complicated business of illness and recovery, is fine as far as it goes. But the best models can take things a stage further, and help us turn understanding into control. With one further refinement, the cusp catastrophe model can incorporate more determinants of illness and health than just the presence or absence of disease, thereby allowing us to predict the effect on health of more variables than just the purely physical. Specifically, it sheds light on:

- how social, economic, cultural and psychological factors impact on individual patients' susceptibility and reactions to disease
- how people's health beliefs and value systems modify their illness behaviour.

The additional refinement is the notion of what catastrophe theorists call *attractors*. The maths is beyond me, but, as I understand it, attractors are forces that exert a kind of gravitational pull on the wandering variable – in our case, a patient – attracting it towards, and stabilising its position on, one or other of the model's surfaces. As I have been depicting it, 'health attractors' operate (from the origin) outwards, upwards and to the left. 'Illness attractors' operate outwards, downwards and to the right (Figure 5.9).

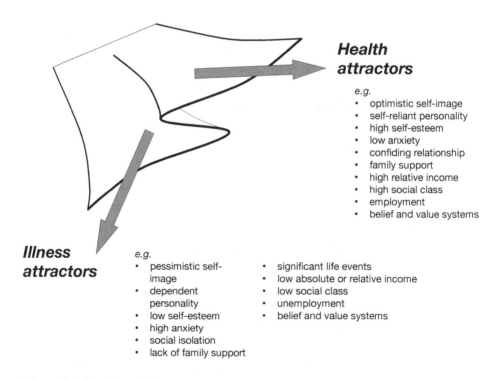

Figure 5.9 Health and illness attractors.

As well as the individual's biological status, a list (nothing like complete) of health and illness attractors would include:

- the 'default self-image': whether one is 'a basically fit person who sometimes has a bout of illness' or 'a never very well person who sometimes feels not too bad'
- health beliefs, e.g. whether maintaining health is primarily one's own business or that of the medical profession; beliefs about what causes or protects against disease (such as 'stress,' or 'getting a chill', or eating an apple a day)
- significant life events, e.g. bereavement, marriage, childbirth, divorce, redundancy[89]
- family culture: tolerance of illness and 'how to enact the sick role' are behaviours largely learned from early role models, usually within the family
- personality traits such as neuroticism, denial, paranoia
- concurrent mental health problems, e.g. anxiety, depression
- the presence or absence of confiding, nurturing or toxic relationships
- strong or weak social support networks
- absolute and relative income[90]
- employment status
- religious or philosophical beliefs.

Any given individual at any given time before a disease process sets in can be located somewhere on the health–illness surface at a position representing the result of health and illness attractors acting in their different directions. The advent of physical disease, for sure, gives the individual a powerful shove in the direction of the illness plane. But, as we have seen with David Wren, whether disease alone is sufficient to pull a previously well person to the edge

---

89 Paradoxically, even 'positive' life events such as falling in love, marriage or childbirth are associated with increased vulnerability to disease, especially infections and malignancies.

90 On virtually every measure, the health of socially and financially deprived people is worse than that of the well-off. Furthermore, health inequalities are most marked in societies where the gradient between the incomes of the richest and the poorest is steepest. For a comprehensive analysis, see *Closing the Gap in a Generation: health equity through action on the social determinants of health* (Report of the World Health Organization's Commission on Social Determinants of Health, Geneva: WHO, 2008).

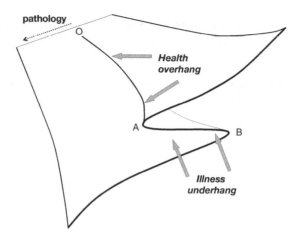

Figure 5.10 Overhang and underhang.

of the health plane and down into illness depends on the strength of other attractors.

This concept of health and illness attractors, operating independently of organic pathology, alerts us to all the factors beyond the purely physical that can be manipulated in the cause of therapy. Strengthening health attractors can be particularly relevant when a patient is in the vicinity of the 'health overhang' (near the edge OA in Figure 5.10), which represents the state of 'being well despite definite pathology', or the 'illness underhang' (OB in Figure 5.10), which is the zone of 'being ill despite having *no* pathology'.

People flip between well-being and illness for more reasons than the science of pathology can account for. Both on an individual and on a mass population scale, resistance to and recovery from illness are profoundly affected by psychological, interpersonal, educational, social and economic considerations. To what extent these fall within the remit of the medical profession is debatable. But the doctor who dismisses them out of hand as 'not my concern' is putting his or her therapeutic potential at a massive handicap. Answers to questions such as 'Why has my patient fallen ill?' and 'What can I do to help my patient get better?' come in more guises than the medical model would suggest.

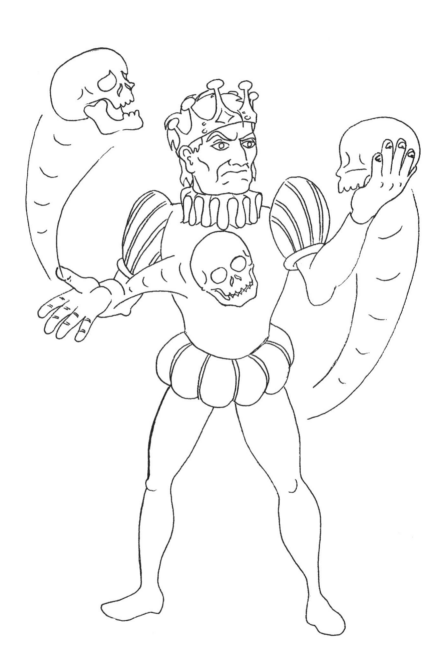

Chapter 6

The case for big picture medicine

In order properly to understand the big picture, everyone should fear becoming mentally clouded and obsessed with one small section of truth.

Xun Zi (c. 312–230 BCE)

Chinese Confucian philosopher

The trick to forgetting the big picture is to look at everything close-up. The shortcut to closing a door is to bury yourself in the details.

Chuck Palahniuk (b. 1962)

American novelist

From *Lullaby*

This chapter is a kind of gathering point. Janus-like, it looks back over previous chapters and forwards to anticipate some themes to be developed later. What I have written so far points to one conclusion, namely that contemporary medicine is in danger of letting itself down through too starry-eyed an infatuation with a narrow specialist way of thinking. A profession that can and did think big has opted to think small. It's as if the medical gaze is in danger of losing its zoom function and of getting stuck in close-up mode. Medicine, I contend, has painted itself into a corner, from which a renewed emphasis on the generalist's 'big picture' perspective offers the best chance of escape. Looking ahead, I want to suggest that the experience of patients and doctors alike can be enhanced if the generalist approach is properly respected in the consulting room, the corridors of power, and – most importantly – in the private inner consciousness of practising clinicians.

I began this book in order to explore some conflicting feelings about the job I had been doing for 30 years. Let there be no doubt: being a doctor remains one of the most worthwhile and exhilarating occupations it can be anyone's privilege to enjoy. But as I approached the end of my own clinical career I was conscious too of an undercurrent of disappointment, a frustration that – for all its triumphs and the esteem in which it is held – high-tech medicine as widely practised wasn't quite delivering on its promise. It felt to be aiming high, yet falling short. There seemed to be a fault line, narrow but deep, dividing what medicine *could* be from what it has become, separating what people want from their doctors from what those doctors in reality provide.

The divide is hard to account for, and, indeed, not everyone accepts that there *is* one. At any rate, it didn't seem to be a gap that could be bridged simply by developing more drugs, or doing more research, or piling on more bureaucracy, or even by shovelling more money into the cuckoo's throat of organised health care. The disappointing gap between aspiration and achievement seemed to have a more philosophical origin – a lack of clarity about medicine's purpose, scope, methods and terms of engagement.

Being by nature and training a generalist myself, I came at my thesis from a variety of starting points.

Chapter 1, 'Beginner's mind', opened with the self-evident truth that no system of health care yet devised has managed simultaneously to satisfy the expectations of its consumers, funders, policy makers and providers. Patients – who are health care's consumers sometimes and its funders always – by and large want to live for ever, or die in the attempt, and to pay as little as possible in the process. Policy makers – by whom I mean politicians and managers in their Don Quixote–Sancho Panza symbiosis – want value for money, and the credit for obtaining it. Providers – doctors, mainly – usually just want to be left alone to treat the sick as they think best and as if money were no object. Acrimony is inevitable: acrimony about what health is; about what value is; about who is master and who servant; about whose priority – science, cash, or choice – trumps whose.

And yet something precious always survives the acrimony, some universal truth about how healing takes place that is left unscathed by the sniping. Whenever a consulting room door closes, and patient and doctor meet each other in mutual trust and trustworthiness, a potential energy is created whose therapeutic power stems from the relationship between the two of them, not from the scientific, social and political frameworks they inhabit. It arises by virtue of who the doctor *is*, rather than what he or she *knows,* and from who the patient *is*, rather than from what condition he or she *has.*

Confusing? Absolutely. Being a doctor *is* confusing – or ought to be.

Ought to be? Absolutely. Medicine is often portrayed as a purely technical exercise, up there with flying a plane or mending a car. Perhaps such comparisons are made in order to discourage doctors from getting above themselves. But the more medical science tries to study human beings as if they were the sum of their mechanical parts, the more their uniqueness, complexity and unpredictability protest that they are not. And when that consulting room door closes, patients expect their doctor to honour their uniqueness, cope with their complexity and tolerate their unpredictability. If that means that the doctor must sometimes make compromises with pure science, or overrule political and financial diktats, then so be it. Add to this the fact that the people who become doctors are every bit as unique, complex and unpredictable as anybody else, and it becomes clear that no single role or skill-set – not even that of 'applied bioscientist' – is sufficient to define everything a doctor should be.

Layers beneath layers, selves within selves. In Chapter 1, I used the metaphor of the nested Russian *matryoshki* dolls to depict the range of identities a fully functioning doctor might need to access. So we met:

> Things should be made as simple as possible, but not any simpler.
>
> Albert Einstein (1879–1955)
> German American physicist

- the doctor as the public face of state-organised medicine, an avatar for the organisation that mass-produces a commodity called 'health care'
- the stereotypical larger-than-life 'doctor as hero' (or villain, or saint, or magician, or devil) of the popular imagination
- the 'doctor as expert in biomedicine', probably a specialist, who practises medicine at arm's length and whose inner life is no one's business but his own
- the generalist 'doctor as expert in the individual patient', for whom medicine is an art as well as a science
- the 'Inner Physician' – the untrained and usually invisible 'raw' human being, the amateur within the professional.

At first, as Chapter 1 got into its stride, I felt I had put my finger on the origin of that gap between ambition and delivery that bedevils modern medicine. The 'biomedical expert' is arguably the most useful of a doctor's possible identities; certainly, if cure rates and longevity are the indicators, it is the most effective. But this role, I reckoned, has become overlaid with unrealistic popular and political expectations of what scientific medicine can deliver. And, in turn, whatever scientific credibility doctors possess has been achieved at the cost of suppressing their most secret and potentially most valuable asset – the frail and fallible human being feeding their compassion from the core – the Inner Physician. So, I thought, the key to bridging the gap between expectation and reality would be to open up successive *matryoshki*, to release the Inner Physician from its carapaces and set it centre stage, blinking in the daylight like a freed hostage.

But it soon became apparent that this was not going to be enough. The fault line that runs through modern medical education and practice is not to be simply healed by a fluffy Aquarian appeal for doctors to get more in touch with their feelings. If the generality of doctors tend to exclude their individuality from their professional activities, it has to be for some reason. Suppressing one's Inner Physician is a symptom, not a diagnosis. But a symptom of what? Confusion over medicine's core purpose? Failure to keep abreast of advances in scientific thinking? Being trapped in persistent but outdated stereotypes? Too simplistic an idea of how healthy people get sick, and sick people get well? A belief that authority requires an outward show of invulnerability? Yes, yes and yes … all of the above, and probably more.

* * * * *

In Chapter 2 we reviewed the history of science and scientific thought, and medicine's place within that tradition. I offered the suggestion that science is how people have tried to convert their initial astonishment at the way the world is into, first, curiosity – the active pursuit of uncertainty – and, then, into sense – the kind of sense that makes us feel we understand how one thing leads predictably to another. What we call the scientific method has evolved as the best way of making the best sense of the natural world.

Until the 20th century, the history of science was one of tension between the rational and the irrational. Intellectually, the rational prevailed, culminating in a scientific paradigm we could call, by way of shorthand, Newtonian. The Newtonian view was that the world was essentially a machine – vast and complicated, but ultimately predictable. And very successful that world view was, establishing once and for all that the Moon was not made of green cheese, nor the cause of madness, but a space-rock that men could walk upon. Medicine's accelerating success began when it, too, adopted a Newtonian view of how the human body functions.

Then in the 20th century everything changed. Einstein and his successors supplanted Newton, offering a more comprehensive account of the universe that was, paradoxically, better at explaining things but increasingly irrational, or at least counterintuitive. Suspending disbelief and rethinking old assumptions proved to be necessary mind-steps for quantum physicists, and a stimulus to innovation in many more mundane disciplines. But medicine, by now firmly established as a Newtonian institution, has found it harder to let go. Medicine's prevailing paradigm remains predominantly mechanistic, with only a few fuzzy mavericks banging the drum for mystery.

But I'm with the mavericks, and it's time to go on the offensive. The charge against biomedicine is not that it is too scientific, but that its science is out of date. There are important lessons medicine has yet to learn from the post-Einstein upgrade. Specifically:

- conventional medical problem-solving relies too heavily on simplistic linear 'cause and effect' thinking to provide adequate analysis in every clinical situation
- conventional medicine's reductionist approach to complex systems fails to take account of their inherent unpredictability, and of the emergence phenomena they can demonstrate
- too many doctors ignore the reality of the observer effect – that what is seen depends on how, and by whom, it is looked at. As a result, doctor-as-scientist and doctor-as-person remain disconnected.

* * * * *

Chapter 3, 'Inchworms and also-rans', charted the traditional but unlovely mutual suspicion between specialists and GPs.

Before the Enlightenment, having little more to dispense than platitudes and hocus-pocus, doctors were (if we overlook the physician's shuddering disdain for the barber–surgeon) not much differentiated by their field of expertise. True, one medical man might cry the supremacy of his leeches and lancets over the other rascal's patent metallic tractors.[91] But either's

---

91 'Metallic tractors' consisted of two 3-inch metal rods, one of brass, the other of iron, which were applied to the affected part to 'draw off the noxious electrical fluid that lay at the root of suffering'. Their invention is usually ascribed to Elisha Perkins (1741–99) of Yale.

claim to greater merit or higher status would have rested more on the force of his charisma and the eminence of his clientele than on any detectable advantage of leech or tractor. Then, as the train of scientific progress began to gather speed, those members of the medical profession with the sharpest elbows – they are destined to become the specialists – jumped eagerly aboard, commandeered the first-class compartments, and prepared to colonise the new territories opened up by medical science. Others, less science-struck, clambered apprehensively into the remaining second-class seats – or else, realising the train had left without them, returned to their provincial obscurity, consoling themselves that at least their patients still loved them.

In terms of prestige and material reward, history has not until recently been kind to the 'left-behinders', who, sceptical or nervous of the rush to scientific determinism, found themselves labelled losers and consigned to a lowly and apologetic life in general practice. It has been the pioneering doctors-as-scientists and their descended tribe of specialists who have established themselves as kings of the medical castle. Until recently …

In 1955 Everett Rogers, an agricultural graduate at Iowa State University, took as his doctoral research topic the question of why, despite clear scientific evidence and strong economic imperatives, some farmers in the American Midwest were reluctant to use chemical weed-killers to boost their corn yields. His conclusion, published in 1962 as the landmark book *Diffusion of Innovations*,[92] was that the advent of a new technology – almost *any* new technology – separated people into categories according to the enthusiasm and speed with which they adopted it.

Figure 6.1 represents how a new idea is gradually taken up by successive cohorts of consumers. In the vanguard are the true innovators, pioneers with genuine originality and creativity. Hard on their heels are the 'early adopters', who at the first whiff of anything novel simply must have it. After the 'must have's come the 'early majority' – the 'keen to have's – followed by the less enthusiastic 'late majority' – the 'might as well have's. Trailing behind we find the 'laggards', the reluctant 'if I have to's and the 'I suppose I must's.[93]

Rogers' analysis is a good deal more thorough than this condensed version suggests. He acknowledges that not every innovation is destined for, or deserving of, universal uptake. Nevertheless, there is a widely held value judgement that 'eager is good, reluctant is bad'. Examples are legion, particularly in the

---

92 Rogers EM. *Diffusion of Innovations*. New York: Free Press, 1962.

93 Innovators and early adopters form roughly 16% of the population; early and late majorities about 34% each; and laggards the remaining 16%.

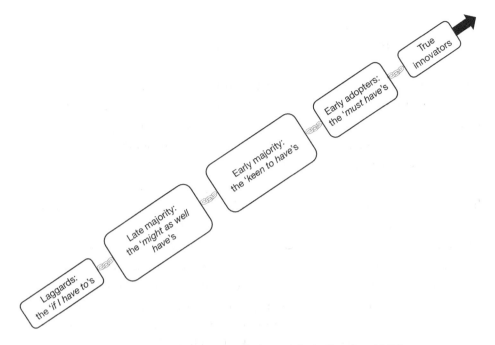

Figure 6.1 How new ideas are taken up (adapted from Rogers, 1962).

area of consumer electronics: computers, mobile communications, digital photography. But wherever there is a rush to adopt novelty there seems inevitably to be a 'laggards' backlash'. Rogers himself understood that individuals are not permanent members of any adoption group. It is possible to be an early adopter in one case and a laggard in another. To the laggard, premature innovation is for geeks, and to be over-eager is to be gullible. There are numerous examples of early adopters getting their fingers burned by rushing to adopt before the technology has evolved its way to stability. In the early days of domestic video recording, those who plumped for the Betamax format as soon as it came on the market wasted a lot of money and looked rather foolish when the later VHS system prevailed. Sometimes the laggard is the person with foresight, someone who can see potential weaknesses in the innovation and is prepared to sit out until a superior solution becomes available.

As a description of how people behave in the face of new technologies, Rogers' theory clearly hits the mark. But we also see very similar behaviour when less tangible forms of novelty – ideas, beliefs, memes – diffuse outwards through a culture from a small core of opinion leaders. The history of most of the world religions follows a Rogerian model, as does the spread of 'big ideas' such as Darwin's theory of evolution or political constructs such as social justice or consumer choice. The medical profession's reaction to the successes of Newtonian science is another example. During the 20th century, the scientific paradigm diffused through the medical fraternity like solvent across a chromatography plate. It separated a once homogeneous profession into a leading edge of clinical scientists (who took their science very seriously, specialising more and more and colonising the hospitals with expensive new gadgetry), and a rump of laggards who, sceptical and perhaps intimidated, concentrated in general practice, protesting to anyone who would listen that 'medicine is an art as well as a science'.

And, here, I'm with the laggards, but not for Luddite reasons. Science itself has changed. The science of which medicine is a subset is no longer the deterministic, atomistic, mechanical and predictable affair it once was. Those who think it is are no longer at the leading edge. The tide of accepted wisdom has turned. Post-Einsteinian science requires a multifactorial view of causality that can incorporate complexity and indeterminacy. We now appreciate that the qualitative disciplines such as psychology, sociology and anthropology can be just as illuminating of the human condition as the quantitative ones of physiology and biochemistry. And we shall see how the arts and humanities can make a contribution to the relief of human troubles no less legitimate than those of surgery and pharmacology. In that the contemporary generalist is a polymath more at home in all these disparate domains than his specialist colleague, yesterday's laggard has become today's early adopter. And vice versa.

There is nothing to be gained by specialists and generalists thumbing their noses at each other and arguing about whose is the better form of practice. The two complement each other. Medicine can be practised in a specialist way and in a generalist way. But it is perhaps best practised by doctors who can do both.

The specialist way of doing medicine currently dominates the profession's corporate mindset, not least because of its spectacular successes in treating the many diseases that yield to a reductionist approach. But it remains my belief that the specialist way is doomed to prove ultimately disappointing unless it can be complemented with the generalist way, which is more responsive to context and complexity. Unfortunately, the generalist way remains poorly understood, under-appreciated, and under-represented in the skills repertoire of many doctors. My immodest hope in this book is to correct this imbalance, and persuade specialism to move over and make equal room for clinical generalism. Later chapters will go into specific features of the generalist way, and suggest how an eclectic mindset capable of accommodating both specialist and generalist approaches can be fostered.

In Chapter 3 I tried to convey, through the metaphor of the *Inchworm* song, some sense of what it can be like to practise big picture medicine. Listening to the mournful refrain as the inchworm measures off the marigolds, 'Two and two are four, four and four are eight ...', it is possible to feel sorry for the specialist, mesmerised by detail and trapped by the compulsion to quantify and calculate. How much more uplifted does the singer–generalist sound, who, while allowing that the inchworm 'will probably go far', nevertheless wishes that it, like him, could 'stop and see how beautiful they are'.

The marigold is no less beautiful for also being measurable. Its interest as an object in the physical world is not diminished if a lyricist sings of its beauty. Lucky the marigold that can be both measured *and* appreciated. Lucky the marigold that holds equal fascination for both inchworm *and* poet. And lucky the patient on whose predicament a doctor can turn both a specialist *and* a generalist gaze.

* * * * *

The idea of a 'medical gaze' – the way doctors perceive and interpret their job and their patients – was further explored in Chapter 4. I compared the specialist's gaze to the view through a fixed-focus close-up photographic lens, which captures only a narrow field of view, but in great detail. The generalist's gaze has an additional wide-angle setting, which can take in a panoramic view of the subject and its surroundings, though with some loss of detail. I suggested that probably the best kind of medical gaze would resemble that versatile hybrid, the zoom lens, able to range continuously between close-up and wide-angle settings.

I remember one of my favourite picture books as a child. The first plate was a photograph of a human hand, life size. As you turned the pages, each image successively zoomed in, magnifying its predecessor by 10. Page 2 showed the surface of the skin, page 3 the pores. Somewhere around page 5 or 6, bacteria became visible; shortly afterwards, as the limit of resolution of the light microscope was reached, the images were electron micrographs of cell structure, culminating in a picture of a lattice of fuzzy dots that claimed to be individual atoms. Halfway through the book we saw the hand again. But this time, page by page the camera pulled back by a factor of 10. You saw the hand's owner, the room she was in, and the neighbourhood. Then the countryside, the landscape, the planet, the sun, the galaxy. What is interesting is that at no stage did you think, 'Ah, *this* is what is ultimately real. *This* is the right level to appreciate what a hand is.'

Our whole scientific endeavour is a response to a sense of awe at what the natural world reveals, whether we explore it with microscope or telescope. Mystery and majesty are to be found at every order of magnitude and in every domain of creation, including – especially – the human condition.

Chapter 4 further complicated the image of the 'medical gaze as zoom lens' by adding a second axis of swivel, allowing the additional option of gazing inwards as well as outwards, attending to the doctor's own inner world as well as the external realm of patients and diseases. This refinement is necessary if we are to understand the importance – crucial to the post-Einsteinian upgrade to the scientific paradigm – of the 'doctor-as-participant-observer'.

Chapter 4 ended with a poet's account of the gaze's zoom and swivel capability. Henry Reed's poem *Judging Distances* illustrates – no, *more* than illustrates: gives a first-hand actually-while-you-read-it experience of – being in the generalist mindset, the gaze moving between close-up and wide-angle, switching between outer and inner worlds. The weapons training sergeant is a solid specialist in his field. His selective attention zooms in upon what, for his purposes, are the salient features in the landscape. He talks of sectors and arcs, and the possibility of dead ground. He is indifferent to – indeed, suspicious of – the distinguishing features of trees and animals. The listening recruit looks at the same landscape, only with a wide-angle gaze. He can tell an elm from a poplar; he can describe the colours of fields and dwellings in the light of the westering sun; and he can recognise an act of human loving when he sees one. Then in the poem's final line his gaze flicks inwards, and he realises with throat-lumpening clarity how wistful he himself is for the intimacy of the now-departed lovers. That awareness of the 'self observing the self' is essential if the totality of the instant is to be captured.

* * * * *

It seems important, if we are to practise rational medicine, for us to have a consensus understanding of what disease is, what causes it, why people get ill, and what influences whether or not they get better. We need to agree how questions like these are to be framed, and what kind of answers will be acceptable. The traditional medical model, rooted in Newtonian science, has established itself as the profession's default paradigm, certainly as far as the specialist way of practice is concerned. And it has an impressive record of clinical success in many areas. But it has its inadequacies too.

The medical model defines disease in terms of departures of biological variables from a limited normal range. It sees the subjective experiences of illness and well-being as correlating closely with the presence or absence of objective abnormality. As for the causes of disease, the medical model prefers them to be physical, recent, and the fewer the better. It gets distinctly uncomfortable if causal claims are made by factors remote in time or from the fluffier areas of life.

Yet patients continue to insist that more can be medically wrong with them than just their biology. Psychological, interpersonal, economic, historic, spiritual, social and cultural influences simply will not be excluded from consideration. And so, with what little mathematical rigour I can muster, I proposed a multidimensional elaboration in the form of the cusp catastrophe model.

The catastrophe model conceives health and illness not as definable conditions but rather as 'inner territories', loosely bounded on most sides, but with a catastrophe edge over which one can plunge precipitately from health into illness, or back from illness into health. The presence or absence of pathology is only one of a multitude of vectors that have the net result of attracting one towards, or holding one back from, a catastrophe transition between well-being and illness. This, I hope, gives a more dynamic, a more comprehensive, a more realistic model of what it is to experience 'the heart-ache and the thousand natural shocks that flesh is heir to'.[94] Specifically the catastrophe model:

- suggests why it is possible to feel well while being diseased, or ill while biologically 'normal'
- explains the often-observed time lag between patients developing symptoms and presenting for attention, or between corrective treatment and resuming normal function
- implies that doctors can intervene therapeutically in more domains than just the purely physical.

* * * * *

I am concerned that my analysis might be taken as an attack on specialism per se, which is absolutely not my intention. Even less do I mean to decry the skill and dedication of my specialist colleagues. But the conventional medical model has no monopoly of the right to explain. And the belief has to be challenged that the specialist way of practice, which is the medical model

---

94 William Shakespeare (1601). *Hamlet*, Act 3, scene 1.

incarnate, is the ideal, fully comprehensive way of doing medicine. Indeed, I think most specialists would agree. There are many hospital consultants who, while thinking and acting within the confines of their specialties, also bring a generalist perspective to their interactions with patients – and are better doctors because of it. What has to be resisted is the pressure to lock the medical gaze in close-up mode. What has to be lamented is that generations of medical students, doctors, patients and policy makers have allowed themselves to be dazzled by the glitz of high-tech reductionist medicine, leaving the more eclectic generalist approach bleached of understanding and appeal.

My unashamed motive for writing this book is to see clinical generalism revalued, rehabilitated in popular and professional esteem. Generalism deserves to be at the leading edge of medical thought. Clinical decision-making, healthcare policy making, the relevance of research and – most importantly – the experience of patients would all be better if it were. So why is it not?

I would have to concede that, if we weigh the achievements of specialism against the generalism of the past – up to the midpoint of the 20th century, let us say – there is no contest. Specialism would win, and would deserve to. During the glory years of scientific medicine, generalism could all too often provide a refuge for also-rans. Lord Moran in 1958, while insensitive, was largely right; the best doctors usually *did* want to be specialists, and general practice often *was* where you landed if you fell off the promotion ladder to hospital consultancy. Clinical standards in general practice *were* often unacceptably low. Protesting that 'medicine is an art, not a science', too many family doctors managed to conceal their ineptitude with a pat on the head for all and a platitude for every occasion. The new specialism could well do with being better at generalism; but too many generalists of the old school had such poor specialist knowledge that patients were too often put at risk.

But now a new generalism is on the march – rigorous, exhilarating, and unfazed by post-Newtonian complexity.

As we saw in Chapter 3, a group of British general practitioners in the 1950s, stung by the hubris of specialists such as Lord Moran, began the process of rescuing general practice from the mediocrity it seemed headed for. They reassured with their insistence that GPs should deliver high-quality clinical care. They impressed with the thoughtful way they could articulate the many points of difference between medicine as practised in hospital and in the home or surgery. They argued persuasively for a healthcare system in which strength in its hospital services was matched by excellence in its primary care. They negotiated a place for general practice on countless committees. They pioneered postgraduate vocational training for general practice, developing educational skills unequalled in specialty training. They opened the way for an influential general practice presence in the medical schools and the undergraduate curriculum. Spurred by their example, increasing numbers of GPs regained a sense of pride in generalism as a clinical and academic discipline.

Though the historical processes were different, a similar renaissance of clinical generalism has taken place in many countries across the world over the last 50 years. Family medicine is now strong in most of Europe, in Canada, Australia and New Zealand. It is developing rapidly in the Middle East, in the subcontinent and in South East Asia. In Japan it is still in its infancy, but healthy, vociferous and growing fast. It is strong in the USA, though only amongst the well-off. There is wide international agreement about the hallmarks of the new generalist. He or she is a clinical polymath who:

1   makes diagnoses in wider terms, and by more diverse methods, than the medical model suggests
2   recognises psychological, social, family, economic and cultural determinants of disease
3   can handle complexity and 'fuzzy logic' in problem-solving and decision-making
4   deals with co-morbidity (having more than one condition simultaneously), where optimal overall treatment may not be the sum of the optimum treatment of each condition
5   manages clinical uncertainty, including atypical presentations, undifferentiated illness and individual variation
6   can improvise safely in situations where firm guidance is not available
7   undertakes a 'gatekeeper' role, facilitating and guiding patients' access to secondary care
8   balances the requirements of the individual patient with efficient use of available resources
9   understands the importance and psychodynamics of the doctor–patient relationship and its contribution to effective care
10 manages the process of the consultation, using specific consulting skills as an adjunct to clinical skills
11 can make effective diagnostic and therapeutic use of the doctor's own thoughts and feelings.

What unites this apparently disparate litany is the mindset of the doctor. Items 1 to 8 are how you find yourself practising if you zoom your medical gaze between close-up and wide-angle, and take in context as well as detail. The last three items (9 to 11) require you in addition to become alert to your own internal thoughts and feelings, and open to the promptings your Inner Physician. There should perhaps be an extra item on the list – the generalist:

12 acknowledges that the 'doctor-as-participant-observer', the 'self observing the self', is inescapably a part of the clinical process.

This 12th item, briefly stated but subtle and complex in its implications, is what converts generalism into what I have chosen to call 'big picture medicine'.

To practise just in a specialist way is not enough. To practise just in a generalist way is not enough either. Better is to practise in both generalist and specialist modes, moving cleanly and elegantly between each, and knowing which is appropriate to the clinical circumstances. But even this is still not enough. Even a composite gaze, competent in scientific detail and sensitive to every context, remains externally focused unless it can also make the inward swivel and allow the Inner Physician into the consultation process. This additional degree of freedom is needed if the fullest extent of the doctor's resources is to be gifted to the patient's service. Anything less, and the practice of medicine becomes like a performance of Hamlet where the lead actor has spent most of the rehearsals learning to juggle skulls.

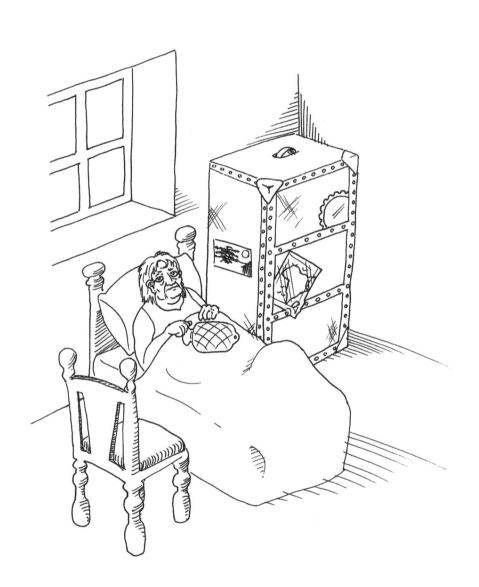

Chapter 7

'What's the matter?'

Everything is vague to a degree you do not realize till you have tried to make it precise, and everything precise is so remote from everything that we normally think.

Bertrand Russell (1872–1970)

English philosopher

The Philosophy of Logical Atomism, 1918

If you wish to gain knowledge of a problem, begin with learning to see it in many different ways.

Leonardo da Vinci (1452–1519)

Italian polymath

Try to be one of the people on whom nothing is lost!

Henry James (1843–1916)

American writer

From *The Art of Fiction*, 1884

This chapter is the first of two exploring diagnosis in the context of big picture medicine. It proposes that diagnosis is 'insight on the verge of action', and that the process of reaching a diagnosis is best understood as bringing meaning to a predicament that was hitherto mysterious. It goes on to examine how far the traditional approach to diagnosis is fit for this purpose, and concludes that, while effective in a narrow range of physical disease, the medical model has blind spots and false assumptions that limit its usefulness to the clinical generalist. Diagnosis, like every other part of the medical encounter, is subject to the observer effect; it is crucially affected by the personality and tactics of the diagnostician.

This is a true story. I once had a patient, a well-to-do lady in her mid-70s – let's call her Alice – who requested a home visit almost every week. She didn't *need* a home visit; I often saw her out shopping, and I'm sure she could quite easily have come to the surgery. She complained in doleful tones of a multitude of symptoms: abdominal pain (she called it 'belly ache'), tiredness, being 'just not right' – but mainly of belly ache. Over the years I had quizzed her, examined her, arranged every relevant test and a good few irrelevant ones besides. Nothing ever showed up. Biologically she was well, but she acted ill. Each week she would tell me that she had tried last week's suggestions, but now her symptoms were slightly different … .

On one occasion I let my frustration show and said something like, 'It's a waste of time, coming to see you. I never seem to find out what's the matter with you.' 'What's the matter with me?' Alice retorted. 'You have no idea what it's like to be me!' 'Okay,' I said, '*tell* me what it's like to be you.' And this is the story she told.

Fifty years earlier and newly wedded, Alice had gone with her husband, a missionary, to a posting in central Africa. She fell pregnant – but so remote was their location that she received no antenatal care whatsoever. After 6 months of pregnancy she stopped gaining weight and the baby stopped moving. It was another 3 months before she reached a hospital, where she had an operation to remove her uterus and the dead child it contained. For 3 months she had known she was carrying a corpse inside her. Imagine that. Then the surgeons had taken away her womb, and with it her chances of motherhood, and also, as it turned out, the tenuous bonds that had kept her and her husband together. And now here she was, 50 years later – lonely, childless and unhappy in a village in the English Home Counties – suffering chronic, apparently inexplicable, symptoms that made her miserable and her doctor cross.

'So,' said Alice, 'that's what it's like to be me.'

(To be continued.)

* * * * *

Almost every encounter between a doctor and a patient begins with an anecdote. There will often be a ritual exchange initiated by the doctor saying, in effect, 'Tell me the story.' And the patient, or a spokesman, will take this as the cue to begin a narrative. The narrative can be quite brief, a few terse monosyllables – 'I've got this rash on my hand.' Or it might be a bit more elaborate, the beginnings of a story – 'Last week I tried some new detergent, and now my hands have come up in this rash.' Sometimes the anecdote has the makings of a full-blown saga, a soap opera if you like – '... and I can't stop scratching it, so at work they think I've got scabies, and then what with the children ...' Even if the patient is unconscious or mute, the body tells its own non-verbal story: a collapse, a wound, a gush of blood.

It is fashionable in scientific circles to sneer at anecdote as a source of reliable information. Science, it is rightly considered, should proceed on the basis of verifiable data. And anecdote is thought to be incapable of providing the necessary objectivity. 'You rubbed some cream on and it got better, you say? That's not proper evidence. It's just anecdotal.' Yet what *is* data, what *is* research evidence, if not lots of individual anecdotes pooled together and their particularities averaged and filtered out?

If you were to ask a doctor, drawing out a patient's narrative, 'What are you doing now?', that doctor would probably reply, 'I'm taking a history.' 'Why?', you might enquire. 'It's the first stage in making a diagnosis,' you would be told. But you persist. 'What's a diagnosis?', you ask, 'and why do you want one?' At this point the doctor's eyes are likely to roll; life is busy enough, without having to explain the bleeding obvious. 'That's how we doctors work,' comes the reply. 'We try to identify the problem, starting from what the patient tells us. Finding out what the matter is, identifying the problem – that's what diagnosis means. I listen to the patient's story, ask some questions to clarify it, probably examine the patient, maybe get some investigations done. That way I arrive at the diagnosis. And I need the right diagnosis in order to decide what the right treatment should be.'

Yes-ish. As an answer, that's partly correct. One has the feeling that what this doctor secretly longs for is a Star Trek-style 'diagnostimeter', some kind of hand-held scanner that when run over the body produces a print-out of its biological malfunctions without all the hassle of interrogating and examining the patient.

We can accept that the doctor needs an understanding of the patient's predicament in order to intervene effectively in it. But we must challenge the assumption that true understanding can be reliably obtained by an uninvolved doctor, even one clutching a magic scanner, operating objectively at arm's length. There is no such thing as an uninvolved doctor operating objectively at arm's length. As we have seen in Chapter 2, the observer (in this case the listening doctor) is never without impact. How you frame a question conditions the answer you get. Even in the first few moments of the consultation, the doctor's precise wording of the invitation to 'tell me the story' modifies the story that is told. And as the narrative gets under way, every comment or intervention the doctor makes further constrains the details and emphasis that the patient presents. It follows that any inferences about the patient's problem that the doctor may draw from the narrative he himself has partly constructed will not necessarily be the pure cold facts such as those the diagnostimeter might reveal. No matter how objective and unintrusive the doctor intends to be, there must always be an element of interpretation – of 'reading between the lines' – in the diagnostic process.

Consider some of the different ways a doctor might prompt the patient to begin, and how their implications could distort the patient's version of events.

- *What can I do for you?* seems a fairly neutral offer, but it subtly encourages the patient to disclose, perhaps prematurely, what is expected by way of outcome.
- *How can I help you?* paradoxically sounds, to my British ears at least, slightly condescending.
- *What's the problem?* may come across as implying that the patient should not really be bothering the doctor.
- The *seems* in *What seems to be the trouble?* suggests that the doctor half expects the 'trouble' to be imaginary; the patient may respond with an overstatement in order to emphasise its genuineness.
- Few doctors nowadays use the phrase I was taught as a medical student: *What are you complaining of?* But imagine the patient's indignation if they did.
- Even a gentle *So ...,* said with an encouraging smile and an open-handed gesture, might to some patients feel like a priest's invitation to begin confession. To others, its very open-endedness could be paralysing.

Admittedly I am reading my own interpretations into these probably innocuous remarks; you, the reader, may interpret them differently, or not at all. Clearly there is no 'right' way of beginning the consultation. The point is, some degree of distortion is inevitable whenever data is transmitted through the medium of language. So diagnosis – which is based on interpreting a narrative jointly authored by patient and doctor – will always rest on information that is to some extent corrupted by the process of eliciting it.

* * * * *

We doctors are sometimes accused of thinking we are gods. I don't mind that – as long as the god we think we are is Hermes. In Greek mythology,

Hermes (or Mercury, as he was known to the Romans) is the go-between god, the winged messenger who imparts the will of the senior gods on Mount Olympus to earthly mortals. Hermes is the god of communication, the inventor and master of language. And so his name is associated with the translation of what is beyond human comprehension into a form we humans can understand. Hermes is the great explainer, the interpreter whose business it is to render the unintelligible intelligible. At Delphi, site of the ancient Greek oracle, the priest who translated the incoherent ramblings of the smoke-intoxicated priestess was called the *hermeios*. The Italian writer Italo Calvino described Hermes as operating 'between universal laws and individual destinies, between the forces of nature and the forms of culture, between the objects of the world and all thinking subjects'.[95] He points out that, according to the psychoanalyst Carl Jung, Hermes represents 'individuation', the process whereby separate components become integrated into stable wholes. To Calvino, Hermes represented the function of literature; we could also take him as a symbol for the role of medicine and for the clinical generalist. The generalist truly does aim to discover, initially through language, the connections between the universal processes of pathology and the destinies of the thinking, feeling individuals they affect.

Hermes also gave his name to the discipline of hermeneutics, into which territory we need briefly to stray.

> **hermeneutics:** the branch of knowledge that deals with interpretation, especially of sacred or literary texts.

Hermeneutics – working out how things are to be interpreted – originally developed as the study of ancient religious texts. It took as its starting point the possibility that what the authors of the texts wrote down may have been less than, or different from, what they actually meant. In other words, things get distorted or left out as ideas are translated from thought into language and back again, from the brain to the lips of the speaker, and from the ears to the brain of the listener. Starting from the written text, hermeneutics would endeavour to work back and recreate the author's 'real' meaning. By analogy, medical hermeneutics proposes that what the patient says and what the

---

95 Italo Calvino (1923–85), Italian writer. From *Six Memos for the Next Millennium* (written for the 1985 Charles Eliot Norton Lectures at Harvard, but undelivered owing to Calvino's death).

doctor infers may be incomplete guides to what is 'really' the matter, and that some degree of interpretation is always necessary.

A wish for things to make sense runs very deep in the human psyche. Much of our conscious life is taken up with trying to convince ourselves that we know what's going on. We try desperately to make every new experience fit with what we think we know already. So it is unsurprising that, when illness strikes, both the patient and the doctor from whom a cure is expected try to understand what is going on in terms of what they each think they know already. Medicine therefore is, at least in part, a hermeneutic activity. Some, indeed, would go so far as to say that the diagnostic part of medicine is 'hermeneutics all the way down'.

One cannot look very far into the literature of medical hermeneutics before encountering such august and intimidating names as Heidegger,[96] Gadamer[97] and Svenaeus.[98] Svenaeus summarises his analysis in these terms:

> *Clinical medicine is not a theory, not even an applied theory, but a practice. This practice ... can best be understood as an interpretive meeting between health-care personnel and patient with the aim of healing the ill person seeking help.*[99]

An 'interpretive meeting' between doctor and patient: so far, so obvious, you might think. But the ideas of hermeneutics become more interesting if we ask ourselves what is the 'text' that the clinician tries to interpret.

Illness expresses itself in several different forms of text, each of which requires to be interpreted in different ways. What we might call the 'first

---

96 Martin Heidegger (1889–1976), German existential philosopher. Heidegger's key idea can apparently be summarised thus: 'The Western philosophical tradition since the Greeks has forgotten the "question of being", and has been interested only in the present, thereby ignoring the temporal dimensions of past and future.' No, I don't understand that either. Heidegger's membership of the Nazi Party from 1933 to 1945 has tarnished his reputation.

97 Hans-Georg Gadamer (1900–2002), German philosopher and pupil of Heidegger. Gadamer argues that the process of understanding a text involves two perspectives: those of the author and of the interpreter. Interpretation is thus a two-way process in which these perspectives merge in a 'fusion of horizons'. The text is always open to new interpretations, so that no single investigative process can guarantee a definitive conclusion. This I think I *do* nearly understand.

98 Fredrik Svenaeus, Associate Professor of Philosophy, Department for Health and Society, Linköping University, Sweden.

99 *The Hermeneutics of Medicine and the Phenomenology of Health: steps towards a philosophy of medical practice.* New York: Springer, 2001, p. 2.

draft' exists only in the patient's felt experience, in the form of symptoms. This subjective 'experiential text' is accessible only to the patient, who must initially interpret the nature and significance of the symptoms in the light of his own medical knowledge, fears, assumptions and health beliefs. If the patient is unsatisfied with, or alarmed by, his own inter-

> Despise no new accident in your body, but ask opinion of it.
> (i.e. Ask yourself what the symptom is trying to tell you.)
>
> Francis Bacon (1561–1626)
> English statesman and pioneer
> of the scientific method
> From the essay *Of Regimen of Health* (1597)

pretation of the symptoms, he is likely to turn to a doctor to interpret them for him. This requires the transformation of the non-verbal experiential text into words – a 'narrative text' that the patient offers and which the doctor can interrogate.

The relationship between symptoms and narrative is highly complex. Lacking vocabulary, the patient may find it difficult to describe physical sensations and emotional states. He may use ambiguous language such as 'tired all the time', 'out of sorts', or 'something between a pain and an ache'. Or, trying to help the doctor, he might make clumsy use of medical terms – 'depressed', 'projectile vomiting', 'crushing chest pain' – which have particular but possibly misleading implications for the listening doctor. The patient's narrative may hint at unexpressed or inexpressible fears, through remarks such as 'I'm probably just wasting your time,' or 'You read all sorts of things in the papers'. A doctor versed in communication skills will be adept at reading between the lines, encouraging and prompting where necessary, and detecting cues to deeper layers of meaning in the unfolding story. Yet, however gentle the doctor's interventions, they will inevitably distort the patient's exposition even as they seek to clarify it.

During this interpretive listening, moreover, the doctor-as-scientist's priority must necessarily be to detect 'the disease that underlies the illness' and thus to remain alert to medically relevant information lurking within the narrative. The clinically trained part of the doctor's attention is on red alert, ready to seize upon, and pursue, clues in the patient's story to possible pathology. Yet the danger of rushing to premature conclusions or overlooking more subtle cues is ever-present. It seems that what is required of the doctor is a kind of divided awareness in which he can listen to the narrative attentively and selectively at the same time. It takes a tricky mental balancing act to be both passively empathic and actively analytic simultaneously. So it is tempting for the doctor to downplay the importance of a patient's narrative and to focus more on the 'physical text'[100] – the disease as documented by the patient's body.

From the doctor's point of view, the physical text written in the patient's body can be easier to interpret than the narrative text, let alone the experiential text – the illness as felt first-hand by the patient – which he can only imagine. For one thing, physical signs tend to be more durable than the spoken word. The physical text is more likely to keep still while the clinician interrogates it with eyes, ears, hands, instruments and investigations. The patient's verbal account of his problem is more wrigglesome than the steady, silent testimony of his body.

For most doctors, their undergraduate medical training will have equipped them better for interpreting the physical text of disease than for unpacking the narrative in which patients describe their illness. The opening, history-taking, stage of clerking a patient, with its battery of closed and leading questions, is designed to filter out the patient's linguistic idiosyncrasies. Like an over-zealous policeman massaging a witness statement into the officialese he thinks will impress a jury, the organically minded doctor paraphrases the patient's account into the language of pathology, tuning out whatever won't translate easily. (Patient: 'When I saw what I'd brought up, it was all black lumps, and I thought Oh God!' Doctor: 'So you vomited some altered blood.') It is the same with physical examination; the doctor selectively latches on to findings that he can readily interpret in terms of biological malfunctioning. And when it comes to ordering special tests and investigations, we see most starkly the doctor's preference for interrogating the patient's body rather than his words. Doctors like ordering tests. The world of technicians with white coats and expensive machinery, with its implied promise of unchallengeable objectivity, is a beguiling one. And, let's face it, it is fun. The ability with a simple signature or mouse-click to bring high-tech resources to bear on an awestruck patient, and to read both past and future in a few drops of blood or a burst of invisible radiation, appeals to the show-off in us all. Most doctors will maintain that, while the patient may indeed be more than just a collection of organs and biochemical processes, he is such a collection at the very

---

100 The terms 'experiential text', 'narrative text' and 'physical text' are those proposed and popularised by Drew Leder, from the Department of Philosophy, Loyola College, Baltimore [Clinical interpretation: the hermeneutics of medicine. *Theoretical Medicine and Bioethics* 1990; **11**(1): 9–24]. Leder also refers to an 'instrumental text' disclosed by diagnostic technologies; however, in this chapter I have subsumed the 'instrumental' within the 'physical' text.

least. And, many will further insist, it is in the interpretation of this physical text that doctors' expertise largely resides.

Be that as it may, the search for meaning in both narrative and physical texts – diagnosis – is arguably the most important part of the clinical process. Misinterpret either, and the doctor will waste time and skill in trying to solve the wrong problem. It is also the most likely part of the clinical process to go wrong, depending as it does on a sequence of translations – from experiential to narrative texts, and from narrative to physical. Chinese whispers may be fine as a party game, but when played out in the consulting room, decisions, even lives, hang on it.

Perhaps as a reaction against a perceived over-reliance by their colleagues on the physical text, some doctors are keen to reassert the importance of narrative in the medical process. Indeed, there are now journals and conferences devoted to 'narrative medicine' as if it were a separate specialty in its own right. In broad terms, the idea of narrative medicine is that people's first instinct, when illness strikes, is to perceive it as an episode in the ongoing chronicle of their lives, each fresh twist becoming part of a developing storyline that will, in hindsight, come to be interpreted as one instalment in the longer saga of the individual's lifespan. This narrative view of medicine recognises our universal fear of the haphazard. We dread the possibility that we are the impotent butts of pointless events; we long for coherence, meaning, direction, significance.

The literary genre that most nearly represents the medical world is the mystery thriller. A potential victim (the patient) goes unsuspecting about the daily round; a villain (disease) lurks, stalks, pounces; there is the threat or the reality of danger and disaster; the detective (doctor) is called in; clues are identified, evidence painstakingly sifted, until a combination of diligence and insight unmasks the villain; the mystery is solved, calamity is averted, and some form of justice or tragedy (for they are closely related) prevails.

Detractors of narrative medicine ask whether this analysis, neat though it may be, adds anything of substance to an essentially scientific discipline already crowded with models and theories. However, its proponents argue that to view a clinical situation from a narrative perspective is to be reminded of just those important ways in which medicine is more than a scientific discipline. Its most powerful effect, they would claim, is to nudge the medical gaze towards its wide-angle setting in which the context and meaning of the doctor–patient interaction can be better appreciated. As no less august a publication than the *Lancet* wrote in a 2003 reference to the work of the late Cecil Helman:[101]

> *The art of medicine is a literary art. One that requires of the practitioner the ability to listen in a particular way, to empathise, but also to imagine. To try to feel what it must be like to be that other person lying in the sick bed, or sitting across the desk from you. To try to understand the storyteller, as well as the story.[102]*

It seems to me that the narrative and the scientific accounts are inseparable and complementary. What the patient experiences on falling ill, and reports to the doctor, is an event in an ongoing story. The process of diagnosis converts – translates – that report into an understanding from which medical action can flow. In the treatment phase of the encounter, the results of medical action are assimilated back into the patient's story, to be passed on to its next round of listeners.

Who needs a diagnosis? This is not such a silly question as it might appear. Both doctor and patient need one, though not necessarily the same one, nor for the same purpose.

Clearly the doctor requires a working diagnosis as a prerequisite for management or treatment. Moreover, that diagnosis needs to be couched in language that fits with how the doctor understands the patient's problem to have been caused, and with how any proposed intervention is expected to work. For example: Esther, a middle-aged office worker presents with worsening headaches. In her narrative text she tells of being 'unable to concentrate on my work', and 'getting hauled up before my line manager for a reprimand'. The physical text discloses no neurological or other abnormality apart from some soft tissue tenderness around the occipital condyles. An organically minded doctor might diagnose 'tension headache' – and if asked to elaborate on this diagnosis might suggest, 'Muscle tension around the neck and shoulders is transmitted to the scalp fascia, producing pain.' Diagnosis in such language is the prelude to an organically focused treatment package that might include

---

101 Cecil Helman (1944–2009), GP, medical anthropologist, author and poet. His best-known work is *Culture, Health and Illness* (2nd edition). London: Hodder Arnold, 2007.

102 From an article publishes in *The Lancet*, 2003; **361**: 2252. © Elsevier. Original syntax preserved.

prescription analgesics, a programme of neck exercises and the general advice to 'relax more'. A more psychologically orientated doctor might make a diagnosis of 'stress-related headaches', explaining how unresolved worries at work are becoming, literally, 'a headache'. In this 'organic-lite' frame of reference, suggested treatment might include over-the-counter analgesics in the short term and, for longer term relief, advice that Esther should discuss her work problems with her manager and renegotiate some of her duties and expectations.

For doctors, diagnosis is a prelude to action.

Patients, too, need a diagnosis; and theirs is, if anything, a more complex need than the doctor's. They need their doctor to have a medically framed diagnosis from which medical intervention can flow if appropriate. But patients also need a diagnosis for their own peace of mind, and it needs to be framed in language that will contribute to that peace of mind. The patient's diagnosis needs to answer their own questions, bringing the reassuring feeling that what is happening to them makes sense, and that they are in safe hands.

Cecil Helman, referred to earlier, reminds us in what has become known as his 'folk model of health and illness' of the importance of factoring the patient's perspective into our medical assessments. He describes how people, ever driven to search for meaning, struggle to put their illness experience into a coherent narrative thread. He lists six questions that the patient entering the consulting room has formed or half-formed in her mind, and which will leave her unsatisfied if they go unanswered:[103]

1   *What* has happened?
2   *Why* has it happened?
3   Why to *me*?
4   Why *now*?
5   What would happen if nothing were done?
6   What should be done about it?

Imagine how the thoughts of Esther, the lady with work-related tension headaches, might be running as she awaits her turn to go in to the doctor. *These headaches can't be anything serious, surely? I suppose they could be*

---

103 Helman CG (1981). Diseases versus illness in general practice. *Journal of the Royal College of General Practitioners* 1981; **13**: 548–52.

migraines. But I've never had migraines before. I'm probably just overtired. Or maybe I need new glasses. I'll book in with the optician on the way home. But you do read about brain tumours starting with headaches. Or a stroke. God, if I had a stroke, and had to give up my job, we'd never manage for money, not on Bill's wage. But at least I wouldn't have her at work criticising me all the time. Perhaps I could get the doctor to write a letter to get me put on light duties. I wonder if he'll want me to have a brain scan. If he does, I'll worry he thinks it's something serious. But then I'll only worry if he doesn't. I mean, he couldn't really tell without a scan, could he? Maybe I'll suggest it ...

Neither the physical diagnosis nor the more psychological alternative does full justice to the range of Esther's anxieties. Given a purely physical diagnosis, she may fail to see the connection between her 'illness' and the work problems that are contributing to it. The psychological diagnosis, while making this explicit, may leave her worried that the doctor thinks her symptoms are 'all in the mind'. So what would be a more comprehensive diagnosis of Esther's condition? Something like this, perhaps: 'Stress and possible bullying at work is causing chronic muscle tension in the shoulders, neck and scalp, resulting in headaches. These are made worse by financial worries and the fear of underlying serious disease.'

Diagnosis in these terms, combining physical with psychological and social elements, is far removed from the one- or two-word pathological diagnoses we were taught to make during our medical school training. It reads, you might think, more like a plot outline for a television soap opera.

Exactly! This is what a good diagnosis is from a patient's point of view – a plot outline: the framework of a narrative strand causally linking past events and present challenges to future developments. We are each of us the lead character in our own personal soap opera, and we need a sense of narrative coherence to play our role convincingly. Without such a sense, everything that happens to us is no more than an unsettling sequence of random events.

In his collection of essays *Aspects of the Novel*,[104] E.M. Forster makes an astute distinction between 'story' and 'plot'. A story, as defined by Forster, is:

a narrative of events arranged in their time-sequence. A plot is also a narrative of events, the emphasis falling on causality. 'The king died and then the queen died' is a story. 'The king died, and then the queen died of grief' is a plot. The time-sequence is preserved, but the sense of causality overshadows it.

---

104 An elaboration of his series of Clark Lectures given in Cambridge in 1927.

Story on its own – *This happened, then that, then the next thing* – can quickly become boring, and is ultimately unsatisfying. Forster likens it to 'a tapeworm, for its beginning and end are arbitrary'. Acknowledging the primitive origins of story-telling, Forster imagines a Neanderthal 'audience of shock-heads, gaping round the camp-fire, fatigued with contending against the mammoth or the woolly rhinoceros, and only kept awake by suspense. What would happen next? The novelist droned on, and as soon as the audience guessed what happened next they either fell asleep or killed him.'

I suspect that rare is the doctor who, listening to a patient's unfolding story of banality succeeding banality, has never stifled a yawn or entertained fantasies of violence. To this day, I cringe when I recall the inoffensive bank clerk who told me, 'I must just tell you the fascinating saga of my catarrh. And I play little tunes to myself on my teeth.' But, unlike the Neanderthal listeners, we smart professionals are not a passive audience for our patients' stories. In addition to sleep and murder as responses, we have the hermeneutic option. From the patient's narrative text, we can infer the thread of causality that elevates story to plot. If the patient–narrator cannot explain why B should follow A, the listening doctor perhaps can. The role – indeed, the duty – of the doctor is to reframe the patient's puzzling predicament into just another example of how we know one thing leads to another.

Plot – the story interpreted and set in context – is an altogether more satisfying form of narrative. Plot is story with a point. If story is events seen in close-up, plot is the wide-angle view. Our preference for plot rather than simple story perhaps explains the perennial appeal of jigsaw puzzles and crosswords. We get a frisson of relief when we see how something fits into a larger picture. The feeling that events do, after all, make sense is intrinsically rewarding. 'Of course!', we think, and relax into our destiny. In Forster's terms, the patient enters the consulting room to tell a story, but should leave knowing the plot.

The psychotherapeutic literature often refers to 'narrative competence' as one of the hallmarks of mental well-being. Healthy resilience in the face of life's vicissitudes correlates with being able to tell the tale (or 'plot', as Forster would have it) of one's own life in a way that makes sense of one's experiences, decisions, values and anxieties. If on the other hand our life lacks connectedness – its story untellable with any convincing sense of explicability, so that we are bewildered as to why we are what we are and why things turn out as they do – then our physical and mental health become precarious. We are more prone to illness, and slower to recover.

I don't know whether or not the correlation between narrative competence and health is a causal one. It could be, I suppose, that the plot lines of a healthy life are easier to discern and describe post hoc than a life battered with affliction, as is the lot of many patients. But it does seem to be the case that an important prerequisite for getting better is understanding what it was that made us ill. In Chapter 5, when we were looking at the multidimensional nature of *health* ↔ *illness* transitions, I introduced the concept of 'attractors' – factors that tend to stabilise an individual in a state of health or illness. Knowing what's going on is a powerful health attractor (see Figure 7.1).

So, for the patient, diagnosis is more than a medical label. It is a vital step in the process of shifting from bewilderment to the insight from which active participation in recovery can flow. The patient needs a diagnosis for narrative reasons – in Forster's terms again, to elevate story to plot.

We should judge the merits of a diagnosis not just by its pathological accuracy, nor even by how much of the patient's narrative it explains, but also by the effectiveness of whatever action it leads to. Diagnosis needs to have a point. For the doctor, the point of the diagnosis is to pave the way for treatment; for the patient the function of diagnosis is to convert the disconnectedness of story into meaningful, actionable plot. These two emphases are symbiotic, mutually nourishing. Medicine is conducted at what the novelist Sebastian

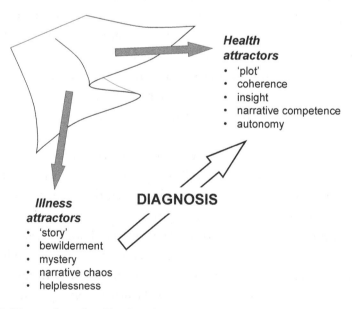

Figure 7.1 Diagnosis as health attractor.

Faulks calls 'the meeting point between thought and flesh'.[105] The consulting room is where biology and biography entwine.

> Diagnosis is insight on the verge of action

A good diagnosis demystifies what was hitherto mysterious to both doctor and patient. It brings to each on their own terms the comfort of understanding, a sense that things make sense, a partial evaporation of uncertainty. It leads each to an indication of what ought to be done next. A *really* good diagnosis is so full of insight that effective management, and the patient's embracing of it, cannot fail to follow.

Is this a realistic ambition? Doctors for the most part are scientists, not novelists or clairvoyants. The biomedical diagnosis of a doctor-as-scientist cannot be expected to illuminate every part of a patient's inner world. Without a novelist's knowledge of the patient's back-story, without a clairvoyant's access to every ramification of the patient's hopes and dreams, are we not bound to disappoint?

What we should remember is that before we became scientists we were, and still are, persons. We are no less doctors-as-persons just because we are also doctors-as-scientists. However much medical school may have encouraged us to ignore the fact, we know at first hand what it is to have a back-story and an inner life, to have fears and dreams. We have our 'Inner Physician'. And it is the Inner Physician that allows us to empathise with our patients as, through their narrative texts, they struggle to tell us their own fears and dreams. We also have bodies of our own, with failings and shortcomings that periodically present their own subjective texts for our attention. Our medical training equips us for the medical part of diagnosis. Our personal life experience, if we are willing to abandon the fallacy that we are non-participant observers in the clinical process, can contribute the rest. We risk short-changing our patients and impoverishing our diagnoses if we try to keep the Inner Physician out of the diagnostic process.

* * * * *

---

105 Faulks S. *Human Traces*. London: Hutchison, 2005, p. 55.

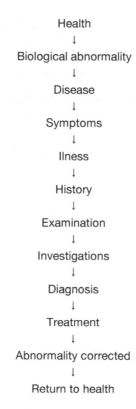

Health
↓
Biological abnormality
↓
Disease
↓
Symptoms
↓
Ilness
↓
History
↓
Examination
↓
Investigations
↓
Diagnosis
↓
Treatment
↓
Abnormality corrected
↓
Return to health

Figure 7.2 The medical model.

In Chapter 5 we looked at the traditional medical model (Figure 7.2). In summary, the conventional view is that 'Disease arises from biological abnormality, which systematic verbal and physical enquiry can identify, and which, if corrected, results in cure.' In the medical model, diagnosis is the process of deducing the underlying biological abnormality from the patient's narrative and the body's physical evidence. With a long history and an impressive track record of clinical effectiveness, this conventional view of diagnosis permeates contemporary medical thought so universally that in everyday practice it usually goes unchallenged. But challenged it must be.

Now that we have seen some of the wider expectations, particularly those of the patient, that a diagnosis ought to satisfy, we have to ask whether the traditional diagnostic process is fit for purpose. Sadly, it is not. Newtonian in its thinking, the traditional method of diagnosis is equally Newtonian in its usefulness – fine as far as it goes, but failing to match up to all the nuances and complexities of the real, lived-in, post-Newtonian world where there are few absolutes and where the observer is inseparable from the process of observation. While for many straightforward medical problems the traditional approach is sufficient, when pushed it can prove impracticable, restrictive, even damaging – not least to the mental agility of the doctor.

First, though, I need to make a disclaimer.

Disclaimer

The following sections are a critique of the traditional method of medical diagnosis, and a challenge to any claim it might stake to intellectual monopoly. However, my account of some of its blind spots, fallacies and false assumptions, and of the consequences of following it too slavishly, should not be taken as a wholesale rejection of its role in medical practice. I do not wish to downplay the importance of science and scientific thinking in medicine. Least of all do I intend any disrespect for the skill and professionalism of the many colleagues who use systematic rational analysis of solid evidence to the clear benefit of their patients. If I myself develop some serious or puzzling organic disease, I want to be treated by a doctor whose clinical repertoire includes as adept a command of the formal diagnostic method as it is possible to get.

Let's begin with a rueful tribute to the great physician Sir William Osler.[106] It is to him that we owe much of the conceptual and organisational fabric of our teaching hospitals – clinical clerkship, the teaching ward round, meticulous record-keeping, systematic postgraduate training. Appreciating the crucial importance of diagnosis, Osler insisted on careful history-taking, accurate observation and thorough physical examination as its basis. He recognised the patient as the focus of all medical attention, the ultimate textbook wherein the answers to all medical conundrums were to be found. 'It is much more important,' he taught, 'to know what sort of patient has a disease than what sort of a disease a patient has.' If only more of the heads of the world's medical schools had been as enlightened as Sir William, all might have been well. As it was, lacking Osler's humility and humanity, many of them trained their students to see the patient as a textbook only of morbid anatomy and pathology, a source only of symptoms, signs and samples, an anonymous representative of some particular class of disease

---

106 Sir William Osler MD CM (1849–1919), Canadian physician and educator. After postgraduate training in Europe, Osler became a Professor at McGill University in 1874, and in 1889 physician-in-chief at Johns Hopkins Hospital, Baltimore. In 1905, following an episode of what we should now call 'burnout', he was appointed to the Regius Chair of Medicine at Oxford University.

sufferers to whom the generalisations of therapeutics could be applied. Sadly, the version of the diagnostic method that has come down to us from Osler's time exactly reverses his 'patient before disease' priority – with some fallacies and unfortunate consequences. Two of the medical model's assumptions in particular I want to expose as false.

Fallacy 1: 'Illness is caused by specific identifiable biological abnormalities'

Many illnesses are, but plenty are not.

Implicit in the medical model is an assumption that the subjective condition of illness should arise only if there is an objective physical disease to cause it. 'No sickness without pathology' is its maxim. And if disease is a crime against biological normality, there must be a criminal – hopefully a single criminal, not a gang of them – to be hunted down and brought to book.

Often, the clinical presentation does indeed have an unambiguous underlying biological cause. Examples might be: chickenpox, scabies, diabetes, testicular torsion, Huntington's chorea. Also common are situations where a presentation may have several possible causes, all of them physical, such as stroke, haematemesis, polyarthritis, pulmonary oedema, the acute abdomen. These conditions are medicine's bread and butter. They form a large part, and arguably the most important part, of a doctor's work. Doctors know – are trained and paid to know – what to do about remediable biological aberrations. It would be a dereliction of responsibility not to use a systematic diagnostic process to identify them.

But there are many more illness conditions, legitimately falling within medicine's remit, where the role, even the existence, of a biological cause is not so clear-cut. As I write, for instance, there is no agreement over what basis, if any, post-viral fatigue syndrome has in biological abnormality. That the clinical presentation exists is generally accepted. But as to aetiology: no infective agent satisfying Koch's postulates has so far been identified. Some of the condition's alternative names – 'neurasthenia', 'chronic fatigue syndrome' – suggest that some clinicians are willing to stay mystified, whereas others, disparagingly calling it 'yuppie flu', view it as just an excuse for indolence. A third group give it the medical-sounding name 'benign myalgic encephalo-myelitis', locating it firmly in the organic disease camp, where it sits between 'benign intracranial hypertension' and 'encephalopathy, unspecified' in the

International Classification of Disease.[107] Equally confusing are conditions where organic disease is only one possible part of the causal picture, such as hypertension, depression, headache, irritable bowel syndrome, and, that bête noire of the harassed GP, 'tired all the time'.

There are even some conditions whose very existence is the subject of international disagreement. It is almost a matter of honour for a self-respecting Frenchman to suffer a periodic *crise de foie* – 'a crisis of the liver' – but only a Frenchman.[108] Peculiarly French too is the condition, much diagnosed in the 1970s, of 'spasmophilia' – a feeling of imminent doom accompanied by an abnormal Chvostek sign, probably attributable to hyperventilation. Cross the border into Germany, and GPs there can be found diagnosing 'hypotension' (pathologically low blood pressure) in up to 17% of their patients. Predictably, most patients are young; worryingly, a quarter of them take prescribed medication to raise their blood pressure, unsurprisingly with little clinical benefit.[109] In the UK the condition does not officially exist; German patients visiting the UK will presumably therefore be cured as soon as they clear passport control. But before we laugh too smugly at the medical follies of our European neighbours we should examine our own track record. There is a long list of conditions widely believed in and frequently diagnosed but lacking convincing evidence of a biological foundation: hypoglycaemia; temporomandibular joint syndrome; fibromyalgia; intestinal candidiasis; total allergy syndrome. Whatever drives the mass consumption of probiotics,

---

107 World Health Organization. *International Statistical Classification of Diseases and Related Health Problems* (10th Revision). Geneva: WHO, 2007, Chapter VI, block G93.2–4.

108 A popular online French medical dictionary, *Vulgaris-Médical*, offers the following definition: *La crise de foie est une entité très française qui n'est pas reconnue comme pathologie au sens vrai du terme dans les pays anglo-saxons entre autres. La crise de foie se manifeste par l'apparition d'un inconfort de l'appareil digestif associé à des vomissements et à des maux de tête le plus souvent. La crise de foie laisse de nombreux médecins perplexes. En effet, celle-ci ne s'explique par aucun dérèglement ni aucune atteinte de l'appareil digestif, notamment d'un organe tel que le foie ou la vésicule biliaire.* ('Crisis of the liver' is very much a French condition, not recognised as pathological in the true sense of the word in the Anglo-Saxon countries and others. It presents with digestive discomfort accompanied by vomiting, and very often headache. 'Crisis of the liver' leaves many doctors puzzled. Indeed, it cannot be explained by any imbalance or disorder of the digestive tract, notably of the liver or gall bladder.)

109 Donner-Banzhoff N, Kreienbrock L, Baum E. Hypotension – does it make sense in family practice? *Family Practice* 1994; **11**(4): 368–74.

antioxidants, multivitamins and dietary supplements, it is not a rational response to firm scientific evidence. It is understandable that physically minded doctors are sceptical about what seem to them to be wacky unevidenced pseudo-diseases. But if their response is simply to walk sulkily away saying, 'This makes no sense biological sense, so it's not my business,' a great many suffering individuals will be denied the comfort of understanding that they are entitled to expect from the medical profession.

Doctors who cling too stubbornly to the 'no sickness without pathology' view are at risk of trapping themselves in an intellectual blind alley. The trap is to think, 'If no organic cause for the illness has been found, it's because we haven't looked hard enough – so we should look all the harder.'

> When all you have is a hammer, all your problems start to look like nails.
>
> Abraham Maslow (1908–70)
> American humanistic
> psychologist
> From *The Psychology of Science: a reconnaissance* (1966)

The dangers to the patient of having a doctor who doesn't know when to stop looking for physical pathology are well recognised, chief amongst them being over-investigation. The patient most at risk is the one with organic-sounding symptoms but negative first-line investigations: the 'tired all the time' patient with normal blood count, glucose and thyroid functions; or someone with low back pain but no neurological signs and a normal ESR. Such patients can find themselves hustled on to an accelerating escalator of diagnostic tests, each more complicated, invasive and expensive than the last. The law of diminishing returns makes a diagnostic breakthrough increasingly unlikely. The law of averages, on the other hand, makes it increasingly likely that sooner or later some test or other will randomly throw up a result marginally outside the normal range, which can be seized upon and given a spurious explanatory significance. The misguided pursuit of clinical will-o'-the-wisps probably accounts for most cases of the iatrogenesis – ill-health produced by medical activity – against which Ivan Illich has so persuasively inveighed.[110] Second- and third-line investigations, such as biopsies, X-rays

---

110 Ivan Illich (1926–2002), Austrian priest, philosopher and social critic. In a series of powerfully argued tracts, Illich attacked the emasculating effects of the organised professions on the autonomy and self-reliance of their clients. His 1975 book *Medical Nemesis: the expropriation of health* explored the medicalisation of ordinary life, and opened with the claim, 'The medical establishment has become a major threat to health.' Finding it hard to refute Illich's critique, the medical establishment defended itself with the limp riposte, 'It's a fair cop, but we didn't mean to.'

or examination under anaesthesia, cause additional anxiety for the patient and are not without physical risk.

A second danger to the patient of an over-investigative doctor is somatic fixation. For various reasons, patients sometimes present with physical-sounding symptoms whose basis, and therefore whose appropriate diagnostic framework, is emotional. Someone who recognises an ill-focused need to see a doctor but who is unclear or embarrassed about the reason may cast about for a physical complaint to justify making the appointment – the so-called 'ticket of admission'. Imagine this:

Yvonne is the mother of two teenage sons, one of whom has recently been charged with drug offences. Struggling to pay off the debts of her unemployed husband, who has a gambling problem, she works days as a cleaner, and evenings and weekends as a barmaid. She can just about cope, until she discovers that her husband is having an affair with her only close friend. This is the final straw. Angry, humiliated, trapped and unsupported, she realises she cannot deal with the situation on her own. She needs help – but what, and from whom? She books an appointment with the GP, not with her usual GP, who has known her since her childhood – that would be too embarrassing – but with another doctor she has not consulted before. 'What can I do for you?', the doctor asks, after the opening niceties. Yvonne's mind goes blank. How can you tell a stranger all the ways life has kicked you in the teeth, or how much of a failure you feel? Inexpressible distress hovers just out of reach of her tongue. 'I, er,' she begins. 'I just feel anyhow. I've got no energy. Tired, that's it. I feel tired all the time.' The doctor asks whether she is breathless, whether her ankles swell, if she is sleeping well? Losing or gaining weight? She sometimes feels she can't get enough air to breathe, she answers. She can't always get off to sleep; she has put on weight, but that's probably the chocolate she guzzles for comfort. 'Is everything all right at home?', comes the question. 'Not brilliant,' she says. And her eyes fill with tears. Leaning forward, the doctor notes not the incipient tears but the possible pallor of her conjunctivae. And her thyroid gland might be slightly enlarged; it's hard to palpate through the fat. Blood pressure a bit on the high side. Anaemia, the doctor thinks. Or hypothyroidism. Or depression, but that could open a whole can of worms. Let's hope it's anaemia, or myxoedema; they're easy enough to treat. But why the raised blood pressure? Renal failure? 'We need to get some tests done,' the doctor tells her; 'I think you may be suffering from iron deficiency anaemia. Or possibly an underactive thyroid gland, or a kidney problem.' Blood test request forms are filled in. The doctor says, 'Come and see me again when the test results are back. If they don't give us the answer we may need to do some further investigations. But I'm sure we can help. Oh, and we'd better check your blood sugar.' And off goes Yvonne to have blood taken and to book the follow-up appointment. In the meantime she will likely read up about thyroid disease on the internet, which will lead her to think she needs a 'scan' ...

What is going on here? The doctor, in the name of thoroughness, has prioritised physical possibilities above emotional or situational in his diagnostic strategy. If challenged he would maintain – probably rightly – that this is the correct priority; to miss a treatable physical condition is arguably a greater sin than to underestimate an emotional one. Attributing non-specific symptoms to psychological causes should be a diagnosis of exclusion. He would say that in his mind the possibility of a non-physical diagnosis is not denied – merely deferred. He will come back to it if he must. But he rather hopes he won't have to. Delving into emotional, social or psychological problems is messy, with no guarantee of success. It would be so much neater if the blood tests were to throw up something abnormal. Fingers crossed ...

Something more insidious, meanwhile, is happening to Yvonne. She is quite relieved not to have to tell the mortifying tale of her personal life. The opportunity to link her symptoms with her predicament has been missed, and is now closed off by the doctor's implied certainty that she is sick, not just sad. She entered the consulting room a worried and unhappy woman, whose body is reacting as worried and unhappy bodies do; she leaves it believing herself to be suffering from a soon-to-be-identified disease. She arrived a victim, and departs a patient. There is some consolation in this change of role. Victims get pitied and, quite often, blamed. But patients get sympathy; patients get help. The price of sympathy and help is that her 'disease' becomes real. The doctor's focus on her physical symptoms has given her a vested interest in keeping them.

We don't fully understand why or how in some people emotional or existential distress gets converted into physical symptoms. I think we could imagine that the first tentative draft of a distressed patient's experiential text comprises a whole array of possible forms of expression – some of them physical, some emotional, some behavioural, but all representing the distress's attempts to reach out for help. On this population of possibilities a kind of Darwinian natural selection operates. If the sufferer lacks a sufficiently nuanced health vocabulary, or has been brought up talking only the language of physical illness, it is likely that only a few tentative non-physical strands will survive the transition from experiential text to the narrative text presented to the doctor. And if that narrative text is further interpreted by a doctor primed by training and inclination to favour the physical, it will be predominantly the somatic expressions of distress that survive and flourish. In a narrative environment biased towards the physical, non-somatic forms of expression swiftly become extinct. The physically minded doctor conditions his patients to present with physical symptoms.

Most acute or serious medical conditions – a heart attack, urinary retention, a broken bone – announce themselves with an experiential text couched in unambiguously physical language, often the language of pain. But, more often, particularly in general practice where problems tend to present less dramatically, the experiential text is not so explicit. To patients developing more subtle and complex problems, the experiential text – those jolts in the stream of consciousness that suggest that something is not right – can be a faltering, shimmering, flickering thing. Awareness of altered physical sensations is accompanied by a fragile kaleidoscope of unfamiliar thoughts, fantasies, imaginings, spasms of emotion, stabs of terror, phrases that reverberate in interior monologue … Dwell too soon or too insistently on the physical, and the kaleidoscope is shattered. To be sure, the shimmering will cease and the confusion of detail subside. But something less than complete, less than true, remains. It is as if, panning for diamonds, one were to throw away nuggets of gold.

None of this is Yvonne aware of. Somatic fixation is a pre-conscious, pre-linguistic process. By the time the doctor starts talking about glands and kidneys and suggesting blood tests, it is too late. The moment has passed when the insight might have dawned that it is her life letting her down, not her body. All she knows, now that the doctor appears to be on to something, is that some aspects of her symptoms feel unimportant, while others – the physical – feel more real. She is experiencing the comfort of understanding. That the understanding may be illusory, and the comfort short-lived, she has no way of knowing.

The over-organic over-investigative doctor is also in some personal danger. Every time a fondness for the medical model selectively emphasises the physical features in a patient's narrative, something is reciprocally closed off in the doctor's own mind. Those parts of his own powers of perception that might have detected and responded to the fullest spectrum of a patient's experience begin to undergo disuse atrophy. His own sensitivity, curiosity, complexity and capacity for insight are all diminished. He is reduced by his own reductionism. The doctor biased towards physical diagnosis is at risk of becoming blind to anything else. This is the most tragic of self-betrayals – like Oedipus, to put out the eyes that cannot bear what they see.

I need to keep myself in check here: I am in danger of over-stating my case. The best doctors are well able to function as zoom lenses, their gaze alternating between close-up 'attentive to the biological' mode and wide-angle alertness to cues to the illness's emotional and psychosocial components. But one of the saddest sights is a professional colleague becoming frustrated and disillusioned because more and more patients cannot – *will* not – be forced into the physical mould, and perversely insist on presenting problems that defy analysis with the medical model.

Fallacy 2: 'Diseases affect every patient in the same way'

One Wednesday evening, John Brown, director of an IT software company, dines at an expensive restaurant. As luck would have it, one of the oysters he enjoys on the half-shell is contaminated with norovirus. On Thursday evening he begins to feel sick and feverish, then to vomit. He spends much of the night on the toilet in his en suite bathroom. First thing Friday, JB phones his PA. 'I've got some damned tummy bug,' he tells her. 'Cancel my meetings, get Tristan to sort out the Yuno-Hoo contract. I'll probably take next week off, get myself properly better, don't want to come in to work and pass it around.' *Yes*, she thinks, *get better on the golf course; it's all right for some.* 'Of course, sir,' she says. 'Hope you feel better soon.'

Later that Friday morning, JB's cleaning lady Yvonne (yes, her again) arrives for her twice-weekly stint of domestic chores. She is surprised to find her employer at home and still in his dressing gown. After the briefest explanation he gives Yvonne her instructions: 'a thermos of China tea, please, and the bathroom could do with a bit of extra attention.' On Saturday evening Yvonne, now working at her second job as a barmaid, begins to feel sick and feverish, then to vomit. Somehow she makes it through to closing time without embarrassing herself, then dashes home, where she hammers on the door of the bathroom where one of her sons is up to something she'd rather not know about. On Sunday morning she phones the pub where she should be back on duty in 2 hours. 'I'm not feeling too good,' she tells the publican. 'Not you as well,' says the publican crossly. 'It's our busy day. I need you on lunches. Just as long as it's not catching – you'd get me closed down.' Yvonne is paid cash in hand; if she doesn't work, she isn't paid. 'No no,' she says, 'just a bit of a headache. I'll be in to work as usual.' And she takes another Imodium tablet. And another, for good measure.

It is almost axiomatic in the medical model that, at the biological level, patients all react in much the same way to a given pathological challenge. The symptoms and signs of a myocardial infarction, for example, though they may differ in detail from one case to the next, are sufficiently consistent for the condition to be recognisable beneath the diverse social, emotional and psychological characteristics of individual victims. Undergraduate medical training has to make this assumption – that from a theoretical understanding of the pathological processes and the example of a small number of clinical cases observed, the fledgling doctor can learn to diagnose and treat the generality of future patients.

The norovirus is not supposed to be any respecter of persons. At the physiological and cellular level, its effects on John Brown and Yvonne are probably indistinguishable. But clearly an attack of winter vomiting has a very different impact on the life of each. The two patients will have some things in common: the vomiting, the abdominal cramps, the diarrhoea. A fuller account of JB's illness experience, however, will probably include some anger with the restaurant, some satisfaction that here is a chance to illustrate how indispensable he is at work, perhaps a little *Schadenfreude* at how Tristan, his deputy, will struggle to cope in his absence, and a distinctly childish glee that he can take a week's golfing break with no one raising an objection. Yvonne's experiential text, on the other hand, is likely to be a confusion of panic (*I can't afford to lose the money if I'm ill*); paranoia (*Someone up there's got it in for me*); guilt (*I know I might pass it on to the customers, but I can't help that*); and resignation (*I just can't win*).

Suppose, now, that Yvonne and John Brown decide to consult a doctor. (In Yvonne's case at least, this is not unlikely; her doctor's medicalisation of her tiredness has already acclimatised her to the 'patient' role.) And let's assume that they consult the *same* doctor. The narratives they present will be scattered with oblique references to the very different implications the norovirus infection has for their daily lives. John Brown, perhaps planning to complain to the restaurant, will emphasise the role of the dodgy oyster. Hearing the call of the golf course, he might well prompt the doctor: 'So you'd agree I definitely shouldn't go back to work until I feel fully fit?' Yvonne, already at her wits' end with family and financial problems, will probably be less articulate than JB. 'Just give me something so I don't have to stop off work,' is probably as much as she might be able to say about her reasons for coming.

The doctor interested only in an underlying biological diagnosis is likely to concentrate on the physical symptoms and to screen out as irrelevant the non-physical hermeneutic cues in each patient's narrative. When, history taken, he comes to examine them, this selective attention will seem to be justified. Both patients will be slightly feverish; both will have soft abdomens, with noisy bowel sounds and no localising signs. If this is the full extent of his curiosity, the doctor's gaze shifts into close-up mode. The questions he ponders will be predominantly posed in physiological and cellular terms. And, as a rule, the further you zoom into close-up gaze, the less individual variation you notice. It is not in their gastrointestinal tracts that the important differences between JB's and Yvonne's cases are to be found. Their individuality resides at higher orders of complexity – their personalities and their life circumstances – which can only be perceived and understood with a wide-angle gaze. If each were to ask '*Why* me?', the answer 'People with blood group O are more prone to norovirus;[111] we can test to see what group you are' would not satisfy.

So – diagnosis confined to the biological domain does not always allow the necessary degree of discrimination between individual cases. Diagnosis is insight on the verge of action; the usefulness – one might almost say the accuracy – of a diagnosis is judged by asking 'To the verge of what action does it lead the clinician?' If all that is required to bump the patient from illness back to health is a surgical or pharmacological intervention, then a diagnosis in anatomical, physiological or biochemical terms is adequate. But if, as is usually the case, the patient's return to well-being is best achieved by intervention on a range of fronts, the diagnosis needs to be couched in no less comprehensive a range of terms. John Brown, it would appear, is perfectly capable of sorting out the consequences of his illness on his own. He has non-medical minions to cushion his temporary incapacity. In his case, a narrow diagnosis of viral gastroenteritis, needing no medical intervention beyond a prescription to alleviate his symptoms, will suffice. Yvonne, by contrast, is in a much more vulnerable position. The ripples of her illness spread wider. There are public health implications for the pub's licensee and customers if she continues to work with a norovirus infection. But any loss of earnings will put extra strain on Yvonne's already precarious marriage. Real despair is not far away. In her case, prescribing symptomatic relief is not sufficient action for her doctor to take. If he sees her situation with wide-angle gaze, he will want in addition to take a persuasive line on her fitness for work and offer at least a sympathetic ear to this latest crisis in the soap opera that is Yvonne's life.

It is clearly wrong for a doctor to act as if a given pathological abnormality affects all those who suffer from it in the same way. Management based on this false assumption will sell the individual patient short. Every patient needs

---

111 Apparently this is true: possessing blood group B or AB confers partial protection against norovirus.

a diagnosis that reflects their individuality, their coexisting medical conditions, their home and work situation, their state of mind, their hopes and fears. A diagnosis of appendicitis is not a sufficient prelude to comprehensive management if the patient has a severe learning disability. A diagnosis of simple dyspepsia does not do proper justice to the worries of a patient whose father recently died of stomach cancer. A diagnosis of hay fever, if the treatment that follows is as routine as the diagnosis, is not sufficient if the sufferer is a student about to take exams on which a university place depends.

* * * * *

One difficulty facing doctors is the lack of a convenient vocabulary to encapsulate the non-physical components of a wide-ranging multi-domained diagnosis. To sum up all the myriad malfunctions that can afflict the physical body we have the language of pathology – all those *-itises, -omas, -oses* and *-opathies*; the *dys-* things and *pseudo-* things; all the *intra-*s and *extra-*s, the *hyper-*s and *hypo-*s that trip so glibly from the tongues of those of us who have learned the code, but which are so satisfyingly impenetrable to the layman. In one or two words of bastardised Greek or Latin – *pneumothorax, hallux valgus* – someone who knows the code can instantly convey to a fellow initiate a detailed mental hologram of the salient features of a patient's medical condition. But we lack an equally comprehensive shorthand for summarising the non-physical (but diagnostically no less relevant) uniquenesses of the patient's mental, emotional, motivational, environmental and social worlds with which their physical disease interacts.

To be sure, we have a basic lexicon of the emotions, some of which has been appropriated for clinical use: *depressed, anxious, demanding, compliant*. But does it help to label Yvonne 'anxious' about her domestic life, or 'non-compliant' if she wants to keep working? Such over-simplifications, far from encouraging the doctor to the verge of action, may well have the opposite effect of justifying *dis*engagement and *in*action.

The medical vocabulary for diagnosing the non-physical dimensions of illness is not fit for purpose, if that purpose is to identify where therapeutic intervention could usefully be made. There is no nuanced equivalent of the International Classification of Disease to capture all the ramifications and implications of disease on a patient's life outside the consulting room.[112] Yet the doctor who would practise big picture medicine somehow needs to articulate his patient's social predicaments within his diagnosis, as part of bringing his insight to the verge of action. We struggle for words to capture succinctly our patients' complicated personal relationships; their loves and longings; their Sisyphean struggles to amount to something. What an irony, given how in thrall we are to the hermeneutic imperative – the quest for meaning – how impoverished is the professional language at our command to express the answers.

Others outside the medical profession have been more successful in finding words to convey insights into human vulnerability. They are our story-tellers – our novelists, poets, playwrights and film-makers. As doctors, we could envy these masters of narrative their wide-angle gaze; but their insights are if anything more profound than our clinical tasks require. In the space of a brief consultation, there is not time for psychosocial diagnosis on the panoramic scale of a Shakespeare or a Tolstoy. We need something at the nutshell level, something less than a novel but more than a couple of words of jargon. It is entertaining to imagine the diagnostic category to which the International Classification of Disease would have assigned, say, Hamlet or Macbeth. Would the troubled Prince of Denmark, his father murdered by the uncle who then marries his mother, be coded as Z63.7 – 'Other stressful life events affecting family and household'? Or perhaps, as evidenced by his 'To be, or not to be: that is the question' soliloquy, Z73.5 applies – 'Social role conflict, not elsewhere classified'. To be fair, Macbeth does seem to fit Z73.1 – 'Accentuation of personality traits: Type A behaviour, characterized by unbridled ambition, a need for high achievement, impatience, competitiveness, and a sense of urgency.' And, again to be fair, the great writers can do nutshell as well as panorama. Tolstoy's *Anna Karenina*, for example, opens with the razor-sharp observation that 'Happy families are all alike; every unhappy family is unhappy in its own way.'

* * * * *

In this chapter I have argued that the purpose of diagnosis is to sharpen the doctor's understanding of the patient's problem until points of possible

---

112 We should, nevertheless, give it credit for trying. The *International Statistical Classification of Diseases and Related Health Problems* (10th Revision), Chapter XXI, includes (Z64) 'Problems related to certain psychosocial circumstances' and (Z65) 'Problems related to other psychosocial circumstances'.

therapeutic intervention can be identified. Diagnosis is an exercise in interpretive listening, in which the doctor interrogates the patient's experiential, narrative and physical texts and massages them into a form to which he can apply the resources at his disposal. If, as is always the case, the doctor can potentially intervene in more domains than just the purely biological, then his diagnosis must likewise be made in broader terms than the purely biological.

Judged according to these lights, the shortcomings of the traditional medical model of diagnosis become apparent. Not knowing how to deal with a patient's ill-formed and often ambiguous narrative, it relies disproportionately on the physical text. It is Newtonian in its simplistic view of cause and effect, in not recognising the interconnectedness of causal factors, and in ignoring how the process of questioning itself changes the story that is elicited. It is wrong for the medical model to assume that the subjective experience of illness always indicates the presence of objective disease. This fallacy leads to over-investigation, to somatic fixation, to the medicalisation of psychosocial problems, and to the blunting of the doctor's own sensitivities. It is also wrong if it down-plays the different ways a single pathological process affects its individual victims. In these differences reside the opportunities for management to be fine-tuned to the individual patient's unique situation.

I freely concede the impressive strengths of the medical model and its approach to diagnosis. It remains the best way of analysing a clinically serious situation, and it provides a valuable fall-back strategy when one has no idea what, medically, is going on. My chief quarrel with the medical model is attitudinal. I charge it with arrogance, with being smugly but mistakenly confident in its own rectitude. As Voltaire observed, 'Some doctors make the same mistake for twenty years and call it clinical experience.' If it could speak, I'm sure the medical model would defend itself: 'These are details. Of course people can feel ill even though they are not diseased. Of course people differ in their reactions to disease. And of course it matters how a doctor takes a history from a patient.' But there is a note of irritation in this response, as if to say 'Don't bother me with these trivialities.' Yet they matter. They really do matter. We betray the trust of our patients, and corrupt our medical students, if we continue to train doctors as if dispassionate science was all there was to the practice of medicine.

So what is to be done?

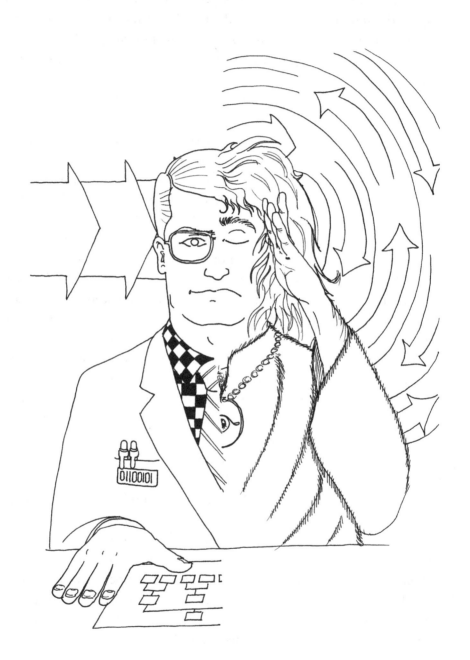

Chapter 8

As long as you think of it[113]

> Not everything that can be counted counts,
> and not everything that counts can be counted.
>
> > Attributed to Sir George Pickering (1904–80),
> > Regius Professor of Medicine, Oxford,
> > and reputedly kept chalked by Albert Einstein
> > on his blackboard at Princeton University

> True genius resides in the capacity for evaluation of uncertain,
> hazardous, and conflicting information.
>
> > Winston Churchill (1874–1965)
> > English statesman and Prime Minister
> > of the UK, 1940–45 and 1951–55

This second chapter on diagnosis reviews some refinements of, and alternatives to, the traditional medical model, in an attempt to overcome some of its conceptual and practical inadequacies. It will conclude that the personal experience and psychology of the doctor cannot be excluded from the diagnostic process, and are potentially valuable sources of insight.

* * * * *

On 29 January 2010 Tony Blair, the UK Prime Minister from 1997 to 2007, gave evidence in public to the Chilcot Inquiry, which had been set up to examine the political decision-making that led in 2003 to the UK, together with the USA, launching a military attack on Saddam Hussein's Iraq despite

---

113 'A diagnosis is easy as long as you think of it'. Remark attributed to Dr Soma Weiss (1899–1942), Hungarian-born American physician.

the absence of authorisation by the United Nations. He was pressed to explain why he had taken his country to war largely on the basis of intelligence, which he knew to be sketchy, that had convinced him – wrongly, as it later turned out – that Saddam was actively developing weapons of mass destruction. 'It's not about a lie, or a conspiracy, or a deceit or a deception,' Blair told the Inquiry, 'it's a *decision*.' He went on to describe how at the time he had asked himself, 'Given the background, can we take the risk?'

Here – regardless of the politics – we see a nice example of the diagnostic dilemma. The ideal (Mr Blair seemed to be acknowledging) would have been for irrefutable facts to lead to an incontrovertible assessment and hence to inevitable action. But the real world is rarely so obliging. In reality it was a case of having to weigh up incomplete and inconsistent information, setting it in a complex context, balancing it with other, often confusing, factors, and deciding whether or not a tipping point had been reached where the evidence of Saddam's villainy amounted to a critical mass sufficient to trigger military action. That tipping point could not be precisely defined. It was a matter of judgement. Someone else might have had a different tipping point, or have weighted the evidence differently, or have differently assessed the relative dangers of action and inaction. Politicians and doctors are equally familiar with the difficulty of having to base their decisions on unreliable information. A dozen times a day the practising clinician wonders, 'Given this degree of uncertainty, what is the best thing to do?'

One thing *is* certain. In ordinary practice, where a doctor's time with a patient is severely limited and the problems presented are seldom purely physical, pursuing a diagnosis *à la* traditional medical model is often *not* the best thing to do. It would be nice if patients only presented problems caused by clear-cut biological abnormalities; but they don't. It would be nice if time and resources were limitless; but they are not. It would be nice if patients and doctors alike were logical, transparent and consistent; but they aren't always. To be successful, the medical model assumes relentless rationality on the part of both doctor and patient. Non-physical problems don't show up on its radar. So – since imprecision, uncertainty and ambiguity are givens in most clinical situations – alternative diagnostic strategies have to be found to bring doctor and patient to 'the verge of action'. The linear rationality of the medical model, while useful in a crisis, is not well suited to unpacking the fuzzy complexities of many workaday consultations.

Most medical consultations resemble those popular television programmes where people bring in items rummaged from their cupboards and attics, possibly antiques, for an expert's evaluation, in the hope that some trinket or family heirloom will prove unexpectedly valuable. When a patient brings a problem for our expert medical attention it is as if, in their narrative, they offer for our appraisal a pile of what might be treasure, or else bric-a-brac or junk. As doctors, we sift through the pile looking for items of significance and value, mindful that we may disagree with the patient about what is valuable, and that what we pass over as insignificant may for the patient have great personal worth. We could see the task of diagnosis as separating out what matters medically from everything that does not; what we can be sure of from what we cannot; what requires action from what does not; what needs to be understood from what can safely remain a mystery. Layers of uncertainty and irrelevance in the patient's narrative and physical texts have to be peeled away to reveal the reliable facts on which diagnosis, and therefore intervention, should be based.

Ideally, successful diagnosis requires two things of the doctor. The first is encyclopaedic and up-to-date medical knowledge. The second is forensic and uncompromising logic in its application. At least in principle, acquiring the knowledge is the easy bit, supported as we are by all the infrastructure of training, continuing education and information technology. It's in the requirement for logical, computer-like analysis that we fall short. For there is a saboteur at the heart of our reasoning processes, called *cognitive bias*. And like every effective saboteur, cognitive bias is so familiar a part of everyday life that it goes unnoticed about its subversive work.

* * * * *

Cognitive bias

The human brain, being made of protoplasm rather than silicon, would – were it to function as a completely logical computer – take an impracticably long time to analyse and respond to a complex situation. We often have to decide faster than we can think. And so, in the interests of efficiency, we develop a repertoire of shortcuts – cognitive bias – to speed up our interpretation of sensory input. We achieve this by selectively ignoring, distorting or misinterpreting some information that, in the interests of objectivity, really ought to be factored into our analysis. Cognitive bias is a largely automatic process taking place below the threshold of conscious awareness. It is hard to overcome it simply by an effort of will. The following are common forms of cognitive bias, with clinical examples of some of the risky conclusions they can lead to.

- **Anchoring**: latching on to one feature of a situation and relying on it too heavily as a basis for decision. 'The patient's ECG is normal, so the pain in the left arm must just be muscular.'
- **Confirmation bias**: looking selectively for findings that will reinforce one's preconceptions. 'No, I can't feel an enlarged thyroid gland. You're overweight because you eat too much. We don't need any blood tests to establish that.'
- **Selective perception**: screening out information we don't think is important. 'This child has a simple upper respiratory tract infection. Rash? What rash? Oh, it's just a heat rash.'
- **Premature termination**: accepting the first alternative that seems plausible. 'The child is running a temperature. Oh, his eardrum is a bit pink. He's got otitis media.'
- **Inertia**: unwillingness to change habitual thought patterns that seem to have worked well in the past. 'I can tell when someone's depressed; I have a nose for it. I don't need a questionnaire!'
- **Optimism bias** (wishful thinking): forming an impression in line with what one would like to be the case, rather than what the evidence suggests. 'I really like this patient. She's too nice to have cancer. The rectal bleeding is probably just haemorrhoids.'
- **Reactance**: the urge to do the opposite of what someone wants, in order to assert one's independence or authority. 'No your swollen knee does not need an X-ray, whatever it says on the internet and even if you do have private health insurance!'
- **Irrational escalation**: continuing to do more of the same thing, even though it is clearly not working. 'Your sore throat hasn't responded to a standard course of penicillin. So we'll double the dose.'
- **Framing effect**: being swayed by the context in which information is presented rather than the information itself. 'It's flu! The waiting room is full of people with flu.'
- **Normalcy bias**: failing to consider something that has never happened before. 'I've gone 20 years without seeing a proven case of food allergy, and I don't propose to start now!'

While mental shortcuts such as these are a universal feature of human cognition, they can be dangerous. In 2003 cognitive bias took the UK to war. Anchoring and confirmation bias led Tony Blair to convince himself, fallaciously, that *Saddam is a bad man, therefore intelligence reports that he has weapons of mass destruction poised for deployment must be true,* a misinterpretation of the evidence that, in the opinion of many, cost the lives of many thousands of Iraqis. His subsequent protestation to the Chilcot Inquiry that he only did what he believed to be right further emphasises the insidious nature of the threat to rational thinking posed by cognitive bias. Data will always bear more than one interpretation and generate more than one hypothesis. Which particular interpretation or hypothesis is settled on depends on the decision-maker's own beliefs and values as much as on a logical process.

It seems that the brain's operating system leaves no option but for diagnosis to be a process in which the biased quiz the vague in search of the absolute. As long as diagnosis is carried out by a human doctor, the observer effect, whereby the very act of observing changes what is perceived, simply will not go away. But surely we have to try and make it? Surely diagnosing meningococcal septicaemia or Perthes disease or suicidal depression cannot be allowed to hang on whether the doctor is rushed, complacent, irritable or over-friendly? Riddled with cognitive bias and frequently less than rational though we doctors are, surely we must so far as possible immunise the process of diagnosis against our individual human foibles, while preserving the insights that human intuition can sometimes provide?

Ah, but how?

That the process of diagnosis is susceptible to human error is not news. Much research and philosophical thought have gone into proposing derivatives of, and alternatives to, the traditional medical model in order to try and make diagnosis more reliable in the hands of an inevitably rushed and inconsistent clinician. Current approaches divide into two mutually suspicious camps, taking different views of how the psychology and bias of the doctor should be dealt with.

One, which we could call the *rationalist* camp, attempts to eradicate the observer effect from the diagnostic process. Rationalists aim to bypass the human factor as far as possible. The other, which we could call the *intuitive* camp, accepts that the human element in diagnosis is inescapable, and can be a source of insight rather than error. Intuitives aim to tame and harness the doctor's psychological idiosyncrasies, seeing them more as potential allies than enemies in the diagnostic process.

Neither camp has an explicit manifesto, and each resists formal definition. Nevertheless, each has its own distinctive rhetoric, its own common currency of values and ideas, and its own favourite vocabulary. To an intuitive, rationalists can look like geeks and nerds; to a rationalist, intuitives are fuzzy romantics. Figure 8.1 tries, by means of 'word clusters', to convey a sense of

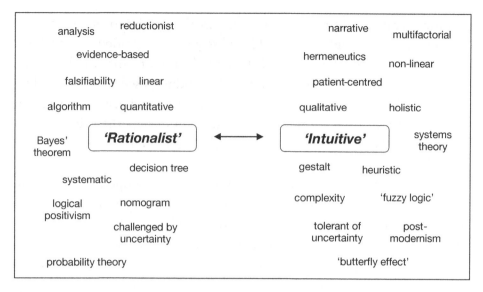

Figure 8.1 'Approaches to diagnosis' word clusters.

how rationalist and intuitive approaches to diagnosis differ. Bearing in mind that what is being depicted is a spectrum of preference rather than a sharp dichotomy, you the reader might like to consider in which direction you find yourself naturally drawn. It doesn't matter if not all the terms in the figure are familiar; the associations carried by the various words and phrases should be sufficient. Probably – indeed, I hope – you will have a foot in both camps.

* * * * *

'Rational' approaches to diagnosis

Algorithms

An extreme example from the 'rationalist' camp is diagnosis by algorithm. The principle is familiar: an algorithm is a predetermined linear sequence of decisions – each triggered by the one immediately preceding it and itself having a limited number of alternative outcomes – leading to one of a predetermined range of conclusions. In the medical setting that concerns us here, the starting point will usually be a clinical presentation, and the endpoint either a diagnosis or a plan of action. As an example, Figure 8.2 shows an algorithm for managing obesity in adults.

Medical algorithms are popular. Their advocates imply, as if it was something to be proud of, that any and every clinical problem will yield to an

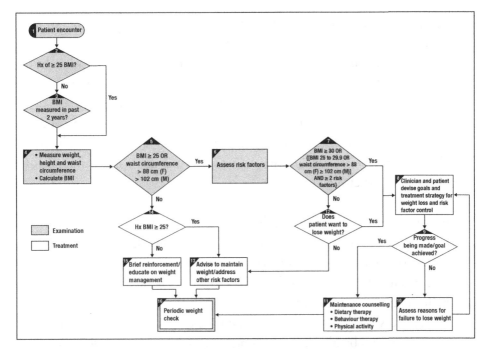

Figure 8.2 An example of a clinical algorithm.

onslaught of sequential unambiguous questions. There are some grounds for this optimism. Algorithmic thinking is what underpins the phenomenal success of the computer software industry. Complicated problems can be successfully analysed, and many human activities convincingly simulated, by breaking them down into chains of binary *either/or* decisions. So why not medicine? Given the enormous advantages that information technology has brought to the infrastructure and organisation of health services, there is every reason, one might think, to encourage computer-based thinking to infiltrate the clinical process. Specifically, there is much to be said in favour of the clinical algorithm or 'decision tree' as a basis for diagnosis.

- The knowledge and evidence base on which contemporary medicine relies continues to grow exponentially. No human doctor, however conscientious, can possibly keep on top of all the advice and recommendations put out by journals, advisory bodies and policy makers, and with which the doctor is expected to comply, on pain of being sued for negligence. Algorithms, which can be swiftly updated and disseminated, look like a lifebelt tossed to the doctor overwhelmed by a torrent of information. Through their use, every clinician – and therefore every patient – stands to benefit from the latest research and the best of expert opinion.

- As doctors are busier than ever and their time more expensive, an algorithmic 'step by prescribed step' approach makes it possible for medical decision-making to be delegated in comparative safety to other health professionals who are quicker to train and cheaper to employ, such as nurses, paramedics, physician assistants and call centre staff.
- Algorithms, which reliably highlight 'red flag' warning signs and key discriminating features in a clinical presentation, are educationally useful for doctors in training, and provide a safety net against misdiagnosis for inexperienced clinicians.

But the strongest argument in favour of an algorithmic approach is that it protects against perhaps the most insidious cause of misdiagnosis – cognitive bias. Constrained by algorithms, the diagnostic process runs a mechanistic and pre-ordained course and is less likely to be led astray by the inadequacies of the individual practitioner.

Nevertheless, there are downsides that have to be considered before we can embrace diagnosis by algorithm as fondly as its advocates would urge.

A circular argument is at work, ironically itself a form of cognitive bias. The more we rely on algorithmic thinking to solve clinical problems, the more we limit ourselves to accepting as problems only those that will yield to algorithmic analysis. Abraham Maslow deserves to be quoted again: *When all you have is a hammer, all your problems start to look like nails.* Anything too complex or too subtle to be understood in stark *either/or* terms is likely to be ignored or – worse – dismissed as 'not medicine's business'. The clinician who thinks predominantly in algorithms risks gradually coming to view the patient simply as a data-set to be interrogated, thereby diminishing both patient and doctor. To see only black and white is to become blind to colour and shades of grey.

Even their most ardent advocates concede that algorithms depend for success on a degree of certainty that is rarely encountered in practice. The algorithmic approach abhors ambiguity. It does not like fuzziness. It is frustrated by *It all depends; I'm not sure; possibly this, possibly that; sometimes the one, sometimes the other.* And it can be derailed if information is not presented in the form, or at the time, that the algorithm requires it. Again, unfortunately, illness and patients' accounts of it unfold over time; data arrives sporadically, not necessarily in the order best suited to rational analysis. Many medical conditions, particularly in general practice, present at an early stage before the full-blown clinical picture has had time to develop. A fleeting rash; a spike of temperature; a niggle of pain; an alteration in sleep pattern; a vague feeling of being unwell – none of these is precise enough to kick-start an algorithmic approach to diagnosis. Add to this fuzziness the fact that virtually no physical finding, no investigation, no rapier-like question is ever 100% conclusive: they all have a margin of error, false positives and negatives. The most we can expect of each new piece of information is that it will shift the balance of probability from one interpretation to another. Diagnosis has to be thought of as a hunt not for the definite but for the most likely.

Bayes' theorem

Those who like a rationalist approach to diagnosis yet are mindful of the inevitable uncertainties of clinical medicine are attracted to Bayes' theorem, which combines probabilistic thinking with the seductive rigour of the algorithm.

The Reverend Thomas Bayes (c. 1702–61) was an English Presbyterian minister and mathematician. An admirer of the scientific methods of Isaac Newton, he made his reputation (and won election to the Royal Society) on the basis of *An Introduction to the Doctrine of Fluxions*, a defence of Newtonian calculus. Bayes' contribution to probability theory, *An Essay Towards Solving a Problem in the Doctrine of Chances*, was published posthumously in 1763.

Bayes' theorem is a means of quantifying uncertainty. It gives a rule for modifying the probability of a hypothesis by factoring in fresh evidence and background information. According to Bayes, if you want to update the odds that a hypothesis is true in the light of new evidence, you multiply the odds that it was true *before* the new evidence by the weight of that evidence (the 'likelihood ratio').[114]

Mathematically, Bayes' theorem for re-evaluating hypothesis A in the light of evidence B is expressed as:

$$P(A \backslash B) = \frac{(P(B \backslash A) \times P(A))}{P(B)}$$

where

P(A\B) is the revised probability that hypothesis *A* is true, given that we now know *B*;
P(A) is the prior probability that *A* was true, before we knew *B*;
P(B) is the probability that *B* is the case, before we applied it to *A*; and
P(B\A) is the probability that *B* is true in situation *A*.
P(B\A) ÷ P(B) is the likelihood ratio (the weight of evidence *B*).

---

114 The 'weight' of a piece of evidence refers to how *much* it changes the odds. It is quantified by the *likelihood ratio*, which reflects how reliable and conclusive the evidence is, and how relevant it is to the situation in question.

(For the reader who, like me, is easily scared by mathematics, an example may help.[115])

In a medical context, when the diagnosis of a particular disease is being considered, new evidence often comes in the form of a test result, such as a physiological measurement, laboratory report, radiological finding or biopsy result. All such tests have both *sensitivity* (i.e. how reliably the test is positive in known cases of the disease) and *specificity* (i.e. how reliably the test is negative in the absence of the disease). The likelihood ratio (the factor by which the test result changes the odds in favour of or against a diagnosis) combines information about sensitivity and specificity. The likelihood for a positive result (LR+) tells you how much the odds in favour of the diagnosis increase when the test is positive. The likelihood ratio for a negative result (LR–) tells you how much the odds decrease if the test is negative.[116]

Here is a practical example of Bayesian thinking applied to a common clinical scenario.[117]

A middle-aged woman presents to her GP with dysuria. On the history

---

115 Of the teenagers in the town centre, 60% are boys and 40% girls. Half the boys (50%) are wearing hoodies, but only one girl in five (20%) does so. You notice one particular teenager wearing a hoodie, but you can't tell his or her gender. What is the probability that it is a girl?

- Event A is that this individual is a girl.
- Event B is that the individual is wearing a hoodie.
- $P(A\backslash B)$ is the probability that the person you are looking at is a girl, given that he or she is wearing a hoodie.
- $P(B\backslash A)$ is the probability of wearing a hoodie, given that she is a girl, i.e. 20% (0.2).
- $P(A)$ is the probability that you are looking at a girl, i.e. 40% (0.4).
- $P(B)$ is the probability of any particular individual's wearing a hoodie. Of 100 teenagers, 30 boys (50% of 60) and 8 girls (20% of 40) are hoodie-wearers. So $P(B)$ is 38/100, i.e. 0.38.

Given all this, Bayes' theorem calculates the probability that the teenager in question is a girl as:

$$P(A\backslash B) = \frac{(P(B\backslash A) \times P(A))}{P(B)}$$

$$= \frac{0.2 \times 0.4}{0.38}$$

$$= 0.21 \ (21\%)$$

116 For a positive test result, LR+ = sensitivity/(1 – specificity). For a negative result, LR– = (1 – sensitivity)/specificity.

117 Doust J. Diagnosis in general practice: using probabilistic reasoning. *British Medical Journal* 2009; **339**: b3823. Data quoted with the kind permission of the author.

alone, it is about 55% likely that she has a bacterial urinary tract infection (UTI). The doctor tests a urine sample with a dipstick for the presence of nitrites and leucocyte esterase. The *sensitivity* of each test is 90%, i.e. it will be positive in 90% of patients who do have a UTI. The *specificity* if both tests are negative is 60%, i.e. 60% of patients without a UTI will have negative tests.

Of 1000 women presenting in this way, 550 (55%) will have a UTI and 450 (45%) will not. Of the 550 with disease, 495 (90% of 550) will test positive for either nitrites or leucocyte esterase. The remaining 55 will be false negatives. Of the 450 women without disease, 270 (60% of 450) will rightly have negative tests; the remaining 180 will be false positives (see Table 8.1). The dipstick test has a positive predictive value (proportion of true positives to total positive results) of 495/675, i.e. 73%. If both tests are negative, it is 83% (270/325) likely that there is no infection, and there is only a 17% chance that infection is present. So – if either of the dipstick tests is positive, the probability of bacterial UTI rises from 55% to 73%, while if both are negative, it falls to 17%. The results of testing are shown in Table 8.1.

Table 8.1 Dipstick testing results

Dipstick results in 1000 women presenting with dysuria	UTI present	UTI absent	Total
Either nitrite *or* leucocyte esterase +ve	True positives ($n=495$)	False positives ($n=180$)	675
Both tests –ve	False negatives ($n=55$)	True negatives ($n=270$)	325
Total	550	450	1000

These figures, and the weight of research evidence underlying them, lend a reassuring sense of scientific respectability to what might otherwise seem a rather sloppy piece of everyday clinical decision-making. It is good to know that a simple rule of thumb – *Test a urine sample with a dipstick, and if anything shows up treat as an infection* – would detect 90% of patients who have a UTI, and will leave only one woman in five without the treatment she needs.

Bayesian thinking seems to bring a welcome objectivity and discipline to what can easily be an unstructured and haphazard process. We are offered the beguiling prospect of the doctor as bloodhound, hot on the trail of a diagnosis as if it were a suspect on the run. At each fork in the diagnostic trail the doctor applies a test to sniff the evidence and decide – *No, not that way; this way. Down here!* – in which direction the quarry is most likely to be hiding, until, with one final clinching investigation, he has the definitive diagnosis by the throat.

But the Bayesian method has an important weakness. It stands or falls on whether or not the evidence that can be adduced at each nodal decision point *(a)* exists at all; *(b)* is reliable; and *(c)* can be quantified. Depressingly seldom are all three conditions satisfied. Of all the ailments that can assail the human frame, lamentably few have been sufficiently researched to support a rigorously Bayesian approach to their diagnosis. Bayes is really helpful if we have to decide whether a chest pain is of cardiac origin or a testicular lump likely to be malignant. But ask Bayes to tell us whether this back pain is genuine, or whether this depressed patient would benefit from counselling, or even whether this sore throat is viral, and he struggles. There simply isn't the evidence to go on. Researchers, understandably, tend to find better things to do with their time and their grants than study conditions where the complicated psychology of individual patients and doctors significantly affects diagnosis and management.

When we refer to a 'diagnostic test' we are usually thinking of a piece of formal science such as a blood test, a radiological procedure or a biopsy. The specificity and sensitivity of tests such as these can be calculated and published. But, in effect, every question asked and every physical examination performed in the course of a consultation is also a test in its own right, in the sense that every response the patient makes, every physical finding, constitutes fresh evidence that changes the relative probabilities of the various possibilities the doctor is entertaining.

However, unless we can know the sensitivity of every casual physical finding and the specificity of every fragment of narrative, it is impossible to quantify the ever-shifting probabilities. Here is a brief extract from a typical general practice consultation, showing how a succession of diagnostic possibilities is cued by the patient's successive remarks.

The consultation	The doctor's thoughts
Patient: I feel tired all the time.	*I need to do a full blood count, blood sugar and thyroid function tests to screen for physical causes.*
Doctor: Do you?	
Pt: Yes. I'm just not sleeping.	*Anxiety? Depression? Ask about sleep pattern.*
Dr: Do you not get off to sleep for a long time, or are you waking up very early?	
Pt: I lie awake thinking about mother …	*I don't know anything about the mother? Is this a bereavement reaction? Is there a family history?*

… because I'm now the age she was when she had her stroke.	*Ah, stroke. I must check for risk factors – hypertension, smoking, cholesterol.*
Dr: I'll just check your blood pressure … It's 170/95.	*The diagnosis is probably hypertension and anxiety …*
Pt: And now there's this business with our daughter. *(Begins to weep)*	*… or depression. But I think I'll concentrate on the hypertension and the stroke risk.*
Dr: I think we'd better check your cholesterol.	

We have the feeling that the doctor here would *like* to be Bayesian, i.e. to explore each cue in enough detail to give it its due weighting as he homes in on a working diagnosis or action plan. But because the narrative is poorly sequenced and fast moving, and because to interrupt too frequently would distort it, he is thrown back upon his own internalised and uncalibrated impressions of the significance of each remark or finding. And, as we have seen, these are notoriously susceptible to cognitive bias – the doctor's own experience, his memory of recent or vivid events, his own likes and dislikes, preferences and assumptions.

Even where there is good clinical evidence allowing a more precisely Bayesian approach, its too rigid application can result in some uncomfortably robotic clinical behaviour that has to be humanised in the interests of good doctor–patient relations. Later in the study of UTIs described above, for example, we read that 'the benefits outweigh the harms of treatment when the probability of a UTI is greater than about 60%. If a woman (*with a history of UTI*) has a pre-test probability of disease of 90%, even if the dipstick test is negative, her post-test probability of disease is above 60%. In this case the dipstick test does not contribute to the decision on management and should not be ordered.'[118] Note that '*should not be ordered.*' In other words, if you're going to treat her anyway, don't bother testing the urine. Well why not? It's cheap; it reassures the patient; and it reminds the doctor to at least try and look like a scientist. Withholding a simple test from a patient who expects it may be evidence-based insensitivity, but it is insensitivity all the same. And it is possible that a remark by the doctor such as, 'That's odd – it sounds as if you have an infection but there's nothing showing up in your urine sample' will provide an embarrassed patient with just the opening needed to ask, 'Do you think it could be anything to do with our sex life?'

In real life, the clinician is multi-tasking throughout the history-taking and examination stages of the consultation – tracking several diagnostic possibilities and adjusting their likelihoods as each piece of fresh information

---

118 Doust J. As footnote 117.

arrives. Eventually (and without its rivals being necessarily dropped from consideration) one possibility reaches a critical mass of likelihood where action must be taken. For example, a child's listlessness and vague history of a rash make meningococcal meningitis enough of a possibility to warrant hospital admission even though this is probably just the prodrome stage of a viral illness. One simply cannot afford to wait for the Bayesian gold standard test, finding Gram-positive bacteria in a sample of cerebrospinal fluid.

There is no mathematical rule or formula that can establish where to set the action threshold. It is always a matter of judgement. Clinicians, both individually on the basis of their clinical experience and corporately by means of consensus guidelines, have to evaluate the risks of action versus inaction. When the differential diagnosis includes something life threatening, action must be taken in conditions of greater uncertainty than would be tolerated in less urgent circumstances, when a policy of 'do more tests' might be appropriate. This was Tony Blair's credible defence against the accusation that his invasion of Iraq was misguided: 'Given the strong probability that Iraq had weapons of mass destruction, could we afford *not* to invade?'[119]

Evidence-based medicine, first described in the medical literature in the 1990s, has been popularised largely thanks to the commitment of a group led by David Sackett and Gordon Guyatt at Ontario's McMaster University. Hitherto, concepts of best practice had been largely determined either by a sloppy 'anything goes' lobby that thought that the art of medicine lay in ignoring science, or by a sycophantic acceptance of the 'If *I* do it, it must be right' opinions of the profession's most prominent clinicians. That clinical decision-making should incorporate the best available objective evidence is unarguable, and this principle has given focus and impetus to the world's research community. I suspect that, in their secret dreams, the pioneers of evidence-based medicine envisaged a Brave New Medicine where incontrovertible evidence would inform all diagnostic and therapeutic conundrums, and would be applied in a systematic Bayesian way to every clinical dilemma. But, as we have seen, even if the results of research had been as comprehensive and unambiguous as would be needed, the purity of the Bayesian approach is

---

119 This argument could *not* defend Mr Blair against the possibly more serious accusation that cognitive bias had got the better of him and that he had (in the language used at the time) 'sexed up' the dossier of intelligence evidence that he made public in order to make Saddam appear more of a threat than in fact he was. There is a clinical parallel here with the surgeon who, because he loves to operate, disregards the normal blood test results which might stay the hand of a less gung-ho colleague.

always going to be compromised by the fact that it takes place in the context of a conversation between two human beings, each psychologically complex and to a significant degree irrational. The Inner Physician – the sensitive but error-prone human observer at the core of every doctor – is not, and cannot be coerced into becoming, a natural Bayesian.

* * * * *

'Intuitive' approaches to diagnosis

> No, no, you're not thinking; you're just being logical.
>
> Niels Bohr (1885–1962)
> Danish physicist

Clinical algorithms and Bayesian decision-making embody the human capacity for logical analysis. But – and remember, our goal is to improve and speed up the traditional medical model as a method of diagnosis – logical analysis is not the only human capacity that can help. Human beings are also good – sometimes *too* good – at generalising, inferring rules and principles from limited information. We have the ability to see patterns in apparent randomness; to pick out key features amidst a morass of detail; to spot connections between apparently unrelated events; to detect a meaningful signal against random background noise. As well as rational beings, we are also creatures of instinct, hunch and reflex. We sometimes have a 'sixth sense'; we feel things 'in our guts' and see things 'out of the corner of our eye'. We may sometimes be wrong in the conclusions we jump to; and so, to the rationalist, these characteristics of the human mind are the enemy. But to the diagnostician they can be a source of insight, even of wisdom.

Heuristics: the mental shortcuts we all take

> This is the essence of intuitive heuristics:
>
> when faced with a difficult question, we often answer an easier one instead, usually without noticing the substitution.
>
> Daniel Kahneman (b. 1934)
> Professor Emeritus of Psychology and Public Affairs,
> Princeton University

William 'Slick Willie' Sutton (1901–80) was a notorious American bank robber who in the course of his 40-year career stole at least two million dollars. A reporter once asked him why he robbed banks. Sutton famously replied, '*Because that's where the money is.*' This truism has become dignified in medical education as Sutton's law, which states that, when diagnosing, one should first consider the obvious.

Sutton's law is an example of a heuristic – an experience-based rule of thumb, an educated guess, applied common sense. Occam's famous razor is another, cautioning us not to make two diagnoses if one will do.[120] In everyday life we regularly use heuristics to try to simplify matters that in reality are bafflingly complicated:

Red sky at night, shepherd's delight; red sky in the morning, shepherd's warning.

I before E, except after C.

The one thing we learn from history is that we never learn from history.

And so on. In medicine, which is at least as complicated as real life, doctors constantly find themselves being asked questions of bewildering complexity in situations made paralysingly uncertain by the number of variables to be taken into account. But regardless of how complex the question or how unreliable the data, in the clinical situation a decision is always required, and preferably a clear-cut one that can be actioned in time to be of use to the patient. *Shall I or shall I not administer intrathecal antibiotics to this child? Do I or do I not prescribe steroid cream for this rash? Shall I or shall I not refer this patient for counselling?* It simply won't do to answer, 'Come back when the research has been carried out, peer reviewed and published – and I've got around to reading it.' It is when we have to make a quick response under pressure that heuristics come into their own.

For 200 years, the study of human decision-making was haunted by the ghost of the Reverend Bayes brandishing his classical model of rational

---

120 William of Ockham (1285–1348), a Franciscan friar, was one of the major philosophers of his day. His principle of 'explanatory simplicity' is summed up in the Latin phrase *entia non sunt multiplicanda praeter necessitate* – 'Entities should not be multiplied more than necessary', i.e. the simplest explanation is to be preferred. In the medical context this underpins a heuristic called 'diagnostic parsimony', i.e. 'Go for the single diagnosis that explains most of the clinical features.'

evidence-based choice. According to this, the 'rational actor' (the phrase by which Bayes liked to refer to the ordinary person) chooses which of several options to pursue by assessing the probability and usefulness of each possible outcome, and opting for the one of likeliest benefit. *And what if the ordinary person is not all that good at calculating probabilities or predicating outcomes?*, we might timidly enquire. *Then he had better learn!*, would come the Reverend's stern reply. It was not until 1957 that Herbert Simon, an American political scientist, acknowledged that the unswerving logicality required by the rational choice model could not be assumed in matters of human judgement, and proposed a more pragmatic alternative – 'bounded rationality' – that took account of the inherent limitations of the human mind. By and large, people think and choose rationally, Simon contended, but only within the constraints imposed by their limited search and computational capacities. Then in the 1960s and '70s Daniel Kahneman and Amos Tversky[121] systematically described how ordinary people exercised their everyday judgement in situations where they didn't have the time, information or skill to behave with computer-like logic. Collating their research in their 1982 book *Judgment under Uncertainty*,[122] Kahneman and Tversky showed how our ability to make predictions and take decisions in complex or uncertain conditions often rests on a limited number of simplifying heuristics rather than extensive algorithmic processing.

In their early studies, Kahneman and Tversky identified three heuristics that underlie many intuitive judgements under uncertain conditions, including medical ones:

- availability
- representativeness
- anchoring and adjustment.

The 'availability' heuristic

We tend to assume that possibilities that most readily spring to mind, or which we can imagine most vividly, are most likely to be right. The more easily we can think of relevant examples, the more we are inclined to accept one particular explanation as true.

In the course of my career I have seen a good many people in the early

---

121 From the Department of Psychology at the Hebrew University, Jerusalem.

122 Kahneman D, Slovic P, Tversky A, eds. *Judgment under Uncertainty: heuristics and biases*. Cambridge: Cambridge University Press, 1982.

stages of appendicitis. They didn't all give the same history, or have the same look about them, or the same physical signs – but it means that if I see a patient with worsening abdominal pain, lying rather still and looking rather more worried than I would have expected, appendicitis is the first thing I think of. And because I've seen lots of cases, I have a low index of suspicion and so probably don't miss this important diagnosis as often as I did when I was newly qualified. Indeed, I probably tend to *over*-diagnose it, and send more people into hospital with suspected appendicitis than necessary. On the other hand, I have seen only two children with acute epiglottitis. One was the daughter of a close personal friend, and I possibly saved the life of the other by passing an endotracheal tube while waiting for the ambulance. Epiglottitis may be – *is* – rare; but, because of the vivid memories I have of these two cases, it comes high up my differential diagnosis whenever I see a child with wheeze and a fever.

The availability heuristic underlies such sensible medical aphorisms as 'Common things are common' and 'When you hear hoof-beats, think horse not zebra'. It is the reason we sometimes reassure patients by telling them, 'There's a lot of it about.' But it also can lead us to over-weight some possible diagnoses simply because of the dramatic examples we have encountered.

The 'representativeness' heuristic

'Representativeness' is a measure of how far the characteristics of an individual are typical of the group to which it belongs.

To save time when we encounter some new situation, we try to fit it into one or other of the various categories of things and events we have experienced in the past. The representativeness heuristic then makes us react to the new situation as if it had all the characteristics typical of whatever category it seems to belong in. Perhaps the best-known version of the representativeness heuristic goes *If it looks like a duck, and walks like a duck, and quacks like a duck – it's probably a duck.* If what we are dealing with does not fit exactly into a previously known category, we nevertheless allocate it to the nearest plausible category and deal with it accordingly.

The representativeness heuristic is widespread and often useful in diagnostic thinking. The more closely a particular presentation matches our internalised template of a typical case, the more confident we feel that we have the correct diagnosis. *If it looks like urticaria, and itches like urticaria, and the patient has a history of urticaria – it's probably urticaria. No need for challenge tests or skin biopsies – it's urticaria, and to be treated as such.* The representativeness heuristic is at work whenever we say, 'In my experience …', or

'I know a case of so-and-so when I see one.' The representativeness heuristic underpins notions of 'diagnosis by pattern recognition' or 'diagnosis by key features', which experienced clinicians, especially GPs, use to justify their instant diagnosis of conditions ranging from acne to zoster. In safe hands, this particular diagnostic shortcut is invaluable, saving the time, expense and inconvenience of confirmatory investigations.

Many diseases and pathological conditions produce a signature cluster of key features – elements in the history, typical physical findings, a pattern of investigation results – that remains recognisably constant from one case to another. Doctors gradually build up a collection of these disease templates or gestalts, which are perceived all at once and at a glance. Psoriasis almost always looks like psoriasis. Almost every patient with polycystic ovary syndrome gives a similar menstrual history, has a particular body shape, and shows a male-pattern hair distribution. In the days before immunisation, experienced GPs could reliably diagnose measles days before the rash appeared merely by spotting the child's red conjunctivae and hearing the typical cough.

As with all heuristics, diagnosis by pattern recognition is fast and often accurate, but sometimes wrong. What if the duck-sized, duck-shaped bird paddling on the lake looks only *quite* like a duck, its beak being black and pointed rather than orange and blunt; and on land it staggers rather than waddles; and it goes 'kwao' rather than 'quack'? Is it still a duck? Actually, no; it's a Pacific loon. Or what if our fledgling ornithologist only knows three categories of birds – ducks, vultures and little brown ones? What will be his reaction on spotting his first ostrich? He will struggle to suppress his expectation, fostered by the representativeness heuristic, that at any moment it will take to the water, fly circles over a dead badger, or go 'tweet'.

When it is being helpful, the representativeness heuristic can lead us to conclude correctly that the listless and uncoordinated child of Ashkenazi Jewish parents has Tay–Sachs disease, or that the young woman with small joint polyarthritis and a high titres of IgG (immunoglobulin G) antibodies is suffering from rheumatoid arthritis. On the other hand it may throw us off the scent if the Jewish child actually has a brain tumour. It may cause us to downplay the significance of the dry mouth and eyes reported by the young woman who is actually developing Sjögren's syndrome.

It would be nice to believe that our internal catalogue of diagnostic templates had been built up solely on the foundation of the most reliable evidence and the most objective clinical experience. Ideally, our representative concept of, say, a patient with alcoholism, against which we are assessing the real patient in front of us, should consist of the diagnostic key features of the condition and nothing but the diagnostic key features, derived from sources as authoritative as possible. But things are seldom so pure. The representativeness heuristic can degenerate into stereotyping and prejudice. Our own subjective elements creep in and contaminate the idealised representation – our own assumptions and prejudices; the idiosyncrasies of our own previous alcoholic patients; perhaps emotional responses to any of our own friends or family members who have had drink problems. Ask yourself what, in *your* mind, are the key descriptors of someone you would place in the diagnostic category 'alcoholism'. Weekly intake of alcohol exceeding a specified number of units? Two or more 'yes' responses on the CAGE questionnaire?[123] Compulsion to drink, increasing tolerance, physical symptoms on withdrawal? Drink-related legal or financial problems? History of disrupted work, social or family life? So far, so non-contentious. When you see a patient with all or most of these features, the representativeness heuristic will swiftly and accurately speed you to a sound diagnosis. But maybe your own stereotypical alcoholic – based on your personal experience and perhaps your own assumptions, even prejudices – is male, working class, ill-kempt, smelly, and disruptive in the waiting room. As a result, it is possible you may jump to the conclusion that this homeless, unemployed and lonely man, who happens to match several of your non-evidence-based criteria, is an alcoholic, and miss the depression from which he is really suffering. Or you may fail to recognise that this articulate and well-groomed businesswoman who wants something to help her sleep is not suffering from anxiety but in fact has a drink problem.

Attempts have been made to immunise the representativeness heuristic against corruption by doctor-derived bias by devising structured questionnaires, such as the PHQ-9 widely used to diagnose depression. This invites the patient to self-rate their mental state on 10 parameters such as mood, sleep disturbance, impaired self-image and suicidal ideation. Such standardised heuristics combine the 'key features' approach with the apparent rigour of an algorithm, and will be invaluable if ever the day comes that medical care is delivered by robots rather than sentient human beings. Even today, they are a useful prop for a disorganised or inexperienced physician.

---

123 Ewing JA. Detecting alcoholism: the CAGE questionnaire. *Journal of the American Medical Association* 1984; **252**: 1905–7. Four questions are posed, relating to alcohol consumption; a score of two or more positives suggests problem drinking.

The 'anchoring and adjustment' heuristic

The name is clumsy but the concept is familiar: 'Shoot first, ask questions later'. If ever we have to make a decision in a hurry, or decide the best thing to do in an impossibly complicated situation, we tend to come up with a 'first best guess' at the right answer ('anchoring'), and subsequently modify it in the light of further thought ('adjustment'). An example from everyday life would be: *Quick! Which exit do I take at the roundabout to get to the motorway? Don't know. I'm not sure, but I don't think it's on the right. I'll go straight on, and look out for a sign.* A medical equivalent might be: *That's a horrible-looking tonsillar exudate! It's probably streptococcal, so I'll prescribe penicillin. That'll do no harm even if it's viral, and we can always do a glandular fever test if it doesn't get better.*

As a way of navigating through a complex world, anchoring and adjustment is a tactic deeply ingrained in many people, myself included. We 'anchorers' prefer to move from the general to the particular, from the approximate to the precise, from wide-angle view to close-up. In medicine, we are probably better suited to general practice, which is more tolerant of initial inaccuracy than, say, neurosurgery. Anchoring and adjusting allows GPs to work faster, so that we get more things right in the course of a working day. Neurosurgeons (I hope) do their assessing and planning and double checking before they make the first incision; that way, they may not see many patients, but they make fewer mistakes.

The danger in the anchoring and adjustment heuristic lies in being too quick to anchor and too slow to adjust. We are too much swayed by the first data we encounter.[124] We tend to over-value and become too fixated on the first tentative idea we come up with. We find it easier to make up our minds than to change them. We rely on too little information at first, but then are willing to ignore too much subsequent evidence if it would mean us having

---

124 A group of school children was asked to estimate within 5 seconds the product $8 \times 7 \times 6 \times 5 \times 4 \times 3 \times 2 \times 1$. A second group was asked to estimate $1 \times 2 \times 3 \times 4 \times 5 \times 6 \times 7 \times 8$. The correct answer in both cases is 40,320. But the median answer from the first group was 2250, while the second group's median answer was 512. Because corrective adjustments are likely to be insufficient, both groups underestimated the actual result. But the group given the ascending sequence of terms $(1 \times 2 \times 3 \ldots)$ estimated an answer much lower than those given the descending sequence $(8 \times 7 \times 6 \ldots)$. They were both disproportionately influenced by the early stages of their computation.

to backtrack from our first impression.[125] Once we have a plausible diagnosis in our minds it is hard to let go of it, even in the face of further evidence that, had we known it earlier, might have led us to a different conclusion.

Getting the balance between rationalism and intuition can be tricky. The default position for many doctors, especially when tired or stressed, is towards the 'intuitive' end of the spectrum; and this can result in avoidable misdiagnosis. In the words of Pat Croskerry, 'Our intuition will always override analytical reasoning. We prefer to be in the intuitive mode; it is comfortably numb, but it gives you a misplaced feeling of security ... [Diagnostic errors occur] not because a doctor didn't know enough about a disease process to make that diagnosis but that they simply didn't think of it, or something diverted them – something the patient said, or something in the context – from the fact that this was an atypical presentation ... Our intuitions mostly serve us well, but they are occasionally catastrophic.'[126] It is hard to disagree with this assertion. However, an excess of rationalism can also be catastrophic, if it diverts the doctor's curiosity away from the bigger picture of the patient's illness of which physical pathology is only one part.

---

125 A chastening example is to be found in the wildly disparate advice various nations give their citizens about safe levels of alcohol consumption. A 'unit' of alcohol is 6 grams (g) in Austria, 8g in the UK, 12g in Denmark, 14g in the USA and 19.75g in Japan. Recommended weekly maxima for men are 168g (UK), 196g (USA), 252g (Denmark) and 280g (Japan). For women, weekly maxima are 98g (USA), 112g (UK), 168g (Denmark) and 210g (Italy). [Data correct at January 2012.] All this advice is based, presumably, on the same internationally accessible database of research evidence.

I suspect that what happened, in the UK at least, is this. In 1987 a group of self-styled experts, charged by the Department of Health with producing guidelines but lacking much hard evidence to help them, sat around and sheepishly discussed what was a sensible daily intake for the average British male. 'Two pints of beer a night', someone suggested. 'A bottle of wine shared between two', said another. 'OK', said the Chairman, 'that's 28 units a week. What about the ladies?' 'Oh, less for them, obviously.' 'Shall we say 21 then?' 'Agreed', chorused the committee. And these figures, once published, have taken on an almost religious unchallengability.

126 Patrick Croskerry MD, Professor of Emergency Medicine, Dalhousie University, Halifax, Nova Scotia. The remarks quoted were made at a conference on patient safety at Great Ormond Street Hospital for Children in 2010 (Think rationally rather than intuitively to avoid diagnostic errors, doctors are told. *British Medical Journal* 2010; **341**: c6705).

Composite approaches

Civil war is never pretty, even between two such well-mannered rivals as the rational and intuitive approaches to diagnosis. One of my favourite books as a child was *1066 and All That*, an irreverent parody of a textbook of British history. In it, the English Civil War of 1642–51 is described as an 'utterly memorable Struggle between the Cavaliers (Wrong but Wromantic) and the Roundheads (Right but Repulsive)'.[127] In the battle for intellectual control of the diagnostic process we could characterise the Rationalists as the Roundheads, having reason and logic on their side but unedifyingly po-faced in their earnestness. The Cavaliers would be Intuitives: flawed, fallible, but somehow engagingly human.

In real life, of course, working clinicians don't adhere exclusively to either extreme doctrine. As they talk with their patients, trying to make medical sense of what they are hearing, doctors keep a foot in both camps, or oscillate between them. We would hope that diagnoses are arrived at by a combination of the algorithmic and heuristic approaches, neither reducing the doctor to an automaton nor putting the patient at undue risk through untempered cognitive bias.

Academics, as is their wont, have devised theoretical models to capture the essence of what good diagnosticians do in practice. One long-established example is the hypothetico-deductive model, which is held to mirror the more general process by which scientific advances are conventionally made.

The hypothetico-deductive method

The hypothetico-deductive method – science's idealised way of working – is little more than a formalised version of the anchoring and adjustment heuristic: *Have a first best guess at what's going on, then modify it in the light of further evidence.*

Starting with an observation that is not fully understood (in the medical context, the patient's account of a symptom or problem), the scientist (doctor):

- gathers as much data and information as possible, then
- comes up with a first tentative explanation (differential diagnosis), and

---

127 Sellar WC, Yeatman RJ. *1066 and All That: a memorable history of England, comprising all the parts you can remember, including 103 good things, 5 bad kings and 2 genuine dates*. London: Methuen & Co., 1930, new edition 1998. Quoted passage from Chapter XXXV.

- formulates it as a hypothesis which, if true
- makes predictions that
- by a process of deduction
- suggest experiments or tests (further questions, examination or investigations)
- that will either support or refute the initial hypothesis
- this further information leads to a 'second draft' hypothesis (diagnostic shortlist)
- which can in turn be questioned and tested, until
- the hypothesis is either refuted or becomes sufficiently credible to be treated as if it was 'true' (the working diagnosis).

Figure 8.3 shows how this iterative cycle of *hypothesis–prediction–test–refine* gradually spirals in on a diagnosis that is sufficiently probable for the doctor to act on.

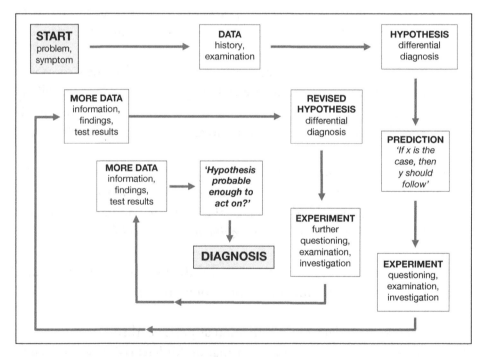

Figure 8.3 Hypothetico-deductive diagnosis.

In the consulting room, the hypothetico-deductive method of diagnosis, despite its mouthful of a name, is so familiar that a brief everyday example will serve.

Process	Doctor's actions and thoughts
START *Patient:* 'I'm tired all the time, and I get breathless, and my periods are heavier than usual.'	
Data-gathering	Establishes that 'breathless' means 'short of breath on moderate exertion'. Obtains history of menorrhagia. Notices patient looks pale.
Hypothesis (1)	Could be anaemia or hypothyroidism.
Prediction	If anaemia, then conjunctivae should be pale and serum haemoglobin level reduced. If hypothyroidism, there may be a goitre, and serum levels of thyroid-stimulating hormone (TSH) would be raised.
Experiment	Enquires about symptoms of hypothyroidism. Examines conjunctivae. Palpates neck. Arranges full blood count and thyroid function tests.
Further data	Conjunctivae are pale. No goitre present. Haemoglobin 9.5 g/100 ml, microcytic picture. Normal thyroid function tests.
Hypothesis (2)	Iron deficiency anaemia. Hypothyroidism excluded.
DIAGNOSIS (insight on the verge of action)	Iron deficiency anaemia, secondary to menorrhagia, cause so far unknown.

Crucial to the hypothetico-deductive method is the notion of 'falsifiability', associated with the name of Karl Popper.[128] 'You can't prove a negative,' the popular saying goes. 'Yes you can,' Popper would counter. 'In fact, in science a negative is the only thing you *can* prove for certain.'

The essence of the scientific method, Popper maintained, is to subject a theory to testing by an experiment that could, in principle, disprove it. He liked to distinguish 'hard' sciences such as physics and chemistry, in which theories can be tested by experiment, from 'pseudosciences' such as psychoanalysis or the Marxian theory of history, which cannot, their validity being asserted solely by the persuasiveness of their authors' rhetoric.

According to Popper, a theory can never be proved true. The most one can say is that it has not yet been proved false. What we for convenience call 'scientific truth' is just the explanation of events that has so far resisted extinction, as if by a Darwinian process of 'survival of the fittest', in the arena of experiment.

So it is with diagnosis. There is no such thing as a conclusive diagnosis; the most one can say is that one's working diagnosis has not yet been proved

---

128 Sir Karl Popper (1902–94), Austrian–British philosopher of science. Popper also wrote extensively on social and political philosophy, taking a humanist stance in defence of liberal democracy.

wrong. In the clinical example just cited, the doctor cannot be certain that the patient's symptoms are due to anaemia secondary to menorrhagia, merely that the competing possibility (hypothyroidism) has been ruled out. For the doctor to believe that the diagnosis, in some absolute sense, 'is' anaemia is dangerous self-delusion. Remembering that diagnosis means 'insight on the verge of action', the doctor can do no more than act 'as if' the anaemia theory is true, prescribing iron and referring the patient to a gynaecologist. He should nevertheless continue to look for evidence that could refute as well as confirm the working diagnosis, remembering too that alternative explanations may not have been considered.

There is a weakness in the hypothetico-deductive approach, one that begs the question implied by the title of this chapter. The cycle of *hypothesis–prediction–test–refine* can operate only once there is an initial hypothesis for it to work on. What never enters the doctor's head cannot be considered. At the point we left the story, it remains possible that the last patient's tiredness could be the result of depression or Jabberwock's disease; but these alternative explanations remain untested because they have not been thought of. We could forgive the absence of Jabberwock's disease from the differential diagnosis; it is, after all, vanishingly rare. But depression? Probably the working diagnosis is indeed anaemia. But not even to *think* of depression? If we ask ourselves why such a common diagnosis seems not to have been entertained, the answer surely has to be that something subconscious in the doctor blocked it, and prevented it from surfacing and coming within reach of rational examination. Reason is at the mercy of psychology, and needs to be rescued from it.

'Dual system' theories
Whenever we have to make a judgement, decision or diagnosis, we are best served by a collaboration between hunch and logic, between what we 'feel in our guts' and what we 'work out with our brains'. In the literature of cognitive psychology, two complementary systems of decision-making are widely described, usually referred to as System 1 ('intuitive') and System 2 ('rational') (see Figure 8.4).[129]

---

129 See, for example, Kahneman D. Maps of bounded rationality: a perspective on intuitive judgement and choice. Nobel Prize Lecture, 8 December 2002. www.nobelprize.org/nobel_prizes/economics/laureates/2002/kahneman-lecture.html.
   Also Croskerry P. A universal model of diagnostic reasoning. *Academic Medicine* 2009; **8**: 1002–28. http://journals.lww.com/academicmedicine/Fulltext/2009/08000/A_Universal_Model_of_Diagnostic_Reasoning.14.aspx.

System 1 – 'Intuitive'	System 2 – 'Rational'
Hunch, gut feeling	Logic, reasoning
Unconscious or pre-conscious	Consciously invoked
Immediate and spontaneous	Slower and deliberate
Gestalt or pattern recognition	Analytical, algorithmic
Experience-led	Intellect-led
Heuristic	Systematic
Emotionally contaminated	Emotion-free

Figure 8.4 'Dual system' theories.

The intuitive System 1 is usually the first to manifest. It comes up with hunches spontaneously and without conscious thought, based largely on accumulated past experience and pattern recognition. System 1 operates rapidly – so rapidly that its conclusions can be premature. Admittedly useful in an emergency and often impressively accurate, it is nonetheless vulnerable to all the biases and emotional contamination that bedevil any heuristic process and which can occasionally lead to catastrophic errors of judgement. If we are sensible and disciplined, we put System 1's 'first draft assessment' on hold until the rational thought processes of System 2 can kick in. System 2's function is to submit our first impressions to methodical and dispassionate evaluation, using (as best we can) such logic-based strategies as the algorithmic, Bayesian and hypothetico-deductive approaches described earlier.

Researchers from the Department of Primary Health Care at Oxford University have refined the dual process model until it looks recognisably lifelike.[130] Zooming in, they describe three stages in the process of diagnosis, as practised by GPs:

1 initiation of diagnostic hypotheses
2 refinement of the diagnostic hypotheses
3 defining the final diagnosis.

These stages represent the doctor thinking:

---

130 Heneghan C, Glasziou P, Thompson M, *et al*. Diagnostic strategies used in primary care. *British Medical Journal* 2009; **338**: b946. I am grateful to the authors for permission to quote from, paraphrase and summarise their paper, and for our enjoyable discussion of the issues arising from it.

1 what could this possibly be?
2 what docs it look as if it realistically might be?
3 what shall I act as if it actually is?

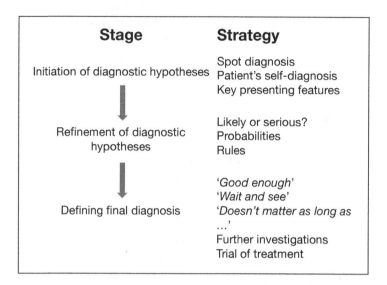

Figure 8.5 Oxford three-stage model.

Heneghan and his colleagues identified various strategies associated with each stage (see Figure 8.5). Among the early 'triggers' that start the flow of diagnostic possibilities into the doctor's mind are:

- instantly recognisable clinical patterns, e.g. facial acne, bacterial conjunctivitis
- the patient's own self-diagnosis, e.g. 'I've got another bladder infection'
- recognising key features or phrases in the presentation, e.g. Parkinsonian tremor, 'crushing chest pain'.

At the 'refining the hypotheses' stage, common strategies include:

- Murtagh's process,[131] in which the doctor considers:
  - what is most likely?
  - what serious condition(s) must not be missed?
  - what conditions are often missed?

---

131 John Murtagh, Professor of General Practice, Monash University, Australia. Author of *General Practice*. New York: McGraw-Hill, 2010.

- could this be one condition mimicking another?
  - could there be hidden agenda, e.g. family or sexual problem?
- probabilistic (Bayesian) reasoning
- clinical prediction rules, e.g. Ottawa ankle rules,[132] CAGE alcohol questionnaire.

Observing how GPs behave during the final 'definition' stage, the Oxford authors remind us that fewer than half of the presentations in routine general practice result in a clear-cut biomedical diagnosis at the first consultation. The strategies they list, therefore, are mainly tactics for managing diagnostic indecision:

- if it's safe, go with your 'best guess, good enough for now' diagnosis
- wait and see what happens next ('the diagnostic use of time')
- be satisfied with knowing what the diagnosis is not
- do some more tests
- give a trial of treatment.

* * * * *

Listen for the creak of the bow, not the rush of the arrow.

Jack Gardner

From *Words Are Not Things* (2004)

This chapter and the previous one have reflected at some length on the nature and function of diagnosis and reviewed various means of achieving it. I make no apology for this. Making a diagnosis – working out, in all necessary complexity, what is the matter with the patient – is the crucial part of the medical encounter. Get it right, and it is usually not too difficult to think what might best be done to help. But get it wrong, and avoidable damage is caused, time wasted, resources squandered and trust betrayed.

In all necessary complexity: this, I suggest, is the measure by which a 'big picture' diagnosis is to be judged. As Einstein remarked, 'Everything should be made as simple as possible, but no simpler.' The factors that impact on people's well-being, bring about their illnesses and contribute to their recovery are more complex than can be captured in the language of anatomy, physiology and pathology alone. A good diagnosis is so much more than

---

132 Guidelines to determine whether or not an ankle injury needs to be X-rayed.

a shorthand label for a physical abnormality. It is a search for meaning on many levels, conducted through a special way of interpreting the patient's narrative, leading to a degree of multidimensional insight from which effective action cannot but flow.

The diagnostic strategies we have examined – from the obsessive grind of the traditional medical model to the more pragmatic dual system approach – all lead to biomedical diagnoses of the labelling, *this, not that* kind. None of them help much to move diagnostic thinking on from the simplistic Newtonian world of *either/or* to the more holistic post-Einstein *both/and* world where, as well as in pathology, individual illness can have roots in psychology, emotion, personality, relationships, family, culture, poverty, literacy, history, economics, religion … Of course the biomedical dimension in diagnosis is necessary – necessary, but not sufficient.

Remember Alice, the exasperating old lady with undiagnosed stomach pains who told me how, when she was a young bride, her first pregnancy had resulted in an intrauterine death and subsequent hysterectomy?

'So,' said Alice, 'that's what it's like to be me.'

I felt a rush of emotion, making me shudder and bringing me to the verge of tears. I had a strong visceral sense of all the sorrow, revulsion, hope and disappointment this poor woman must have experienced. For me, the feeling quickly abated. But Alice had lived with anguish and emptiness literally in her viscera for 50 years.

Back at the surgery, as my System 2 looked back on what I had learned, I was able to put into clever-sounding words the obvious connection between the pain in her life and the pain in her belly. That interpretation came too late, however, for me to share with Alice at the time; and, indeed, I never did. I'm not sure it would have made any difference even if I had. At all events, she continued to complain of the same old symptoms in the same old wearisome way. But something changed – *me*. After these revelations my heart no longer sank when I saw Alice's name on my visiting list, and my teeth no longer clenched in irritation and frustration as I listened yet again to her litany of complaints.

But at the time, when Alice said, 'That's what it's like to be me,' and I found myself struck wordless by the poignancy of her story, there was only one thing I could do. I got up, crossed the room, and gave her a big hug.

(To be continued.)

I don't know what Alice's medical diagnosis was: functional symptoms or somatisation disorder, probably. Or possibly, dared I but enter it in her notes, 'sad lady needing a hug'. But I know that the insight she vouchsafed to me in response to my unprofessional show of annoyance brought about an action more helpful than any amount of further tests or hospital referrals.

In Alice's case, my flash of recognition came without conscious thought on my part. It just happened when something in me resonated with her gut-wrenching tale, as a piano string will resonate in sympathy with its corresponding note sung or played on another instrument nearby. This resonance frequently occurs when a doctor's gaze is in wide-angle mode. We usually 'can just tell' when a patient is unhappy or anxious or embarrassed; or when a marriage has turned toxic; or when a grimace, a silence or an unusual choice of word points to some hidden agenda. In 'dual system' language, our System 1 is pre-loaded with patterns and templates enabling us to recognise in an instant the significance of these cues. We are, as it were, pre-tuned to resonate to them. But how does this pre-loading, this pre-tuning occur? We know how System 1 acquires its repertoire of immediately recognisable physical disease templates; it is the function of our medical schools to install a starter kit, and of continuing medical education to refresh and upgrade them. But how is our repertoire of recognisable emotional, behavioural and psychosocial templates installed?

My contention – to be further developed in the rest of this book – is that this is one of the roles of that medically naïve but worldly wise part of our professional persona that I am calling the Inner Physician.

* * * * *

> I observe the physician with the same diligence as he the disease.
>
> John Donne (1572–1631)
> English metaphysical poet, lawyer and priest
> From *Devotions Upon Emergent Occasions* (1624)

Big picture diagnosis is not without its dangers to both parties.

Diagnosis – extracting understanding from narrative and physical texts – is usually reckoned to be a one-way asymmetrical process; the patient furnishes data, and the doctor interprets it. However, what we might call bio-narrative diagnosis is a two-way transaction. Patient and doctor both tell their own story, and each interprets the other's. The patient too is in search of insight on the verge of action – and to this end is sampling, filtering, intuiting and analysing what is said at least as attentively as the doctor. Moreover, the patient is not signed up to any notion the doctor may have of remaining the uninvolved observer. Like it or not, patients do not differentiate between the doctor-as-healthcare-professional and the doctor-as-fellow-human-being as clearly as we might imagine. The more comprehensively we try to see into the subtleties of our patients' lives, the more we expose of ourselves. Bio-narrative diagnosis renders the doctor more transparent than some will find comfortable.

Transparency can be a danger for the patient, too, as we expand our curiosity beyond the purely physical and into increasingly personal and private domains. No part of the patient's experience or thought is out of bounds to a ruthlessly holistic diagnostician who has assumed a right of access. Time pressure, of course, imposes its own constraints on how much can be explored in a routine consultation. Nevertheless, there is a line to be drawn between curiosity and voyeurism, between the comfort of understanding and the discomfort of total exposure. As Carl Edvard Rudebeck[133] reminds us, 'the diagnosis never needs to be more accurate than what benefits the patient'.

It seems that we have some way to go before bio-narrative diagnosis becomes as universal as the medical model was in the past. Why? Why is it so disproportionally easy to pursue biological malfunctioning and so hard to be curious about the lived experience of the fellow human being who is our patient? Daniel Kahneman, he of 'heuristics' fame, makes the point that it is easier to settle for as little detail as you can get away with:

> *You cannot help dealing with the limited information you have as if it were all there is to know. You build the best possible story from the information available to you, and if it is a good story, you believe it. Paradoxically, it is easier to construct a coherent story when you know little, when there are fewer pieces to fit into the puzzle.*[134]

I think there is more to it than that. I think we are good at the 'bio' part of diagnosis because it has been thoroughly trained *into* us. We are poor at the 'narrative' part because something has been trained *out* of us.

What that something might be is the subject of the next chapter.

But before we move on …

* * * * *

---

133 Professor in the Department of Community Medicine, University of Tromsø, Norway.

134 From Kahneman D. *Thinking, Fast and Slow*. London: Penguin, 2012.

I got up, crossed the room, and gave Alice a big hug. We stood in silence for some moments in the middle of her living room, our arms around each other. It felt – appropriate. Then I heard a click as the door from the hallway opened. Alice's home help stuck her head round the door. 'It's only me,' she said. Then she saw us, client and doctor in mid-clinch. 'Sorry,' she said, 'I'll come back later.'

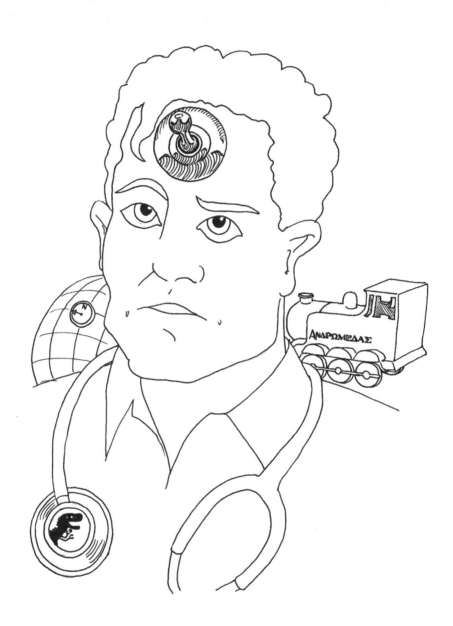

Chapter 9

Crichton's switch

They train bank clerks to stifle emotion, so that they will be able to refuse overdrafts when they become managers.

P.G. Wodehouse (1881–1975)

English humorist

From 'Ukridge's Accident Syndicate' in *Ukridge* (1924)

In the 1998 film *Patch Adams*, set in Virginia Medical University in the 1970s, Robin Williams in the title role plays a mature medical student. Adams[135] is a maverick whose determination to bond with his patients through humour brings him into conflict with the academic and medical establishment. On their very first day at medical school Patch and his fellow students crowd into an old-fashioned tiered lecture theatre to hear a motivational address from the head of the medical school, Dean Walcott (played by Bob Gunton).

Imagine yourself to be one of them. You are fresh from school, and clever, but getting into medical school has been an obstacle course. At various points along the way people have asked why you want to be a doctor, and you've perhaps mumbled something excruciatingly trite about working with people and wanting to make a difference. But now at last the great adventure of actually becoming a doctor is about to begin. Here you sit, eager and nervous, as the white-coated god-like figure of the Dean sweeps into the lecture theatre. There is an expectant hush, and Walcott begins to speak:

---

135 Williams's character is based on the American physician Dr Hunter 'Patch' Adams, born 1945. In real life Dr Adams is also a social activist and an accomplished clown. In 1971 he founded the Gesundheit! Institute in Arlington, Virginia, an innovative hospital and teaching facility that integrates conventional medicine with complementary therapies and the performing arts.

First, do no harm [he declares portentously]. *What is implicit in this simple precept of medicine? An awesome power – the power to do harm. Who gives you this power? The patient. A patient will come to you at his moment of greatest dread, hand you a knife and say, 'Doctor, cut me open!' Why? Because he trusts you. He trusts you the way a child trusts. He trusts you to do no harm. Sad fact is, human beings are not worthy of trust. It is human nature to lie, take short cuts, to lose your nerve, get tired, make mistakes. No rational patient would put his trust in a human being. And we're not gonna let him! It is our mission here to rigorously and ruthlessly train the humanity out of you and make you into something better. We're going to make* doctors *out of you!*

On that note the Dean turns on his heel and departs. At the prospect of being made into something better than a human being, all the students applaud rapturously – all, that is, except Adams.

* * * * *

The late Michael Crichton[136] is best known as the author of science fiction novels such as *Jurassic Park*, *The Andromeda Strain* and *Prey*, and as the creator of the NBC television series *ER*, set in a hospital emergency room. Before becoming a full-time writer, however, he qualified from Harvard as a doctor, though he spent only a short time in clinical practice.

Among Crichton's lesser-known non-fiction books is *Travels*,[137] first published in 1988. It consists mainly of accounts of, and reflections on, his journeys to some of the remotest and most exotic places on Earth. Its first section, however, is entitled 'Medical Days 1965–1969', and tells of a different, more private, journey – his passage through medical school, and the

---

136 John Michael Crichton (1942–2008) trained as a doctor, graduating *summa cum laude* from Harvard College in 1964 and receiving his MD from Harvard Medical School in 1969. While a medical student he began, and later published, a study of patients with pituitary tumours [Crichton M, Christy N, Damon A. Host factors in chromophobe adenoma of the anterior pituitary: a retrospective study of 464 patients. *Metabolism* 1981; **30**(3): 248–67]. Crichton's first novel, *Odds On*, was published under the pseudonym John Lange while he was still a medical student. He later went on to write over two dozen best-selling novels, as well as writing and directing numerous successful films.

137 Crichton M. *Travels*. London: Pan, 1989. Extracts are reproduced with the kind permission of the author.

exploration of his own inner world that it prompted. In the first chapter, 'Cadaver', Crichton describes his experience of dissecting a human body, and begins with this arresting sentence:

It is not easy to cut through a human head with a hacksaw.

When I first read this I thought, *He's right; it's very difficult.* Crichton would have been aged 22 or 23 at the time. I was even younger, 18, when, in the dissecting room at Cambridge University's Anatomy School, I too had to saw through a corpse's head down the mid-sagittal plane, so that two groups of students could have half a head each. Shuddering slightly at the memory, I read on:

The blade kept snagging the skin, and slipping off the smooth bone of the forehead. If I made a mistake, I slid to one side or the other, and I would not saw precisely down the center of the nose, the mouth, the chin, the throat. It required tremendous concentration. I had to pay close attention, and at the same time I could not really acknowledge what I was doing, because it was so horrible ...

Several times I stopped, cleaned the bits of bone from the teeth of the blade with my fingertips, and then continued. As I sawed back and forth, concentrating on doing a good job, I was reminded that I had never imagined my life would turn out this way ...

The eyes were inflated, staring at me as I cut. We had dissected the muscles around the eyes, so I couldn't close them. I just had to go through with it, and try and do it correctly.

And then I came to the passage that, more than any other thought or experience I have had, has prompted the writing of the present book.

Somewhere inside me, there was a kind of click, a shutting-off, a refusal to acknowledge, in ordinary human terms, what I was doing. After that click, I was all right. I cut well. Mine was the best section in the class. People came around to admire the job I had done, because I had stayed exactly in the midline and all the sinuses were beautifully revealed.

Now the key bit:

I later learned that this shutting-off click was essential to becoming a doctor. You could not function if you were overwhelmed by what was happening … I had to find a way to guard against what I felt.

And still later I learned that the best doctors found a middle position where they were neither overwhelmed by their feelings nor estranged from them. That was the most difficult position of all, and the precise balance – neither too detached nor too caring – was something few learned.

This 'click' of something shutting off so that we can bear the unbearable – it is as if there is inside us a switch that can be thrown in order to close off our spontaneous reactions and prevent them from getting in the way of what our professional role requires us to do.

Let's call it 'Crichton's switch'.

* * * * *

Since I came across these passages in *Travels*, I have read them aloud to numerous groups of doctors at every career stage during lectures and seminars I have given. On every occasion, as I look around at the faces of the audience, I see many people turn their attention inwards. Their eyes defocus and their heads droop. If I then ask for a show of hands to indicate who amongst them have been reminded of similar incidents in their own careers when, in order to cope with challenging or traumatic circumstances, they have had to suppress their instinctive reactions, most hands go up. Some people raise their hands rather sheepishly, as if ashamed to admit to strong feelings that sometimes needed to be switched off. Others do so more readily, encouraged by Crichton's story to want to tell their own.

Keen to explore further, I wrote to some of my medical friends and acquaintances, asking them if they had experienced any 'Crichton moments', and, if so, what they had made of them. From their replies it was clear that Crichton's switch is a common and significant phenomenon. Here are some of their stories and reflections, reproduced by the kind permission of the contributors.

Gunnar, a Swedish GP, recalls, like Michael Crichton, being a first-year medical student and dissecting a cadaver:

It was the first time I saw a dead human body. The smell was intense. A few of us shared one 'preparation', as the teachers called it. We made jokes to keep away the feelings of disgust. As I grew tired, the whole setting seemed to shift like Rubin's vase.[138] *It seemed preposterous that we were standing around a dead woman who had donated herself to science, cutting her open.*

I found out that the best way to bring back the medical setting by force was to get in close contact with the corpse. I touched the body with both my hands and tried to observe the detail of the muscles and nerves. It worked. The dead body became once again an anatomical object. I was back on track.

Unsurprisingly, medical students often find that cutting up a body during dissection is a shocking and powerful experience. Paul, a third-year undergraduate, tells how …

I was dislocating the hip joint in order to study its contents and bony structure. My colleague and I spent around 20 to 30 minutes trying to prise the femur from the pelvis, and, with an incredible amount of determination and the application of sheer strength, the bones eventually came apart with a pop.

It was at this moment I realised that, in order to apply so much force in breaking up a part of the body, I had stopped thinking of it as part of the human body at all.

Scenes of mutilation or violent death will often activate Crichton's switch. Xanthe, then a junior doctor working on a surgical firm, remembers:

One day we performed a forequarter amputation on a young woman for the recurrent sarcoma in her left arm. This involved removing the arm and shoulder girdle, leaving just the contour of the rib cage on that side. I was recounting this to a non-medical friend soon afterwards. He asked if there was any support or counselling for the medical staff. I remember that my Registrar had asked if I was OK after the operation, but recalled thinking at the time that this was quite unusual. My friend was horrified that as individual doctors and as a 'caring profession' we were so bad at looking after one another.

138 Rubin's vase: the well-known visual illusion where perception of a silhouette oscillates between a vase and two faces in profile.

David H, an experienced GP, recounts this incident from early in his career:

Just after seven on a sunny summer morning, a call came in from the local police. Would I go out immediately to a local farmhouse where they had found a body?

I drove straight there. Outside the door was a young police constable looking shocked and pale. Inside there was a body – an almost headless body. The farmer had placed a shotgun in his mouth, and blown most of his head off. I recall seeing brain on the ceiling, and a note on the kitchen table. 'I'm losing weight,' it read. 'I know this must be cancer. I can't face it alone, and I am alone. This is the best way. Forgive me.'

I certified death, and distinctly remember having the bizarrely inappropriate thought that I hoped it wouldn't turn out that his scales were faulty. I then attended to the policeman, who had needs I could help with, and drove home.

My wife, who hadn't known what sort of call this was, had cooked me a wonderful breakfast – bacon, eggs, even a sausage. Perfect. I devoured it happily, slurped down my coffee, and drove to the Health Centre to start morning surgery. Life was good.

And sitting in my consulting room at 11 o'clock I went ice cold. An almost painful chill passed down my spine. I thought, 'What sort of bastard have you turned into?' And I cried.

It is hardly surprising, when we are violently confronted with the inner workings of the physical body in all its blood and squelchiness, that some mental mechanism should kick in to protect us from sensory and imagination overload. Unsurprising, too, that the horrors we remember most vividly should date from early in our medical careers, before we have learnt to hide behind professional nonchalance. The dissecting room may very well be where we truly appreciate for the first time the dual nature of the 'person-as-machine' and the 'person-as-sentient-being, like me'.

The 'I' that I feel myself to be doesn't usually seem to have insides. The 'I' of which I am conscious has thoughts, sensations, emotions, memories, imagination – but not entrails. We don't think of our individual uniqueness as defined by the variation of our particular anatomies and physiologies. I think I know, intellectually, that my sense of 'I' is an emergent function of the brain inside this skull; but it doesn't *feel* like that. I can see that this is my skin; I can tell these are my muscles; I know my tongue can taste and my nose can smell. But the squishy inside bits, the vital organs that will snuff out 'me' when they fail, these for the most part I don't identify with. And it upsets me to be forcibly reminded – as by the sight of a laid-open body – that I *must* identify with them. Terrifying though it may be, 'I' is inseparable from the flesh that embodies it.

Paul, the medical student, resumes his story:

> *It is now difficult for me to recall exactly how I felt about the human body before I dissected one. Unlike other 'things', humans have the mysterious qualities of personality, intelligence, the ability to interact with one another etcetera. Taking a body apart, seeing the inside of the body as a complicated construction of machinery and wiring, brought me to see that the human body is not so different from other worldly objects when it does not have these active, energetic, human properties.*

Rather generously (it seems to my cynical mind), Paul concludes:

> *Although the main purpose of dissection is to learn about human anatomy, I suspect that part of the educators' rationale is also to allow students an early opportunity to see the fragility and complexity of human life.*

Sometimes the situation in which Crichton's switch protects us is emotionally harrowing rather than gruesome. Carol, an experienced midwife, was working in the labour ward:

> *I was asked to care for a 35-year-old woman who had a long history of infertility. She and her husband had conceived a child through the process of IVF [in vitro fertilisation], and this child was awaited with great anticipation. In the 24-hour period before she came under my care, this lady hadn't felt the baby moving, and on admission there was no foetal heartbeat detected. Two days before the due date, the baby was confirmed as an intrauterine death.*

> *When labour was approaching the end, and the delivery of this lifeless baby was imminent, I remember having palpitations, sweats and the overarching feeling that I was going to be physically sick. As the head appeared, the mother screamed, 'Carol, please make my baby breathe!' It was at this moment that*

the click, or 'power', kicked in. My physical symptoms vanished, leaving in their place a feeling of numbness which enabled me to conduct the delivery in a professional, caring and compassionate manner, with a strength I did not think I possessed. Something happened to my physical body which I could not explain; my shaking stopped, the palpitations settled and I no longer felt sick. I became suddenly very calm and controlled.

I think this click may be able to be switched on and off. I remember a few days later receiving a card and a gift from this couple, expressing their gratitude and saying how thankful they were that I was there to support them through one of the most difficult times of their lives. At that point, I remember all the emotions that I could have felt during the delivery, flooding in, and I cried in the privacy of my own home. This made me feel human.

Carol's story reminds us that there are circumstances when the flipping of Crichton's switch, bringing much-needed focus and self-control, is of benefit to both patient and doctor. At the time of this next incident, Julian, now an established GP, was a very newly qualified house officer, on call at the weekend for urology and orthopaedics. His senior house officer had gone off sick; an orthopaedic registrar was on call from home. Julian was called to see a rugby player brought in with a fracture–dislocation of an ankle, which the casualty officer thought would need to be reduced as the blood supply to the foot was compromised. He telephoned the registrar, who was playing tennis but would call back, and went down to the Accident and Emergency (A&E) department.

A big chap was lying on a trolley in a cubicle, screaming. While his right foot pointed towards the ceiling, the left one pointed in the direction of the wall. His bloated foot had a pale colour that I realised was not good.

Eventually my somewhat irritated Registrar was on the phone. He told me to get the casualty officer to reduce the ankle, otherwise the foot would be lost. The casualty officer refused as he didn't know how. It was now down to me.

Having been given some telephone advice I headed back to the cubicle. All eyes were on me. The senior A&E sister explained to me what I had to do. I felt a calmness descend. I saw someone's hands — mine, apparently — confidently take hold of the foot. The screaming became a low background hum. As I pulled the foot into a more conventional position I felt a warmth on the palms of my hands, and the foot turned pink. I was aware of a communal sense of relief around me, which I did not share. I was without emotion. In that moment I had changed.

It is interesting to follow the evolution of Julian's feelings through this harrowing episode. Initially, he was panicky, resentful and self-doubting:

To expect a newly qualified house officer to manipulate a dislocated ankle is clearly wrong and hazardous. I didn't realise this at the time. My anger and frustration were purely at myself. I thought this was a task any competent house officer would be able to do. I thought the reason I didn't know what to do was because of idleness at medical school. I didn't want to appear stupid or ignorant, so I just did whatever I was asked.

But as time went by …

… my emotions became increasingly blunted. Patients died left, right and centre, but I became numb to the human suffering. My priorities changed. I was pleased the ankle was reduced, but mainly because it meant I could go and get on with my other work. Only later did I realise I had done something quite amazing. This was a brutalisation, which continued until I began my GP training. Then I gradually changed back. I was given a chance to reflect on what I was doing. I became interested in patients again as people.

Lest we imagine that it is only in circumstances of crisis and drama that Crichton's switch operates, and before we learn how more of my correspondents were affected by it, let us pause and hear from Tom W, who practises in a very different field. Tom is a composer of classical music, but, when I told him about the internal 'blotting out' that could make the intolerable tolerable, he immediately recognised the phenomenon.

I have always thought of composition as a balance of the emotional and the rational. For me, the composing process falls pretty squarely into two phases: one in which I 'lose myself' and try to suspend my critical faculty in order to generate ideas and the other in which I order, edit, accept/reject and refine these ideas.

I asked Tom what might be his equivalent of having to saw a head in half.

Being made to sit down and write a fugue, which, to a musician, is the ultimate exercise in rational ordering. If that's what the whole of composition were to prove to be, I would have to turn off all hope and ambition that music could be moving. I would add that, while learning the nuts and bolts of one's compositional craft can at times be tedious, I can't imagine it involves the same sense of existential trauma as the head-sawing. The main challenge is to keep one's motivation up when the compositional task is pursued in the absence of the oxygen of creative thinking. Anaerobic composition, if you like.

* * * * *

As replies came in from the colleagues I had written to, I was struck both by the power of their stories and by their evident recognition that the experiences they were describing were, albeit sometimes only in hindsight, significant events in the development of their professional personas. They might by now have forgotten the anatomy of the tarsus and the stages in the Krebs cycle, but the memories remained vivid of how they came to learn that their feelings, and their ability to imagine the feelings of others, could be both a help and a hindrance in their work as doctors. It may of course be that, given my own personality and interests, I know only people with a penchant for this kind of navel-gazing. But I don't think so. Check out your own experience: take a moment of introspection now, and I'll warrant you can recall at least one episode in your own career where you too have needed to suppress an instinctive response in order to cope with a gruelling situation.

Thomas B, now a senior GP and unafraid (as we all should be) to acknowledge some ambivalence in his professional values, remembers this:

When I was a medical student I lived in a flat. One evening, the 60-something-year-old man downstairs suffered, as it transpired, a fatal heart attack. His wife, knowing I was a medic, called me to resuscitate him. Sometime during his cardiac arrest he had vomited, but I still had to do mouth-to-mouth. I think I experienced some kind of detachment, otherwise I would have been unable to carry out the task. I knew that the situation was hopeless, but felt obliged – because of the presence of his immensely distressed wife – to carry on until an ambulance arrived. Thinking about it now, I don't know whether, in similar circumstances, I could do the same thing again. It's the repellent nature of vomit that would stop me. But I suspect I probably would do the same again, because the circumstances of a desperate emergency would somehow enable me to overcome my revulsion. Maybe it's something to do with adrenaline, or with empathy for whoever the bystanders happened to be. I think I might not do mouth-to-mouth if I came across the arrest with no family or friends in attendance, and would rationalise this because I've now been taught that it's actually more important to keep the circulation going with whatever oxygenated blood is in the system by means of chest compressions than to do mouth-to-mouth. But I think it would be different if it were a child.

Not sure if this helps.

Yes, Thomas, it helps. It helps to have Michael Crichton's conclusion confirmed, that 'the best doctors find a middle position where they are neither overwhelmed by their feelings nor estranged from them. This is the most difficult position of all, and the precise balance – neither too detached nor too caring – is something few learn.' Difficult it may be; but finding a way to that centre ground between the extremes of emotional involvement and indifference is surely one of the core tasks for an emerging professional. 'Crichton moments' such as those reported by my correspondents are often seen, in retrospect, to be pivotal in the evolution of those values that our subsequent way of practice will come to embody.

That 'in retrospect' is important. Crichton moments make their learning points some time later. 'Poetry,' said Wordsworth, 'takes its origin from emotion recollected in tranquillity'.[139] By the same token, insight and professional growth come not from the flipping of Crichton's switch at a moment of crisis but rather from the realisation afterwards that a switch has been flipped. The self-awareness is all. Remember what David H told us; it was only *after* he had gone out to the suicide at the farm, after he had enjoyed a hearty breakfast, after he had been seeing patients for two hours in his surgery that he suddenly went ice cold, asked himself what sort of bastard he had turned into, and wept.

In another example of enhanced intuition following the reversal of Crichton's switch, Dan describes how when, as a medical house officer, he attended cardiac arrests:

… it was with little emotional attachment and a persistent sense of unreality. Even when I had to break the bad news to relatives, it felt like I was acting

---

139 William Wordsworth (1770–1850), English Romantic poet. Quotation from *Preface to Lyrical Ballads* (1800).

a part. This was the 'switch' that had been shut off. Did it have a functional advantage? I'm not sure. I remember being very clear headed during resuscitation – I knew exactly what needed to be done, and did it. It would have been difficult to remain effective if I was thinking about how upset the grandchildren were going to be.

However, it is the circumstances when the switch was turned back on that I remember with most clarity. I was working in paediatrics and we were called down to A&E. A beautiful girl, at most five or six years old, had been brought in by her distraught parents having stopped breathing. Her heart had stopped as well. She looked so full of life, with that slight chubbiness children have at that age. My consultant, who had previously struck me as entirely pragmatic and imperturbable, was upset as well. Outwardly she remained as level-headed as ever, but her nose went bright red: the only sign that she too was struggling to hold back tears.

Dan seems to have successfully made his way to that elusive middle ground where, combining detachment and empathy, he can recognise the reddening of his consultant's nose as a sign of supressed distress.

David W was also a newly qualified doctor when he told me this.

I am not sure when the light went out, but I remember the day it was turned back on. As a house officer I had precious little time to address the psychological needs of patients, let alone my own. Over a four-week period, I admitted a patient three times for draining of her malignant ascites, performing this quick and uncomplicated procedure with great effect. On the third occasion, however, I began to feel that perhaps there was more I could offer. I discovered she was frightened of dying, depressed at the futility of her plight, but most of all angry, because this inexorable disease was robbing her children of their mother. We both wept. I couldn't believe how selfish and perfunctory I had been, looking after a dying woman no older than my own mother, and I hadn't even bothered to ask her how she felt until now. Now I remember I am a human first and a doctor second.

As we saw earlier, it is often a student's or young doctor's encounter with a broken human body, and the realisation that *I too am made of that stuff* that first activates Crichton's switch. This shock of recognition also has its emotional counterpart when, through the mixed blessing of imagination, we can be set reeling by our ability to empathise with the mental distress of a fellow human being. The empathic *That could be me* reaction is the sharpest of double-edged swords. Without it, we are heartless automata; but, if we feel it too intensely, our own equanimity is at the mercy of every kind of anguish we encounter in our patients. What seems to have affected David W, and what took him several sessions of peritoneal drainage to recognise, is that his dying patient was no older than his own mother. Then the penny dropped – *That could be her!* – and in an instant he reached that middle ground where the symptom relief he could deliver as a good doctor was complemented by the compassion he could offer in the surrogate role of good son.

It can be unnerving, at least the first few times it happens, to witness a patient's psychological vulnerability and to have the distinct impression that we are looking in a mirror and seeing something of ourselves. With growing clinical experience there may come the wisdom that tuning in to the emotional resonances the patient evokes in us is one route to diagnostic insight. This lesson is at the heart of the Balint tradition in general practice; but it is learning of a high order, and on first exposure to it the doctor can feel threatened with a level of discomfort that might prove unbearable.

In the following account, Duncan, a final-year medical student, describes an episode during his attachment to a medium-secure psychiatric unit. He was introduced to a paranoid schizophrenic patient in his early thirties.

Talking to him reminded me of bargaining with a young child. As far as he was concerned he was not ill and needed no treatment; everyone around him was either an impostor or plotting against him. He wouldn't talk to the doctors, but for some reason he seemed to trust and open up to me.

I was cautioned not to buy into his delusions, which was easier said than done. His stories were very elaborate and it was often hard to discern fact from fiction. One of his delusions was that he was a doctor, and he had invented something, though what it was was a closely guarded secret.

It suddenly struck me that this man had been a medical student. His notes confirmed that, indeed, eleven years ago he had been in his second year at medical school when his psychosis became apparent. I initially felt like I should identify with him – but I could not. Talking to him was akin to holding a conversation with one of my younger siblings. Yet I found myself feeling not parental, but judgemental. I was casting elements of his story into either 'true' or 'false', dismissing his claims as the delusional thoughts of a sick man. Who was I to do this? If it were a child, you would find it amusing and play along. There was something in me that made that distinction and drove me to start making these judgements: something I wasn't quite sure I controlled.

We can sense that Duncan is poised on the edge of intuition, perceptive and self-aware, his finger nevertheless hovering, as it were, over Crichton's switch. In his meeting with this disturbed and disturbing patient (a former medical student), Duncan (also a medical student) finds himself facing a common professional ambivalence – *I felt I should identify with him, but I could not.* Emotional resonance leaves him feeling something of the cold and dismissive parent the patient himself may well have had, and something of the indulgent older brother the patient may well have longed for. It is only a short step from these countertransference feelings to valuable insights into the patient's world. But it is a dangerous step; insights like these come at a price, that price being the doctor's vain hope of remaining the uninvolved observer of the patient's predicament. Small wonder, therefore, that Crichton's switch cut in – *Something I wasn't quite sure I controlled drove me to be not parental, but judgemental.*

* * * * *

In a previous chapter, 'The medical gaze', I offered the image of a swivel-mounted zoom lens as a metaphor for how a doctor can view a problem in either close-up or wide-angle mode, and can attend to the internal world as well as the external. Crichton's switch seems to form part of the 'zoom and swivel' mechanism. We find the extremes of human misery hardest to contemplate when, in full wide-angle view, we see them, their ramifications and our own reactions as well – when, for example, we understand the effects of cancer not just on a breast but on the woman whose breast it is; on her partner, her family, the network of her friends; on her destiny and her legacy; and on those who will care for her, ourselves included. Activating Crichton's switch appears to flip the doctor into outwardly directed close-up mode, so that the attention becomes fully taken up with detail to the exclusion of context and self-awareness. Remember how Gunnar discovered in the dissecting room that *the best way to bring back the medical setting was to get in close contact with the corpse. He touched the body with both hands and tried to observe the detail of the muscles and nerves. It worked. The dead body became once again an anatomical object. He was back on track.* Remember too how

Paul, in similar circumstances, found that the sheer effort required to wrench a femur from its socket mercifully blocked his awareness of the gruesomeness of what he was doing.

So maybe it works the other way round as well. Maybe, if we need sanctuary from the pain of excessive empathy, zooming in (or being made to zoom in) on detail will do the trick. Shortly after I had qualified, when I was working as a house surgeon …

> *I admitted a boy of 15 with what looked like peritonitis. I assisted my consultant at the laparotomy. As soon as the abdomen was opened it was obvious that the poor lad was riddled with some malignancy. His liver was almost bursting with secondary deposits, his peritoneal cavity pouring ascites; he was clearly beyond surgical help. As the hopelessness of the situation dawned on everyone in the theatre there was total silence for a moment, and then I heard someone – me – sniff and choke back a sob. I could feel myself on the verge of running from the operating room, past the waiting parents whose world was about to implode, running perhaps from my newly hatched career as a doctor. 'Neighbour,' said the consultant, 'would you sew him up, please?' It was the first time he had asked me to do this; normally he liked to 'sign off' his operations by doing his own closure. Being forced to concentrate on the suturing immediately flipped me into close-up mode, and I was back in control of myself and doing something constructive. I don't know whether the surgeon gave me this task on purpose, but I suspect he did, and it was an act of great kindness.*

Another kind of 'enforced context shift' worked for Margaret as well:

> *Many years ago I was a Senior House Officer in obstetrics. Early one morning I was called to the post-natal ward, where a patient had chest pain. 'I think I'm going to die,' she cried, and collapsed. The crash trolley was on another block, and chaos ensued. Tragically the patient died, leaving a husband and two children. The consultant thought she had had a pulmonary embolism, but I disagreed. I thought she had dissected an aortic aneurysm, a feature of her Marfan's syndrome.*

> *My diagnosis was subsequently proved correct at post mortem. I was told I was presenting her case at the next Obs and Gynae meeting of the Royal Society of Medicine.*

The family's tragedy became my interesting case. I had to research the litera-
ture and make up slides to present at the meeting. The person was forgotten
about as her pathology took centre stage.

Margaret concludes her memoir by wondering, *How many doctors are*
able to hide their feelings in this way? Yet from the very fact that she can ask
this question we know that she has *not* hidden her feelings, and the patient
has not been forgotten. Margaret too has reached the middle ground where
empathy and detachment co-exist, to the mutual enhancement of each.

* * * * *

Using the word 'switch' to describe the suppression of our human responses
when they threaten to overwhelm us rather suggests that this is an all-or-
nothing on-or-off phenomenon. But, for some of my correspondents at least,
Crichton's is a switch of the continuously variable dimmer variety, not the
two-position toggle kind.

Jamie, now a GP and trainer, recalls the first time he was present when a
hospice patient died:

He was only 12 years older than me, with end stage carcinomatosis. We'd
struck up a good relationship as I tried to help him adjust to the steroids,
keep his appetite ticking over, and help his wife and three-year-old daughter
through the process. It was the middle of the afternoon when the nurses called
me to say his breathing had deteriorated. His wife was at his bedside and
his daughter was outside the room, playing with a Star Wars version of the
Mister Potato Head toy called Spud Vader. Funny the bits you remember. He
had stopped breathing and the nurse asked me to certify death. I listened with
the stethoscope, and suddenly he took one deep long gasping breath.

SWITCH. He's Cheyne–Stokesing, I thought, as a normal breathing pattern
returned. His wife looked at me confused, almost smiling, but tortured. I
left the room, telling the nurse I would return in five or ten minutes. Just 12
years older than me. What would I be doing in 12 years' time? By the time
I returned I knew I needed to carry out the necessary clinical procedures but
also acknowledge the feelings I had for him and his family. This time as I
listened to his chest there was a breath, very faint, and his eyes looked straight
into mine. Then – no more breaths. 'He's gone,' I said. It was the good death,
with his wife beside him, that they had wanted.

We talked, his wife and I, about his progress from diagnosis to hospice and the difficulties of facing all this in their 30s. I think it was therapeutic for her, but it certainly was for me. If I had opened up my whole feelings about it all, I would have cried with her, and I don't think that would have been what she needed. So for me it's not a switch, but a dimmer, feeding varying degrees of basic humanity into the clinical knowledge and bedside manner: a dimmer that can be flexibly adjusted depending on the situation.

And Andrew, a registrar in general practice, writes:

The switch is not a switch in the true mechanical sense. For me it's more a dial with no zero. You can turn the dial down to very low levels, so low that it almost doesn't register, but never off. You always react to emotionally difficult situations, whether you choose to acknowledge it or not. You have to in order to survive in medicine but also in order to grow and learn. Have the dial too low and you become emotionally distant; too high and you are too emotionally involved to give the best care. Certainly when I was doing surgery I had the dial too high at the start, but then it was turned down very quickly. My current struggle, as I switch to general practice, is to turn it back up to the right level.

* * * * *

The English language, or rather my grasp of it, is letting me down. If becoming a professional is the goal, how shall we describe the prior condition of the physician-in-training? I want a word or a catchy phrase to denote the untutored state of the brand-new day-one medical student before medical education is applied. *Unprofessionalism*, which implies falling short of some ethical standard, certainly isn't right. *Innocence* makes it sound as if what follows will inevitably corrupt. *Artlessness* is too often the prelude to cynicism. *Naïvety*, although strictly speaking signifying nothing more than lack of experience, is sometimes interpreted as gullibility, a magnet for the attention of those who would exploit, deceive or sneer. I quite like *beginner*, not least for its association with the Zen master's remark quoted in my opening chapter: *In the beginner's mind there are many possibilities.* But to call someone a beginner is to give them an avuncular pat on the head and not much more.

So I think, at risk of ambiguity, I'm going to go with *naïvety*, in its original sense of being unspoiled by too much sophistication. To be naïve is to be natural and spontaneous as opposed to over-complicated and artificial, unaffected as opposed to pretentious. The naïvety of the medical student is to be appreciated for its curiosity and altruism as well as the sponge-like way it can be made to absorb tuition.

Between the naïvety of the novice and the competence of the qualified doctor are many journeys, to be undertaken simultaneously. Some have factual knowledge as their destination, others practical skills. Long though they be, these journeys lie through territory well mapped by educational theorists and curriculum designers. The most difficult journey is a quest for a grail less tangible but arguably more precious – the accumulation of ways of thinking, behaving and practising that, taken as a whole, we call 'professionalism'. Tasked with guiding a young doctor through this foggy domain, many medical teachers find themselves at the edge of their comfort zones, and are tempted to throw up their hands and flee, crying, 'Here be dragons!'

Professionalism is one of those things easier to define in terms of their opposite. We all know *un*professionalism when we see it: the doctor who is inept, unfeeling, inconsiderate, unreliable or arrogant lets down not only his or her own patients but also the generality of colleagues whose integrity is tarnished by association. Professionalism largely comes down to trustworthiness. In 2005 a working party convened under the auspices of the Royal College of Physicians defined medical professionalism as: 'a set of values, behaviours and relationships that underpin the trust the public has in doctors'.[140]

'Trust' was one of Dean Walcott's favourite words. 'The patient trusts you like a child,' he told his impressionable young audience in the scene from *Patch Adams*. 'But, being human, you take short cuts, lose your nerve, get tired, make mistakes. You are not worthy of trust.' The Dean, if you recall, saw his mission as to protect patients from medical error by rigorously and ruthlessly training the humanity out of his students and making them into something better. He said 'doctors', but he meant 'robots'. Walcott's ideal graduate would be a doctor like the third *matryoshka* doll we met in Chapter

---

140 Royal College of Physicians. *Doctors in Society: medical professionalism in a changing world.* Report of a Working Party of the Royal College of Physicians of London. RCP, London, 2005. In February 2005 the RCP working party, of which I was privileged to be a member, took evidence from Dame Janet Smith DBE, a Lady Justice of Appeal and former Chairman of the Shipman Inquiry, the public investigation into the activities of the GP and serial killer Harold Shipman. 'Professionalism,' Dame Janet told us, 'is a basket of qualities that enables us to trust our advisors.' The learned judge is meticulous in her use of English; when she says 'enables' and not 'enable', she is emphasising that the professionalism resides in the totality of qualities taken as a whole, not in any incomplete subset of them.

1 – uncompromisingly committed to the traditional medical model; ruthlessly logical; undistracted by an inner life (his own or the patient's); someone for whom 'care' is a commodity, not a verb. In the language of the present chapter, Walcott's aim would be to flip Crichton's switch in every aspiring doctor, firmly and permanently. You would think he would be pushing at an open door. Given how many young doctors experience Crichton clicks in circumstances of high stress, the task of brutalising the humanity out of them should be easy. All you should need to do is to expose them systematically to scenes of intense physical and psychological trauma; train them to endure extreme fatigue; rehearse them in the role of infallible demigod; and forbid any display of emotion in the workplace.

Now where have I come across a training programme like that? Oh yes, I remember …

No doubt I shall be told that medical schools are not like that any more. And I shall say how pleased I am to hear it, and cross my fingers.

What *is* true, on the evidence of my correspondents, is that Crichton's switch is one stage in a pathway to professionalism that is a good deal more sophisticated than Walcott could ever contemplate. Figure 9.1 attempts to show this graphically, with the optimum route emphasised.

A young person entering medical school, although selected for intellectual ability, has – or should have – nothing special in the way of background or life experience. Neither privilege nor deprivation should confer any advantage. What the majority of students know of life, of families, of relationships, of the roller coaster of emotions is pretty much what most youngsters do. Unsurprising, therefore, that the physical and emotional horrors they inevitably encounter in the next few years will challenge their resilience almost to breaking point.

At moments of such extremity, Crichton's protective switch needs to activate. Should it fail, the student or young doctor may be so traumatised as to abandon medicine as a career, or else become locked into an ineffectual pattern of over-sensitivity and over-involvement that will eventually foster an unhealthy degree of mutual dependency between doctor and patient. Perhaps you can think of a colleague with a non-functioning Crichton's switch. Such a one cannot, indeed, 'switch off', is often overwhelmed by relatively minor problems, and perhaps becomes a compulsive carer, addicted to being needed.

If Crichton's switch operates as it is meant to in a crisis, inhibitory reactions such as revulsion, horror or paralysis are suppressed. Also suppressed is the power of imagination, which in less extreme circumstances confers the ability to empathise and identify with the patient in distress. Perception

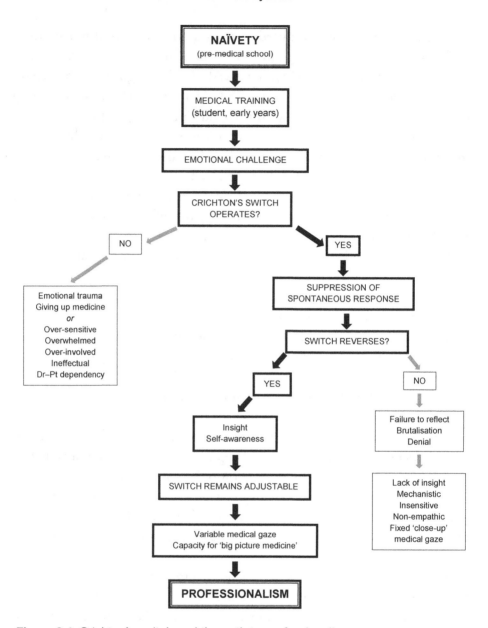

Figure 9.1 Crichton's switch and the path to professionalism.

zooms into close-up mode, focusing on detail rather than context. A kind of tunnel vision sets in, and a bubble of calm concentration is established, inside which the emergency can be managed with almost serene objectivity.

The stress-induced suppression of normal psychological responses is, mercifully, seldom permanent. Whatever it is that Crichton's switch turns off wants to come surging back. It may be soon, it may be delayed; it may be sudden or gradual; but the usual course of events is for the switch to revert, at least in part, to its pre-crisis position. The ability to imagine, to feel, to see things in context and in perspective all reassert themselves. And, as we have seen in many of the stories in this chapter, the reversal of Crichton's switch is followed by a growth spurt in insight, emotional competence and self-awareness. But should the reversal fail, a doctor afflicted with a jammed Crichton's switch – and perhaps you have met one – remains brutalised, unable to leaven the mechanics of medical practice with much sensitivity or human responsiveness.

My informants, whom I consider to be all professionally well-adjusted, report that, having once experienced the psycho-protective effect of Crichton's switch, they subsequently find that they can call upon it almost at will in the course of everyday practice. Situations constantly arise when it is useful to be able consciously to decide how much of one's emotional experience to allow into the clinical process. Patrick, a young GP, gives an example that is not as banal as it might seem, of how he can press the switch …

> *when examining a patient's visual fields. There's a game children play where you have to stare at each other and the first person to laugh is the loser. It is not uncommon for either myself or the patient to start smiling when I ask them to stare at my nose and point if they see a finger moving. I'm aware of the possibility of a smile before I begin the examination but somehow I banish this prospect from my possible reactions – a 'This is no time for joking, I have a job to do' sort of attitude. I'm aware of a switch on my part. Occasionally if a patient starts smiling then I will smile too, but I like to think I have a choice.*

In my own practice, I found that I could stop myself laughing at some nonsense I was being told by calling to mind my childhood memory of my grandmother as she lay dying. And I have certainly had the experience, when brought by the pathos of a patient's situation to the verge of tears of my own, of being able to take a detached decision on whether or not it will help the process of the consultation to allow them to be shed. A fully functioning Crichton's switch allows the doctor to choose how much of his or her own inner life to make available to the patient.

So, after its initial deployment, Crichton's switch is adjustable. Some experience it as like a toggle switch, either on or off; for others it is more continuously variable between the two extreme positions. Another colleague once told me it felt as if his attention was constantly and very rapidly oscillating between the external objective world in which the patient resided and the private subjective world of his own thoughts. This state of simultaneously monitoring both inner and outer worlds strikes me as a very sophisticated but nonetheless highly desirable professional mindset; and it is one to which we shall return before this book is done. I am again reminded of the wisdom of E.M. Forster's observation that 'truth, being alive, is not halfway between anything. It is only to be found by continuous excursions into either realm.'

At all events, one of the corollaries of having an effective Crichton's switch is that the 'bubble of calm concentration' and the big picture view of illness in all its complexity are both available to the self-aware practitioner. Without the switch there can be no variability in the medical gaze; and without that variability of gaze – that capacity to understand the multidimensional nature of human distress – the doctor's professional trustworthiness is diminished.

Michael Crichton was right in his observation that 'the best doctors find a middle position where they are neither overwhelmed by their feelings nor estranged from them'. But I think he was unduly pessimistic in concluding that the balance of being neither too detached nor too caring is a position attained only by a few.

An old story tells of a craftsman who carved exquisite likenesses of elephants from unpromising blocks of wood. Asked how he did it, he replied, 'I just cut away the bits of wood that *don't* look like an elephant.' If our concern is for more of us, at every stage of a medical career, to achieve Crichton's elusive position of balance, our task is like the woodcarver's. We needn't try to force sensitivity, empathy and compassion into people who would otherwise lack these qualities; they have never been absent. We must just guard against their being clumsily chipped away in the frenzy of training and clinical practice, so that the totality of our latent physicianly qualities can be revealed.

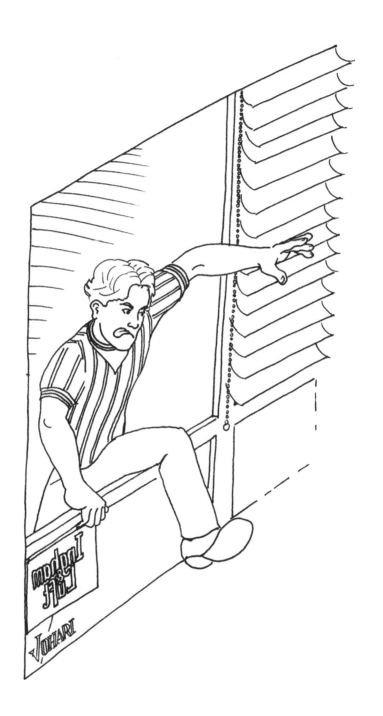

Chapter 10

Through Johari's window

The Outer – from the Inner
Derives its Magnitude –
'Tis Duke, or Dwarf, according
As is the central mood –
…
The Inner – paints the Outer –
The Brush without the Hand –
Its Picture publishes – precise –
As is the inner Brand –

Emily Dickinson (1830–86)

American poet

From poem number 450

Medicine is not only a science, but also the art of letting our own
individuality interact with the individuality of the patient.

Albert Schweitzer (1875–1965)

French theologian and medical missionary

The nibs who study these matters claim, I believe, that this has got
something to do with the subconscious mind, and very possibly
they may be right. I wouldn't have said off-hand that I *had* a
subconscious mind, but I suppose I must without knowing it.

Bertie Wooster in *Right Ho, Jeeves!* (1922)

by P.G. Wodehouse (1881–1975)

The poet Emily Dickinson was a reclusive spinster from Massachusetts whose
concentrated little verses prickle in the mind like popping candy on the
tongue. In one of them (number 1263) she advises:

Tell all the Truth but tell it slant –
Success in Circuit lies

She would, I think, be pleased with the circuitous way I have so far approached my central thesis: namely, that inside every professionally trained doctor there remains an untrained 'amateur' element – an Inner Physician – contributing in crucial but often under-appreciated ways to the doctor's effectiveness.

When we reviewed the history of our profession, we saw that medicine was for many centuries the province of the doctor who, for lack of any science, had nothing but himself to offer his patient. And – with a few notable exceptions such as Hippocrates and William Harvey – the self he had to offer was not a particularly effective one, doctors all too often fobbing off the scared and the gullible with quackery and baloney. But with the Age of Enlightenment superstition began to be supplanted by reason. The scientific method personified in Isaac Newton revealed that the universe ran like clockwork; and so too, it seemed, did the human body, just one more mechanism in a mechanical world. The doctor-who-was-little-but-a-person made way for the doctor-who-is-nothing-but-a-mechanic, and human beings in their grateful millions have lived longer and healthier lives as a result.

Then Newtonian determinism was obliged in its turn to yield to the relativities of quantum theory. With Einstein, science entered the realm of 'it all depends'. What we see, Einstein realised, depends on who it is who looks and on how the looking is carried out. To engage with the world is to alter it; questioning changes the narrative. The observer effect is everywhere, even – *especially* – in our consulting rooms. The idea that one person (a doctor) can study and manipulate another (the patient) in the same dispassionate way that a palaeontologist might chip away at a fossil simply will not stack up. Medicine is impersonal science conducted within a personal relationship, and not the other way round.

As generalists, we know that we draw upon more than just our medically trained selves when we diagnose, treat and relate to our patients. Unknowingly but inescapably, the patient who consults us consults the *whole* of us; and it is the parallel unspoken consultation with our private thoughts and feelings that unlocks our intuition, empathy and insight. The doctor-who-is-still-also-a-person is an advance on the doctor-who-is-nothing-but-a-mechanic. 'You and your arithmetic,' sang Danny Kaye to the inchworm looping its dreary way across the marigolds, 'you'll probably go far. Seems to me,' he mused, 'you'd stop and see how beautiful they are.' By the same token, the doctor with a functioning Inner Physician not only knows how to measure and analyse but can also step back and appreciate the beauty, the mystery, of the person being measured.

When we looked in more detail at the medical gaze, we saw that the price of specialisation is inflexibility. The specialist gaze tends to get stuck in either close-up 'detail' mode or wide-angle 'context' mode. The more reliant the doctor becomes on either one, the greater the risk of disuse atrophy of the other. In contrast, the hallmark of the generalist gaze is its variability, the way it can zoom appropriately back and forth between detail and context. And it goes further. The generalist gaze can also swivel inwards and attend to the internal world of the doctor's Inner Physician in a way that the specialist gaze does not; the observer becomes the self-observed.

Does all this complication matter? Can't medicine just be a question of a person who is sick getting advice from someone who knows what to do about it? Do we really need to embroider this already difficult task with so much introspection and navel-gazing? When my book *The Inner Consultation* first came out in 1987, and I had to start declaring royalties to the taxman, I went to see my accountant. Feeling rather pleased with myself, I asked him, 'Do accountants agonise about the accountant–client relationship like we do about the doctor–patient relationship?' He looked up from his paperwork, sighed wearily, and said, 'Don't be silly.' And he was right. I mean no disrespect to his profession; it calls for years of training and mastery of a body of knowledge way beyond my personal grasp. But ultimately all I want from my accountant is to be told how much tax I have to pay. If that advice comes with courtesy, friendliness, even a touch of sympathy – well, that's nice. But it's not essential. To be brutally honest, if he knows the regulations and can work a calculator, I'm happy. And he in turn can go home happy if nothing has flummoxed him and he's got his sums right. Need medicine be any different in kind?

Well, yes, it must. The relieving of human distress cannot be reduced to regulations, and is so complex that a state of flummox is never far away. There are seldom any clear-cut answers, just what is 'probably the best thing to do'. Illness is not synonymous with disease, nor health with its absence. As catastrophe theory showed us, people flip between health and illness in ways that don't correlate precisely with the waxing and waning of physical abnormalities. What we might call an 'inner patient' is at work, tempering the effects of biological fluctuations with an array of non-corporeal factors such as personality, self-image, family and social networks, moods, emotions, motivations, beliefs, values …

Nor is diagnosis a straightforward matter of fault-finding in the body's machinery. Diagnosis, as we have seen, is hermeneutics – making sense of an illness narrative, told not only in the patient's words but revealed also through the body's language of physical signs and acted out in the patient's behaviour. A comprehensive 'big picture' diagnosis needs to make several simultaneous kinds of sense: biological and pathological sense; emotional sense; sense in the context of the patient's personality, circumstances and world view. We therefore see in practice a tension between, on the one hand, a diagnostic process that is rigorous but of limited scope, exemplified by the Bayesian and algorithmic approach beloved of the specialist, and, on the other, the generalist's widespread use of heuristics – the fuzzier, wider-ranging but error-prone strategy of the educated guess.

Practising clinicians tend to use a combination or composite of the systematic and the intuitive, such as the approach described by Heneghan and his colleagues.[141] It starts with the doctor thinking of a list of diagnostic possibilities that might make sense of salient features in the patient's presentation, then whittling them down by applying scientific logic. But there's the rub; how do we come up with possibilities in the first place? To repeat Dr Soma Weiss's shrewd observation, 'A diagnosis is easy, as long as you think of it.' Some part of our awareness must be scanning the patient's narrative in its various modalities, sifting it for relevance, disregarding some bits of information and weighting others, comparing its salient features against our existing library of diagnostic templates until – *Bingo!* – one of them is enough of a match to deserve inclusion on a shortlist of possibilities. We ignore '… rained on Tuesday …' and '… as I said to Ethel …' But our medical ears prick up at '… knees … stiff … painful …' A mental bell rings: *arthritis*, we think; and a glance at the patient's misshapen joints appears to support this tentative diagnosis. We check: 'May I just have a look at your hands, please?' Heberden's nodes; just as I thought. 'OK, it looks to me as if you might be developing osteoarthritis …'

Coming up with possible diagnoses is an example of the 'figure-ground' phenomenon, where the task for our perceptual mechanism is to distinguish what is meaningful from its irrelevant background. At first sight, Figure 10.1 is just a scattering of random splodges.[142] However, if you know there are such things as Dalmatian dogs, the chances are that you'll quickly recognise that this is a picture of one. But you have to know about Dalmatians (or at least dogs) in the first place, otherwise you'll never see it. And once you've

---

141 Heneghan C, Glasziou P, Thompson M, *et al*. Diagnostic strategies used in primary care. *British Medical Journal* 2009; **338**: b946. This 'Oxford model' of diagnosis was more fully described in Chapter 8.

142 Original photograph by Ronald C. James, first published in *Life Magazine* 1965; **58**(7): 120.

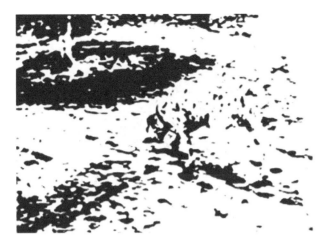

Figure 10.1 Figure – ground A.

seen it (Figure 10.2), you will never be able to not see it; indeed, you'll wonder why it isn't obvious to everyone.

This begs two questions. First, how do we come to build up our library of recognisable disease templates against which to compare the salient features in the patient's story? And, second, how do we decide which features *are* the salient ones?

The answer to the first question is easy, at least as far as organic disease goes. This is what medical schools are for. Training to be a doctor consists largely of having one's knowledge bank populated with clusters of symptoms and signs, each labelled with the name of a disease and underpinned by the associated anatomy, physiology and pathology. My personal 'psoriasis' template, for example, includes: purple plaques with silvery scales; not particularly itchy; extensor, not flexor; may affect joints and nails; possible recent history of streptococcal infection. If my selective attention notices enough features of a patient's rash that fit the template, somewhere in my mind the 'psoriasis' bell rings, and I'm ready to start testing this hypothesis like the rational scientist I am. But the early part of the process – the matching of features to template – is largely subliminal, pre-conscious; the tentative diagnosis 'just comes to me'.

The second question – how we preferentially light upon some features in the patient's narrative rather than others, and deem them to be 'salient' – is more complex. As for the well-known hallmarks of organic disease, such as pain, weight loss, swelling, bleeding, we are professionally trained to be on the alert for them. But, as we saw in Chapter 5, more things are relevant to people's illnesses, and to recovery from them, than just the presence or

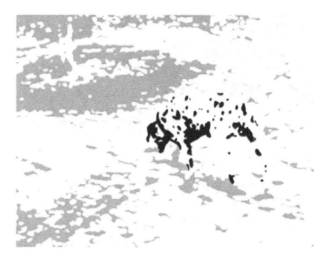

Figure 10.2 Figure – ground B.

absence of physical disease. To the big picture diagnostician, 'salient' features include all those that matter to the patient in their particular predicament: everything that matters within an individual life with its unfoldings and diversions, a life of emotions and relationships, of priorities, beliefs, opinions. Salience has to be defined on the patient's terms, not ours. And if diagnosis is to be more than mere disease-labelling, and is to carry us on to the threshold of helpful intervention, the scope of our competence needs to extend way beyond the usual biomedical territory. We need eyes that can detect an unshed tear or the falsity of a too-bright smile. We need ears that can hear the rattling of skeletons in a family cupboard. We need emotional intelligence that can recognise and empathise with loneliness, or misery or dread. We need the ability to read between the lines of an apparently outlandish presentation and make out its subtext of anxiety.

Such sensitivities were certainly not instilled into us as part of our formal medical education. Indeed, as the stories of Crichton's switch showed in the previous chapter, they have often been actively trained *out* of us. Luckily, we each have our personal Inner Physician, which was pre-installed before we ever went to medical school and is being continuously updated throughout our professional and non-professional lives. Episodes of intense focus on the biomedical aspects of the job, when our medical gaze is at 'maximum close-up' setting, may, Crichton-wise, render us temporarily deaf to our Inner Physician. But in normal circumstances all that is needed is for us to open the 'mind's ear' to its promptings.

Rooting in my memory for an example of the Inner Physician in action, I found myself recalling a patient from many years ago, an irritatingly obsequious little man in his fifties. Let's call him Derek.

'It's ever so good of you to see me, Doctor,' he began. 'I know I get on your nerves.'

'No, no,' I lied.

'Anyway,' he said, 'I must just tell you the fascinating saga of my catarrh.'

I could feel my teeth clench.

'And,' Derek continued, 'I play little tunes to myself on my teeth.'

What went through my mind was certainly *not* a list of the causes of catarrh. My consultation skills training kicked in.

'Tunes on your teeth?' I echoed.

'Yes,' he said, 'like this.' And he began rhythmically tapping his canines, upper against lower, alternating left and right. 'There,' he said, 'that was *The Entertainer*, by Scott Joplin. Is that normal?'

Give me strength, I thought; and exasperation took hold of my tongue.

'Derek,' I told him (I was always 'Doctor', he was always 'Derek'), 'I don't know whether to laugh or throw you out.'

'That's what my wife tells me,' he replied. 'Anyway, it's laugh or cry, isn't it? That's what they say.'

Luckily, exasperation loosened its grip before it could turn to rudeness, and some protective part of my mind asserted itself: *Keep calm; don't say anything hasty that you'll regret*. Behind what I hope was an impassive face, my Inner Physician was in overdrive, monitoring the headlong rush of my reactions, the self observing the self; registering, taking stock, remembering, connecting, wondering, supposing, and whispering – whispering *what*? Rational analysis? Partly. *This is not psychosis*. But mainly my thoughts were less than rational, or possibly beyond rational – associations, intuitions, hunches. *Clenched teeth – that's suppressed anger. Whose anger? Mine, certainly, but maybe his as well. And 'laugh or cry' – what's that about? Why 'cry'? And the wife: does she think he's funny? Does she really want to throw him out?* An idea emerged from the fog. Spoken out loud, it sounded banal.

'You're not happy.'

'No, I'm not,' he said, with some vehemence. And then it all came out: the missed promotions; the less-than-hoped-for salary; the son of 22, recently diagnosed as schizophrenic; the younger daughter, so flawless as a child, now almost crippled by obsessional rituals and bullied at work.

'I can probably help with the catarrh,' I said lamely.

'Oh, that. It's not important. But thank you anyway,' he said. 'No, really – thank you, Doctor.'

It seemed it was more important that Derek's distress be fully recognised rather than partly relieved. He, of course, neither knew nor cared whether he was consulting with the trained physician in me ('I can probably help with the catarrh') or my Inner Physician ('You're not happy'). The distinction exists solely in the privacy of my own head, and then only in hindsight, when I reflect on what happened; in real time, there were just 'thoughts of unknown origin', arising, competing. For his part, Derek knew only that some of the things I said to him seemed to close him down, while others opened him out.

How is that recognition of distress made and communicated? I myself know at first hand – which of us does not? – something of Derek's feelings: something of disappointment; something of what it is like to be helpless while a loved one suffers; something of feeling ashamed of one's own short-comings, yet wanting to be accepted in spite of them. It is as if all our life experiences, not just those at medical school, leave patient-shaped imprints on us, like smell receptors contoured to the molecules they are primed to recognise – imprints, in this case, into which some of Derek's own hurt could nestle and be comforted. For what we know, we can recognise; and what we recognise we can find ways to soothe.

I take no credit for any apparent skill or insight in what proved a pivotal conversation in our relationship. We doctors all have an Inner Physician similarly poised to contribute to our encounters with patients. The issue is whether or not we allow it to.

The Inner Physician is only a metaphor; no tangible neurology underlies it. It is simply a convenient way of referring to some fraction of our totality that is there in our consultations to be drawn upon. A nice way of envisaging the various fractions of our mental totality is the well-known Johari's window.

* * * * *

When I first came across Johari's window in the 1980s someone told me, and for a while I believed it, that its creator was one Ernst Johari, a psychoanalyst from Bucharest. But no; this handy little map of the human psyche is the brainchild of Joseph Luft and Harrington Ingham, psychologists working on group relations at the University of California in 1955.[143] 'Johari' is a portmanteau of their two first names, Joe and Harry.

---

143 Luft J, Ingham H. The Johari window, a graphic model of interpersonal awareness. *Proceedings of the Western Training Laboratory in Group Development.* Los Angeles: UCLA, 1955.

Johari's window invites us to categorise the contents of our mind – thoughts, memories, facts, knowledge, personality, emotions, opinions, beliefs, motivations, intentions, imaginings – according to who knows about them: we ourselves and/or other people. This sets up a simple grid with four quadrants, shown in Figure 10.3.

Some things about ourselves we know to be the case, and other people know them as well, or at least, we don't mind if they know. My name, my shoe size, my marital status, my job, whether or not I can speak French or play the piano (yes and no respectively) – all this I am happy to be public knowledge. Stuff that anybody is welcome to know about us goes in the 'public' quadrant of Johari's window.

Known to self?

	Yes	No
Known to others? Yes	PUBLIC	BLIND
No	PRIVATE	UNKNOWN

Figure 10.3 Johari's window.

Other aspects of ourselves we prefer to keep private, or at least known only to a few close confidants whom we trust with our vulnerabilities. These are the secrets we know about ourselves, but others do not, and we don't intend that they should. Our hidden agendas; our character flaws and peccadilloes; for some of us, our politics, religion or sexual preferences; the traumas that haunt us, the fantasies that excite or scare us; the emotions that perhaps embarrass us and the less-than-noble schemings that drive us – these all go in Johari's 'private' quadrant.

Some things about us other people can see, but we cannot. This, in Johari terms, is our 'blind' area. What in the mirror may look to us like lamb, to the onlookers is plainly mutton. A candid opinion I regard as refreshingly honest might rightly be recognised by its recipient as an expression of my persistent adolescent rebelliousness. The contents of the 'blind' quadrant are not the results of wilful concealment or conscious denial; these belong in the 'private' area. The attributes to which we are blind more often come about through the workings of cognitive dissonance, the unconscious self-protective re-interpreting of unwelcome truths.

Finally, the Johari window has an 'unknown' quadrant – deep, dark, unconscious territory through which psychoanalysts pick their cautious way by Freudian torchlight. Here are located all the psychological drives that, notwithstanding their often far-reaching impact on our thoughts and behaviour, neither we nor anyone else are consciously aware of: our profoundest motivations, the lingering influences of early experience that script our unfolding destiny.

The boundaries between quadrants are movable; they can shift over time and according to whom we are dealing with. The content of our 'public' quadrant, for example, enlarges as we accumulate knowledge and experience. Personal information that I might initially withhold from a new acquaintance I might opt to disclose as we get to know each other better.

The boundaries are also porous, allowing items to cross from one quadrant to another. We might find it can in fact be safe to make public some of the information that previously we kept private. We can gain insight into our blind spots; and hidden motives can be inferred from our actions and choices, and thereby brought to light.

I like Johari's window, not just for its simple elegance, but also for how it suggests that we can change through interpersonal relationships. Indeed, Luft and Ingham developed it originally as a tool in the training of counsellors and group therapists. We are mentally at our healthiest (they suggested) if we can maximise the 'public' at the expense of the 'private', the 'blind' and the 'unknown'. The fewer secrets we feel we need to conceal, the more truths about ourselves we can learn from other people, and the better we understand the forces at work in our subconscious, the more we feel at ease with ourselves and the less likely we are to be unsettled by life's vicissitudes.

To achieve a private-to-public shift (how Marxist that sounds!) calls for self-disclosure. We need to take the risk of revealing something of ourselves hitherto kept secret, trusting – and usually finding – that it will be found acceptable. Any self-disclosure needs, of course, to be voluntary and intentional, so that we are not bullied or tricked into 'letting it all hang out'. With that proviso, life is usually easier if we don't feel compelled to defend the boundaries of our privacy too desperately.

Reducing our 'blind' and 'unknown' areas requires us to become conscious of matters we were hitherto unaware of, generally with the help of a third party (see Figure 10.4). It is usually as a result of constructive feedback on our

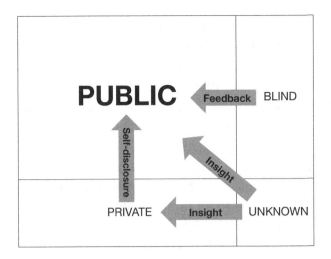

Figure 10.4 Moving the Johari boundaries.

behaviour from someone whose judgement and benevolence we trust that we can make inroads into our 'blind' area. My one-time mentor John Heron[144] had a nice phrase for the kind of feedback that is effective in this context; he called it 'loving confrontation'. Gaining insight into our 'unknown' area calls for more sustained and committed self-exploration, such as is usually undertaken only with a trained therapist.

Self-disclosure, feedback and insight – these are the means whereby the private, blind and unknown sectors of our minds can be helped to see the light of day, and thus make their fullest contribution to our mental well-being.

* * * * *

What has all this to do with the Inner Physician? Actually, everything. Be advised, Emily Dickinson; here is an end to circuit. Through Johari's window we can see the Inner Physician much more clearly.

Although some people view doctors as 'expertise on legs', nothing more and nothing less, the truth is that whenever a doctor sits down to consult with a patient it is the *whole* of the doctor who is present. Both patient and doctor, because they are each human beings, have within their psyches the four Johari quadrants. But, because this is a professional and not just a social encounter, the doctor's Johari's window in this case is a map of all those of the doctor's attributes that potentially have a therapeutic impact on the

---

144 John Heron (b. 1928), humanistic psychologist. See also Chapter 3, footnote 70.

patient, partitioned according to whether or not doctor and patient are aware of them. This allows us to distinguish between those parts of himself or herself that the doctor *intends* to make available to the patient, and those parts that the patient *in fact* draws upon (see Figure 10.5).

Equivalent to Johari's 'public' area – the information we are happy to be in the public domain – is the doctor's huge accumulation of medical knowledge, skills and resources acquired over years of medical education and experience: all the clinical acumen and manual dexterity; the access to all the facilities and networks of colleagues; the familiarity with how the healthcare system operates; the authority to make things happen – everything, in short, that a patient expects, and has the right to expect, from a medical professional. The doctor knows that all this is legitimately and routinely at the patient's disposal, and the patient knows it too.

What the doctor does *not* routinely allow the patient to know – the equivalent of the 'private' box – is the intimate detail of his or her own private life, past and present. To be sure, some personal information may already be in the public domain, or at least not secret – marital status, for example, home address, perhaps the number and names of any children. But, in general, we like there to be limits to what patients may know about the kind of person we are. The patients, after all, are not there as friends, let alone confidants. The emotional demands of the job are so great that we need there to be boundaries behind which we can withdraw to lick the day's wounds and to refresh ourselves for tomorrow. The corollary of 'don't take the job home with you' is 'don't take home in to work'. Perhaps patients, too, need us to maintain a degree of detachment, of mystique; it is part of what Balint calls

Known to doctor?

	Yes	No
Yes	MEDICAL KNOWLEDGE, SKILLS & RESOURCES	PERSONAL ATTITUDES EMOTIONS & HANG-UPS
No	LIFE CIRCUMSTANCES & EXPERIENCES	UNCONSCIOUS

Available to patient?

Figure 10.5 The doctor's Johari's window.

our 'apostolic function', the potency that accrues to us by virtue, in part, of our remoteness.

As Figure 10.5 shows, the 'blind' quadrant of the Johari model is occupied by the doctor's personal attitudes, emotions and hang-ups: specifically, those that the patient recognises but we do not. This needs some explanation.

At the beginning of the chapter about Crichton's switch, I quoted from the scene in *Patch Adams* where the Dean of the medical school addresses the new intake of students. 'It is human nature', he told them, 'to lie, take short cuts, to lose your nerve, get tired, make mistakes … [But] it is our mission here to rigorously and ruthlessly train the humanity out of you and make you into something better. We're going to make doctors out of you!' Many of us will recognise this as a lesson still taught, at least by implication, in our own training. *Don't get involved*, runs the message. *Don't allow yourself any emotional responses to the patient or their predicament. Keep your thoughts and feelings to yourself.* We have learned this lesson so well that we conceal some of our most powerful feelings about patients even from ourselves, especially the more risky ones, such as attraction, loathing or fury.

These responses often have a basis in our past experiences. I myself, for example, used to have a strong dislike of smelly old ladies. Smelly old men were no problem; but if an old lady came in, with a certain 'old lady' smell of sweat, stale urine and liquorice allsort sweets, I would quickly become irritated and impatient, and would try to get her out of the room as quickly as possible. On one occasion a trainee, sitting in with me during such a con-sultation, said afterwards, 'What's the matter with you? You were not very nice to that lady. I thought she was rather sweet.' Then the penny dropped. When I was aged 10, I was shown into the bedroom where my grandmother, of whom I was very fond, lay dying. It was made clear to me that this would be the last time I would see her. That smell was in the room; and it became for ever afterwards associated in my mind with distress and grief. I had been blind to the power it still had, decades later, to affect my behaviour with patients. Once the connection was made, however, I could manage to inhibit my negative reaction by silently reminding myself that this person was not my grandmother.

Patients can be shrewder than we sometimes give them credit for. If we think that they cannot see behind our professional mask, we delude ourselves. Just as we are constantly scanning the patient for verbal and non-verbal point-ers to their inner world, so too is the patient scanning *us*, reading between *our* lines, wondering and interpreting just as we do. The patients who say, 'I hope you don't think I'm wasting your time, Doctor,' have probably, despite our protestations, sensed that we think they are. Derek with the musical teeth knew that he got on my nerves, though to this day I'm not sure I know why I found him so irritating, or how he could tell.

I happened once to be standing in the reception area of my practice, out of sight of the patients but able to overhear what was being said at the front desk. I heard a voice I recognised as belonging to one of my regular patients. She was a troubled lady, trapped in a loveless marriage, constantly worried about her teenage children's brushes with the law. In most of her consultations with me there was a large element of counselling, touching on her feelings of isolation and worthlessness. I prided myself on being a significant part of her support network. But, to my surprise, I heard her ask to make an appointment with one of my partners. 'Don't you usually see Dr Neighbour?', the receptionist enquired. 'Yes,' she replied, 'but I can't always be doing with his big brown eyes looking through me.' How chastening! Without realising it, I had become over-fond of my self-appointed heroic role as the only person who understood her. A painful crack appeared in my complacency. When she next consulted me I was much more cautious, much more respectful of her right to inner privacy. I never did thank her for helping the blind to see, but the feedback she had unwittingly given me made me realise that what I intended to be – believed to be – my sympathetic concern was at least in part my own need to be needed.

Of all the mental territory that makes up the Inner Physician, the 'blind' area of our attitudes, emotions and hang-ups is probably the most significant in the impact it has on our encounters with patients. Some patients seem to have a knack of 'pressing our buttons'; that is to say, they evoke a negative reaction in us that is stronger than, or different from, the effect they have on other doctors. My reflex aversion to 'smelly old ladies' is an example. Many of our buttons have their origins in long-established attitudes that have become so familiar to us that we no longer see them for what they are – opinions, points of view, idiosyncrasies acquired as a result of our personal histories, as uniquely ours as our taste in music. We tend to assume that, because we take our own attitudes for granted, everybody else shares them too. Surely everybody is put off by a smelly old lady? Well – no, actually. My observing trainee found her rather sweet; he hadn't seen my grandmother on her death-bed. Surely everybody is reassured and consoled by the gaze of my big brown eyes? Well – no, actually; too much concern can at times become intrusive. We see patients relating to us in ways we sometimes find challenging or puzzling, but we don't always see the role of our own attitudes and blind spots in causing them.

Finally, the doctor's Johari's window, like everybody else's, has an 'unconscious' quadrant, the locus of all those of our thoughts, reactions and behaviours whose origin remains unknown both to ourselves and to our patients. By its very nature, it is hard to fathom the workings of the unconscious. But we see its effects when, for instance, we find ourselves in the grip of an unexpectedly strong emotion, or taking an irrationally implacable position on a matter of no real significance.

So there we have it: the doctor's totality categorised by Johari's window into public, private, blind and unconscious components, all with potential impact, whether for good or ill, on the patient in the consultation. Subtract the public, set aside the 'trained physician', and what remains – private, blind and unconscious – is the Inner Physician: 'the expert minus the expertise'; three domains of what the doctor has to offer, which in the conventional account of medical practice are ignored, overlooked, undervalued, gagged, shackled and excluded (see Figure 10.6).

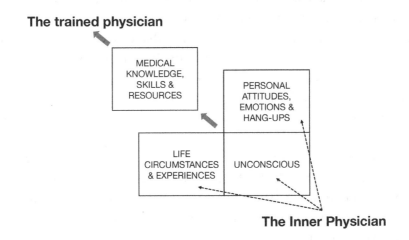

Figure 10.6 The expert minus the expertise.

* * * * *

What these largely submerged parts of the doctor's mind bring to the clinical encounter, complementing the biomedical knowledge that is the contribution of the public 'trained physician', is access to a library of perceptual templates based on personal experience. These templates allow the doctor to recognise non-physical aspects of the patient's condition, and are the prerequisites for the development of emotional sensitivity and empathy.

As we move through the course of our lives from birth to maturity, as events unfold and circumstances change, as our roles and relationships evolve, we pile up memory upon memory and experience an ever-expanding range of all the emotions human beings are capable of feeling. By the time we qualify as doctors we will have learned at first hand something of how families function. We will know what it is like to be a child, an adolescent, perhaps a lover, a carer or a parent. Perhaps by then we will have encountered death or serious illness, and seen how it affects those touched by it. In our own lives we will inevitably have experienced something of anxiety, sadness, pain, fear, bewilderment, loss, hope, resignation, helplessness, rage; almost everything that the patient in front of us might be feeling, we ourselves to some extent will already have felt.

The memories we form of these significant experiences are more than just souvenirs; they act as models or blueprints, encoding the key features and emotional concomitants of situations we will subsequently be able to recognise when they happen to other people. Seeing is made easier by having already seen, as the Dalmatian figure–ground example showed.

One legacy of our personal history is our capacity for empathy. To have, say, a personal memory of grief is to acquire grief-shaped receptors into which the contours of someone else's grief can in future fit snugly enough to trigger our empathic recognition. Our attitudes, too, are fashioned by the cards destiny deals us. Growing up in a family with a domineering parent, for example, might leave a doctor with feelings of resentment that could later surface as a disproportionate intolerance of patients perceived as being over-demanding.

As life experience accumulates we gradually install a library of 'been there, felt that' situations to which, if we allow ourselves, we can resonate when patients encounter them. The result is ... we could call it a kind of wisdom, if you like, though acumen, sensitivity or shrewdness might be better. In the next chapter I shall use its Greek name, *phronesis*.

The phenomenon of musical resonance is a good analogy. When a piano is built, the makers install strings of varying lengths and gauges, each capable of emitting, when struck, a note of a particular frequency. The strings encompass between them the instrument's complete range of pitch, covering more than seven octaves from the lowest bass to the highest treble. Now imagine this: you depress the piano's sustaining pedal, leaving all its strings undamped and free to resonate. Then another instrument – a clarinet, say – plays a note nearby. Softly but unmistakably the piano strings corresponding to this stimulus note, and others related to it, begin spontaneously to vibrate. If the clarinet plays a C, all the C strings on the piano and also, to a lesser extent, the Gs and the Es, begin to reverberate in supportive harmony. It is as if the piano is recognising those frequencies in the stimulus note to which some of its own strings are pre-tuned, and is resonating in sympathy.

The doctor with a properly functioning Inner Physician is able and willing to allow his or her own past experiences to resonate with the emotional timbre of some of the strands in the patient's narrative, and with non-physical components of the patient's predicament. The willingness is important, akin to raising the dampers on the piano strings with the sustaining pedal and putting the instrument into 'ready to resonate' mode. As we learned from the stories in the chapter on Crichton's switch, some doctors all of the time, and all doctors some of the time, switch off their emotional responses and disconnect their Inner Physicians in times of crisis, leaving themselves functioning solely as a vehicle for their purely biomedical skills. Figure 10.7 illustrates this. We also saw how most of my Crichton correspondents felt themselves to be fractured and diminished by this splitting-off, and were relieved when the separated medical and non-medical parts of their identities were re-united. Crichton's switch, it appears, operates as a toggle switch, either excluding the Inner Physician from, or integrating it with, the rest of the doctor's clinical expertise.

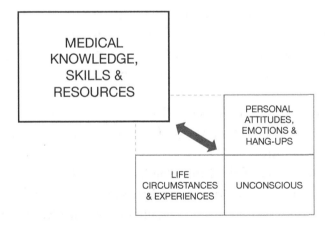

Figure 10.7 Crichton's switch.

To coin a phrase, we could say that a doctor whose Inner Physician is accessible during the consultation has the capacity for 'narrative resonance'. Narrative resonance is the condition of a doctor who is attentive to the text, subtext and context of the patient's story, and is ready to resonate to it. It implies a willingness to allow personal memories and associations to surface from the private, blind and unconscious sectors of the doctor's mind, and to welcome them as a potential source of insight, supplementing the biomedical information being gathered by the 'public' trained physician. Narrative resonance means allowing our memory bank to be stirred on several levels by what the patient communicates, without prematurely censoring what comes up as 'not medically relevant'. Narrative resonance allows us to recognise the patient's emotions, and supplies us with a vocabulary to describe them. Narrative resonance is the state of mind in which we most readily recognise the patient's verbal and non-verbal cues to any covert agenda or hidden depths. It helps us read between the lines, and helps make sense of an account that would, by purely rational lights, be fuzzy or inconsistent.

Narrative resonance is often – indeed, usually – a liminal or subliminal phenomenon, operating on the edges of conscious awareness. It just happens, without any effort on our part, as when the piano strings respond to the clarinet with a chord that just appears, without any keys being struck. It is in a state of narrative resonance that we get hunches, intuitions and 'gut feelings' about our patients. The Oxford three-stage model of diagnosis depends on the doctor coming up with some diagnostic possibilities before the rational brain can set to work evaluating them. When some feature of a patient's story or demeanour fits one of the Inner Physician's library of templates, pattern recognition takes place subliminally, and the thought that 'such-and-such might be the case' spontaneously arises. Both the expert trained physician and the Inner Physician contribute to this process, generating physical and non-physical hypotheses respectively. But if the doctor is in a state of narrative resonance, receptive to messages from parts of the mind usually excluded from the clinical process, both kinds of insight coalesce into a comprehensive 'big picture diagnosis'.

One manifestation of the Inner Physician at work in the consultation is our own internal dialogue: the silent discussion we have with ourselves, the unspoken running commentary we maintain even while, out loud, we and the patient are conversing normally (Figure 10.8).

On a bad day, the voice of this 'second head' is intrusive and distracting: *Oh, get to the point! I'm bored. And hungry. What do I fancy for supper?* But on a good day, when we are consulting with all the fluency and competence we are capable of, fully attentive and ready to resonate to the patient's narrative, then the voice of the Inner Physician (for that is what it is) can be an invaluable ally. *She looks really sad. That's twice she's told me her husband's away a*

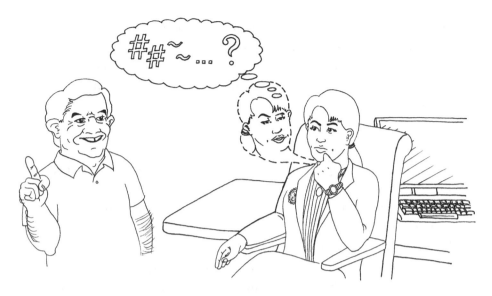

Figure 10.8 Internal dialogue – the voice of the Inner Physician.

lot. I wonder if there's a marriage problem. I've never liked him. But that doesn't mean he's unfaithful. Anyway, I need to ask about depressive symptoms ...

This is the big picture medical gaze in action: alternately scanning the patient's narrative 'out there' in the real-world consultation, zooming between close-up detail and wide-angle context, and 'here inside', where our private stream of thought provides its silent counterpoint – sweep by sweep building up the best understanding we can muster of the complexity in which we and the patient are both embedded. As we monitor our own internal dialogue, we become 'the self observing the self', the participant observer, aware of our own awareness and of how it is subtly but inevitably influencing the course of our interaction with the patient.

I have perhaps given the impression that the Inner Physician's contribution to the consultation is nothing but helpful. This is not the case; there are circumstances where it is not in the patient's interest for the doctor's personal self to intervene. The lesson of Crichton's switch is that in situations of high stress or medical urgency we need, for everyone's sake, to disconnect from our human reactions, lest they overwhelm us and compromise our medical skills. Nor have all our formative experiences been positive. If we ourselves have been caught up in dysfunctional family relationships, say, or have unfinished emotional business after traumatic experiences, the templates these experiences leave behind may not be best suited to our role as professional helpers. My aversion to smelly old ladies and my initial exasperation with Derek of the musical teeth are examples of such 'pressable buttons', which can leave patients at risk from our own hidden agenda. Nevertheless, I remain convinced that a technically competent doctor who is 'inner aware' has more to offer patients than another who is equally expert but 'self-blind'.

* * * * *

Let's explore what happens when one Johari-person talks to another, as in Figure 10.9. (I've re-configured the four quadrants of the windows to look more like the panes in a set of casement doors, in order to show the interactions more easily.)

The text of their conversation, as a microphone might record it, is a spoken exchange conducted at the 'public' level. But, as in all communication between people, there is a subtext of things unspoken, things hinted at and inferred, things to be read between the lines, representing interactions between the private, blind and unknown realms of each party.

Now suppose that the conversation is the special case of a consultation between a patient and a doctor. In this professional setting I have suggested that the doctor's attributes potentially impacting on the patient were distributed among the Johari quadrants as follows:

- in the **'public'** quadrant – the doctor's medical knowledge, skills and resources (the 'trained physician')
- in the **'private'** quadrant – the history and details of the doctor's personal life outside medicine
- in the **'blind'** quadrant – the doctor's personal emotions and values, especially those affecting professional behaviour to a greater extent than we like to imagine
- in the **'unknown'** quadrant – the unconscious forces of the psychological deep ocean.

We could similarly map everything the patient brings to the consultation onto the Johari framework.

From the 'patient's **'public'** quadrant comes the opening narrative, setting out, as it were, in first draft, the symptoms or problem for the doctor's consideration. The problem as stated will usually be couched in biomedical terms, or readily translated into them, in the expectation that the doctor's response will draw upon the medical resources in his own 'public' quadrant. This

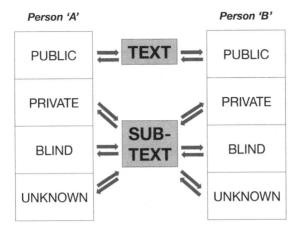

Figure 10.9 A Johari conversation.

public-to-public transaction constitutes what we could call the 'surface con-sultation', where the presenting problem is taken at face value and explored within the traditional medical model.

But just as the private, blind and unknown areas of the doctor comprise the Inner Physician, there is an 'inner patient' similarly constituted.

Known to the patient but kept concealed, at least initially, from the doctor is the '**private**' quadrant containing things the patient hopes the doctor will deal with but that are not explicitly stated. This zone is the source of hidden agenda; of verbal and non-verbal cues to be interpreted and lines to be read between; of 'While I'm here …' and 'I don't like to ask …' and 'I don't sup-pose …'

The patient's '**blind**' area is the seat of emotional needs. Many patients will come to a doctor motivated, at least in part, by a need to be accepted, understood, protected, cared about. They may also have elements of more assertive needs, the legacy of their own personal histories, such as a need to challenge, dominate or frustrate. The patient may not be consciously aware of these needs, but they are powerful drivers of behaviour, impelling some patients to become serial non-attenders, others to 'shop around' from one doctor to another. They may also be glimpsed in involuntary cues such as a moistening eye, a clenched jaw, a restlessness, a grimace, or the use of emo-tionally charged language.

Finally, unconscious forces in the patient's '**unknown**' quadrant come into play, here as in every human interaction. Though these might be discussed in various psychoanalytic dialects – 'life scripts', 'the id', transference phe-nomena – what they have in common is that they give the doctor–patient

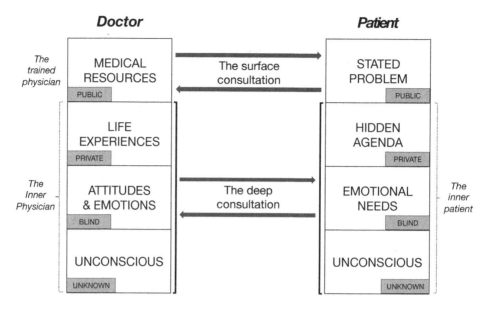

Figure 10.10 A Johari consultation.

relationship a symbolic significance over and above its role as a vehicle for medical problem-solving.

Figure 10.10 represents a consultation *à la* Johari. Beneath the surface, the doctor's Inner Physician, stocked with an accumulation of experience and emotional intelligence, is primed to resonate to nuances and depths in the patient's narrative. But the scrutiny is not one-way. The 'inner patient' is reciprocally on alert, playing us at our own game, reading between *our* lines, interpreting *our* subtext, scanning *our* every utterance, gesture and expression for indications of the life within. Two consultations are under way simultaneously. There is a surface consultation between the patient with a stated problem and a doctor equipped with an array of medical resources. And there is a deeper consultation between inner patient and Inner Physician: murkier, fuzzier, less articulate, but arguably no less important.

'Medicine,' said Albert Schweitzer,[145] 'is not only a science, but also the art of letting our own individuality interact with the individuality of the patient.' Agreed – but it's complicated. Sometimes, however, if things get complicated enough, something akin to a miracle happens. Emergence happens.

* * * * *

---

145 Albert Schweitzer (1875–1965), French theologian, organist, philosopher, physician and medical missionary. He received the Nobel Peace Prize in 1952.

A tourist was being shown round the city of Cambridge.

'This is Trinity College,' said the guide. 'And this is King's, with its famous chapel.'

'Lovely,' said the tourist.

'And here is the Cavendish Laboratory, where Rutherford split the atom,' said the guide.

'Fascinating,' said the tourist.

'And this is The Eagle pub,' said the guide, 'where Crick and Watson first announced the structure of DNA.'

'Most interesting,' said the tourist. 'But, please – I should like to see the University.'

---

emergence: unexpected global system properties, not present in any individual sub-systems ... A surprise-generating mechanism dependent on connectivity ... A system's behaviour and properties that cannot be predicted from knowledge of its parts taken in isolation.

Encyclopaedia Britannica

If you take a fairly simple component, and connect lots of them together, the resulting interconnected network develops properties you couldn't anticipate by studying the individual parts. This is the phenomenon of 'emergence'. For example: a transistor (my geeky friends tell me) is a simple electronic gismo. If you connect up lots of transistors, you get a computer, which can do things you could not possibly have foreseen, no matter how thoroughly you understood how a transistor works. Then, if you connect up lots of computers, lo and behold!, you have the internet, which again does things – Facebook, Amazon, cybercrime – that no amount of poking around inside a PC or a Mac could have predicted. Or take a neurone, nothing special in cellular terms; but connect enough them up, and you have the human brain, possessed of perhaps the most miraculous emergent property of all – consciousness. Connect up enough brains and you have, despite what Margaret Thatcher claimed, society.[146] Or democracy. Or the moon landings ... .

---

146 Margaret Thatcher, UK Prime Minister 1979–90, and, in the opinion of some, myself included, the clearest demonstration of the need for humility and generosity in human affairs. In an interview for *Woman's Own* magazine of 31 October 1987, she famously observed, 'And, you know, there is no such thing as society.'

In this chapter we have been considering the minds of doctor and patient as if each consisted of the four Johari components. If we put the two of them into a consulting room, and allow any part of one to connect and interact with any part of the other, the resulting network (Figure 10.11) is complex enough to allow the possibility that some unexpected and unpredictable phenomena might emerge. Once we concede that medicine goes beyond the simple matching of a biological abnormality to its corresponding corrective measure, the consultation becomes much more than just a shopping trip. If we allow that GPs have to deal with people's hopes and worries and sadnesses as well as their physical diseases, with poverty, inequalities and isolation, and with philosophical issues such as mortality and 'what does it all mean?' – and when we accept that doctors by their very humanity affect and are affected by what they see and hear – then the doctor–patient relationship acquires some near-miraculous emergent properties.

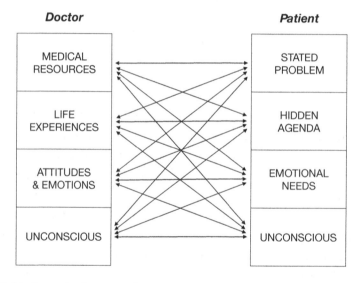

Figure 10.11 Consultation complexity.

Most obvious, least miraculous, and the *sine qua non* of everyday practice is the exchange at the public level between a patient with symptoms and a doctor who can relieve them. 'My knees are swollen and painful.' 'Looks like arthritis; try these tablets.' Beneath the surface, however, at the private, blind and unconscious levels, various surreptitious agendas are being played out. Often the parties – doctor and patient – are oblivious to what is happening in the deep consultation; and not infrequently one or both of them will end up feeling dissatisfied or unsettled as a result.

Many of what have become known as 'heartsink patients' present problems that refuse to be coerced into the strictly medical model, stemming rather from emotional needs that neither patient nor doctor can express. It is all too easy to place responsibility for the doctor's reaction solely on the patient who is 'one of the crosses we have to bear'. The problem may be the feelings that arise within the doctor, but it is the patient who is stigmatised by the derogatory label. Yet not every doctor is equally discomfited by a particular heartsink patient. In his 1988 paper[147] in which he popularised the term, Tom O'Dowd did not perhaps sufficiently acknowledge the role of the doctor as co-author of these narratives of dismay. The heartsink patient may press buttons, and we may not like the feelings that result; but they are *our* buttons, and it is our personal histories, emotions and attitudes that installed them and keep them functioning. In the language I have adopted in this book and this chapter, the heartsink reaction is a special case of narrative resonance, where some features in the patient's narrative (text and subtext) resonate with vulnerabilities in the Inner Physician, triggering, in this case, the opposite of empathy (see Figure 10.12).

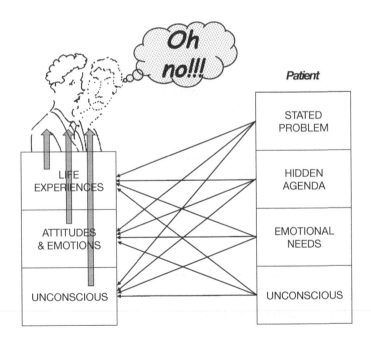

Figure 10.12 The 'heartsink' reaction.

147 O'Dowd TC. Five years of heartsink patients in general practice. *British Medical Journal* 1988; **297**: 528–30.

We could map the Johari transactions of some frequently encountered challenges in general practice. Take the somatising patient with physical-sounding but medically unexplained symptoms, common examples being chronic tiredness or flitting chest pain; most authorities agree that such symptoms represent the bodily expression of underlying tension, anxiety or psychological distress, which are, however, unrecognised or denied by the patient. Figure 10.13 depicts the dynamics of this situation.

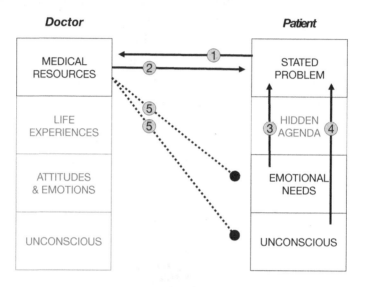

Figure 10.13 Medically unexplained symptoms.

At (1) the patient presents a physical symptom that the doctor assesses using the conventional medical model (2).

> Patient: 'I feel tired all the time.'
> Doctor: 'You could be anaemic.'

The symptoms are initiated and maintained by unexpressed emotional and unconscious 'drivers' (3 and 4), possibly marital disharmony; but the doctor's enquiries about underlying problems are blocked (5).

> Doctor: 'The tests are normal. Could it be that you are worried about something?'
> Patient: 'Absolutely not! It's not all in my mind, you know.'

The consultation is now trapped in unproductive pursuit of nonexistent organic disease until a way can be found of opening the 'inner patient' up to enquiry.

Doctor and patient sometimes collude to ignore a problem they both know exists, but which both, for their own reasons, prefer to overlook, such as obesity or tranquilliser dependency. Figure 10.14 shows the exchanges between a doctor and patient who both drink more alcohol than is good for them.

Doctor: 'Two pints of beer a night? I dare say that's an underestimate.' (1)
Patient: 'It's not every night, of course. And never any more.' (2)
Doctor (thinks): *Actually, I drink more than that.* (3)
Patient (thinks): *And I've no intention of cutting down, whatever he says.* (4)

And so, because neither dares confess their secret thoughts to the other, the issue goes unconfronted.

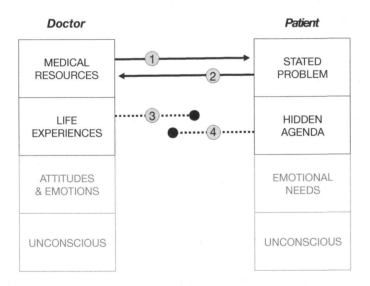

Figure 10.14 Collusion.

Most doctors will have had the experience of being manipulated by a patient into doing something – prescribing a hypnotic, or signing a sick note – against their better judgement, rather than face the argument that a refusal would cause. Here (Figure 10.15) a patient makes what to the doctor seems an inappropriate request (1).

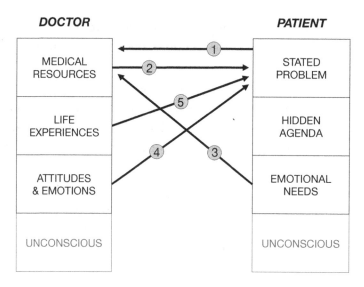

Figure 10.15 Manipulation.

Patient: 'I want a second opinion from a specialist.' (1)
Doctor: 'I really don't think that's necessary.' (2)

When the patient was aged 6, his parents divorced, leaving him insecure and mistrustful of those who ought to take care of him.

Patient: 'It's not that I don't trust you …' (3)

The doctor aims to be popular with all her patients (4). Also, she recently misdiagnosed a case of meningitis and was lucky to avoid a formal complaint (5).

'Okay,' she says, 'I suppose I could refer you.'

Eric Berne in his 1988 book *Games People Play* introduced the ideas of transactional analysis to a wide professional and lay readership,[148] including the concept of 'games' – repetitive behaviours that, although ultimately damaging, are in the short term psychologically rewarding. One game often played in the consulting room is 'Yes, but …', in which the patient rejects every suggestion made by the doctor. The patient's aim is to confirm a

---

148 Eric Berne (1910–70), Canadian psychiatrist and originator of transactional analysis, an approach to psychoanalysis based on a model of the mind as consisting of three 'ego states': Parent, Adult and Child.

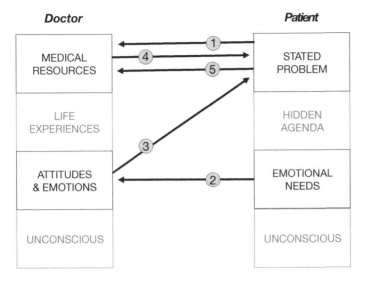

Figure 10.16 A game of 'Yes, but …'.

deep-seated belief that authority figures, perhaps originally a parent, always let you down. The game begins (Figure 10.16) with the patient reporting a treatment failure.

> Patient: 'Those pain killers didn't work either. I need something stronger.' (1)

The subtext of this remark is *I knew it; you've failed me, just like everybody always does.* (2). The doctor, who wants to be a good and effective doctor, is hooked (3), so says (4),

> 'I can certainly give you something really strong,'

to which the patient replies (5),

> 'Yes, but I can't be doing with anything that might upset my stomach,'

and so initiates another round of the same game. The game can continue until both players acknowledge what is going on and – easy to say, but not so easy to do – agree to stop, and communicate at a more rational level.

One particularly important component of the deep consultation between inner patient and Inner Physician, involving exchanges at the emotional and unconscious levels, is the 'as if' phenomenon of transference. While on the surface what goes on between doctor and patient might appear to be a purely practical and emotionally neutral business transaction, as between shopkeeper and customer, doctor and patient may in fact find themselves relating as if one was an emotionally significant figure in the other's life. Feelings and attitudes that might be appropriate in one psychological context become 'transferred' or projected into another.[149] Thus, a consultation that ought to be a meeting of equals could, as often happened in the days when a doctor-centred consulting style was the norm, become a paternalistic relationship in which the patient plays the role – and, indeed, feels the emotions – of the grateful and obedient child of the doctor's father figure. Figure 10.17 depicts this.

At (1), the doctor pronounces his verdict on the patient's problem.

Doctor: 'You're going to have to have an operation,'

to which the patient meekly replies (2),

Patient: 'Whatever you think is best, Doctor.'

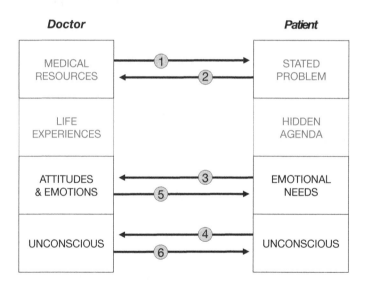

Figure 10.17 Transference and counter-transference.

---

149 Strictly speaking, 'transference' refers to the patient's feelings towards the doctor; the doctor's reciprocal feelings towards or about the patient are termed 'counter-transference'. Much of classical psychoanalysis consists of tracing the origin, evolution and resolution of the transference relationship. The analyst in turn is expected to undergo his own analysis, and to undertake regular case supervision, in order to protect the patient from inappropriate counter-transference.

The transference dynamics now are as between a caring but powerful parent and a compliant child. The patient's acquiescence stems from an ingrained need to be protected (3), just as she had been in childhood by her late father, whom she worshipped (4). Her passivity elicits an authoritarian response from the doctor (5), who feels entitled to the same respect and deference he was made to show his own rather domineering father (6).

As Figure 10.18 shows, transference and counter-transference in the consultation can take many forms. Leaving aside the inevitable knowledge gradient between doctor and patient, even a politically correct 'relationship of equals' is not devoid of transference issues, begging the question, 'Equal in what respects?' Rights? Power? Obligations? And although a parent–child transference is probably the commonest of the psychologically loaded relationships, even here the roles are not fixed. A parent-like doctor could be either a good nurturing parent, with whom the patient-as-child can gratefully cooperate, or else a rigid over-controlling parent, to be challenged and confronted. Or it may be the patient who takes the parent role; many doctors, especially early in their career, will have had the experience of being treated by a patient from an older generation as if they were naughty children needing to brought to heel. In another common transference scenario the doctor plays 'rescuer' while the patient adopts the role of 'victim', whether of disease, misfortune or harsh treatment. While this is often the basis for an entirely healthy professional relationship, some doctors, for their own deep-going psychological reasons, are wedded – even addicted – to the rescuer role, as if their own self-worth has to be constantly reinforced by cultivating a succession of

Doctor	⟷	Patient
Good parent	⟷	Child
Bad parent	⟷	Child
Child	⟷	Parent
Friend	⟷	Friend
Lover	⟷	Lover
Expert	⟷	Amateur
Amateur	⟷	Expert
Rescuer	⟷	Victim
Victim	⟷	Rescuer
Priest	⟷	Sinner
Producer	⟷	Consumer

Figure 10.18 Transference relationships in the consultation.

over-dependent patients. On the positive side, however, many unhappy and damaged patients have been steered back towards mental health through the experience of being cared for by a doctor on whose abiding concern and support they find they can rely.

If we pull back from the detail of all these exchanges, it is clear that the Inner Physician is intimately involved in the depths and subtleties that make 'big picture medicine' so much more than an arm's-length exercise in applied science. The interactions among the private, blind and unconscious domains of both doctor and patient form a network of inter- and intra-psychic connections so complex that the doctor–patient relationship acquires emergent properties; it becomes, in its own right, an instrument of diagnosis and treatment. Narrative resonance, as we have seen, lies at the heart of insight, intuition and empathy. Patient and doctor become partners in a dance choreographed jointly by their histories and emotions. The symbolic roles they adopt in transference determine whether they act in synergy or opposition. As participant observers we see more clearly the patient's humanity; and the patient sees ours. Embracing the Inner Physician, we are no longer inchworms.

* * * * *

Earlier in this chapter we saw how the boundaries between the Johari categories are permeable, so that information can move from one compartment to another. (Figure 10.19 is a reminder.) We can, if we choose, disclose and make public facts about ourselves we have hitherto kept private. Feedback from other people, if we can accept it, allows a blind-to-public shift, so that we can see ourselves more as others see us. Through reflection or more formal therapy we can gain insights into previously unexplored parts of our makeup. In the counselling setting for which Johari's window was first developed, the assertion is that psychological well-being is enhanced the more we can allow ourselves to be self-disclosing, self-aware and self-accepting.

We should perhaps, therefore, ask ourselves this: is it possible that some similar opening-up – a greater degree of self-disclosure, self-awareness and self-acceptance – might have benefits for our patients or for ourselves as doctors? Might it sometimes be useful for us to allow patients to know a little more about our private lives? Might it sometimes be helpful to show or discuss our own feelings a little more in the consultation? Might an ongoing commitment to our own personal development be as legitimate a professional

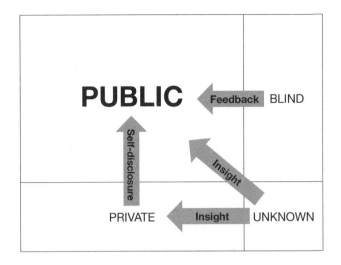

Figure 10.19 The Johari route to psychological well-being.

responsibility as maintaining our clinical competence? Should we, in other words, allow the Inner Physician to make a more prominent – a more overt – contribution to our work with patients? Figure 10.20 makes these suggestions in graphic form.

These are sensitive and contentious questions. On the occasions I have talked about them with groups of GP colleagues, discussion can become heated. The first reactions tend to be negative, even outraged: *My private life is my own! There have to be boundaries. They're my patients, not my friends.*

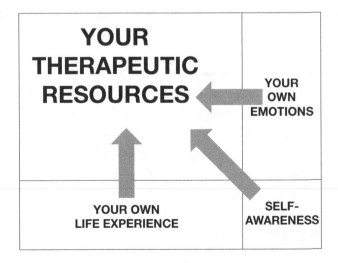

Figure 10.20 Involving the Inner Physician.

Once you start giving of yourself, there's no end to it. They'll suck you dry. I'm a doctor, not an agony aunt. People's attitudes begin to show. *If they really knew what I thought about some of them, I'd be up before the GMC. I haven't got time for all that navel-gazing. Medicine is complicated enough without opening up cans of worms if you don't have to. If you get into all this 'feeling' stuff, you just make a rod for your own back.* All of which is to say, by way of subtext, *I'm scared.* And understandably so; almost from day one at medical school we have been taught not to get involved, trained to don the white coat, wear the mask, flip Crichton's switch.

But then usually someone will tell a personal story, nervously at first, but gaining in confidence as other doctors present start to nod and to recall similar experiences of their own.

> *I was having a really bad day. In the morning one of my children had told me he was being bullied at school, and later I'd had a call to say my father had been rushed into hospital. I couldn't concentrate on the patients, and it must have showed. One patient said I looked at the end of my tether. I just couldn't help it – I broke down in tears, and told her what had happened. 'Oh you poor thing,' she said. 'And here's me going on about nothing.' And she reached into her handbag and gave me a piece of chocolate. I can't believe how much that helped; and not just with her, with all the other patients too. It made me realise I don't have to give, give, give to the patients all the time – I'm allowed to get something back.*

On another occasion, a GP in her fifties told a large group I had been addressing:

> *I have breast cancer. I've had radiotherapy, but it's spread, and ... well, my partners know, of course, but I didn't tell my patients. But I have found it hard dealing with terminally ill patients. One day recently I was visiting a man with advanced bowel cancer, and he said, 'I wake up in the night sometimes, sweating, wondering what it'll be like to die.' And I said, 'So do I.' And he said, 'Do you?', and I said, 'Yes.' So we talked, and then we stopped and just held hands. I don't know who helped whom the most. But I'll tell you this; ever since then, I've not minded talking to dying patients, not just about serious things, but anything – their bowels, their grandchildren, anything.*

And she looked around her and saw the sympathetic faces of the audience. 'This is the first time I've told anybody about that,' she said. And such was the intensity of narrative resonance among her assembled colleagues that they broke into gentle applause.

As an example of how the Inner Physician can enhance our capacity for narrative resonance, let me tell you this.

My own mother, of whom I was very fond, died in 2000. As my grief unfolded over the following weeks and months I recognised all the classic stages of the well-known Kübler-Ross model: denial, anger, bargaining, depression and acceptance.[150] But I, of course, was the observed as well as the observer. To me, bereavement was not a curriculum topic; it was personal. It was what I felt, and, for a time at least, what I *was*. Eventually, once I had (dreadful phrase!) 'worked through' the worst of my grief, I noticed that I was talking to bereaved patients in a different way. As I listened to their narratives, what resonated in me was no longer a theoretical understanding gleaned from textbooks, but rather my own memories and feelings, and the words I had used to express them. I no longer came out with theory-based clichés such as, 'I wonder if you sometimes feel angry about things,' or 'I'm sure you miss her, but time is a great healer.' Instead, I found myself saying, 'Is it like there's a person-shaped hole at the heart of you? In due course, you'll manage to lead your life around it; but the hole will never go, and, in a way, I guess you wouldn't want it to.' It seemed, from patients' responses (and indeed it seemed to me), as if I had found a better, a more recognisable, way of showing I understood; and, if this was true, it was also a legacy to me from someone I loved, and I value it.

These stories illustrate how involving the Inner Physician can sometimes be beneficial to doctor and patient. Perhaps you can recall some similar incident in your own experience; if so, please pause now and reflect on it. Moreover, there are also circumstances where it can prove harmful for the providers of care *not* to disclose some personal information about themselves. One such episode, albeit on a larger scale, made British national newspaper headlines in 2001.

In 1998 *The Lancet* published a paper by Andrew Wakefield suggesting that childhood autism and colitis could be caused by vaccination with the

---

150 Elisabeth Kübler-Ross (1926–2004), Swiss American psychiatrist, specialising in the emotional care of the dying and the bereaved. Her pioneering book *On Death and Dying*, first published in 1969, was subtitled *What the dying have to teach doctors, nurses, clergy and their own families*. Although subsequent authors have quibbled about the nature, sequence and inevitability of the five stages of bereavement she described, Kübler-Ross's work has contributed enormously to end-of-life care, and, by extension, has helped those reeling from other forms of loss, such as of a precious relationship, role or ambition.

combined measles, mumps and rubella vaccine (MMR), then standard practice in the UK. These claims were comprehensively rebutted by subsequent research; the original paper was withdrawn by *The Lancet* and deemed 'fraudulent' by the *British Medical Journal*, and Dr Wakefield's licence to practise was revoked by the General Medical Council in 2010 for serious professional misconduct. Nevertheless, mud stuck; parents of young children took fright, and MMR vaccination rates plummeted from 90.8% in 1997 to 79.7% in 2003, leaving many thousands of children at risk from the serious complications of these previously uncommon illnesses. At the height of the public consternation, the Prime Minister of the day, Tony Blair, was repeatedly asked whether his own 19-month-old son Leo had been vaccinated. If they knew that he had been, many more parents might well have accepted vaccination for their own children. But Mr Blair refused to say, his office issuing a statement explaining, 'In the light of ... a horrible and unjustified attempt ... to drag a member of my wife's family into the issue of MMR, I would like to say the following. The reason we have refused to say whether Leo has had the MMR vaccine is because we have never commented on the medical health or treatment of our children ... Once we comment on one [piece of advice], it is hard to see how we can justify not commenting on them all.' We can sympathise with the Blairs' dilemma, weighing their right to privacy against the lives that might have remained unblighted had they felt less defensive. But the Chief Medical Officer, Sir Liam Donaldson, later made his view clear, namely, that the Blairs' refusal to go public 'caused major problems for public health'.[151] The few straw polls I have taken with British GPs suggest that most would have been prepared to tell a patient what they themselves had done as parents, as well as what as doctors they recommended, or to give an honest answer to the question, 'Well, Doctor, what would *you* do?'

Enfranchising the Inner Physician through such complex and open-ended processes as self-disclosure, self-awareness and self-acceptance is not an all-or-nothing affair. It is a matter of degree, and stretching the boundaries of one's habitual consulting repertoire involves a measure of risk-taking. One must judiciously choose the right patient, the right topic, the right timing, and the right way of saying things. Nevertheless, there are a few general guidelines.

---

151 *The Guardian*, 2 June 2013. Is it cynical to note that Mr Blair's wife, Cherie, in her 2008 autobiography *Speaking for Myself*, and 7 years after it might have been helpful, *did* feel able to reveal that young Leo had in fact been given the MMR vaccine, information that was trailed as part of the book's launch publicity?

We must guard against what I think of as the Sybil Fawlty style of sympathy. Aficionados of the classic British television comedy *Fawlty Towers*[152] may recall Sybil, the hotelier's wife, telephoning a friend, listening to some tale of woe, and, commiserating, say 'Ooh, I *knooooow*' in a *faux*-empathic tone. It does not necessarily help a patient to be told that the doctor, too, has had backache or an operation, particularly if the disclosure seems to carry the implication that the doctor's case was more severe, or was more bravely borne or better managed, than the patient's. There is a danger that self-disclosure can degenerate into point-scoring, game-playing or one-upmanship: *Yes, I've got the 'flu myself; but I, of course, have to keep on working.*

Narrative resonance with the patient's story is just the first stage in a truly empathic response. It is not enough for the doctor, when reminded of some similar experience of his own, simply to regurgitate it unprocessed. The associations triggered by the resonance really need to be combined with other resources, such as prior knowledge of the patient and their circumstances, into a consciously thought-through intervention with a clear result in mind. When the doctor with breast cancer, whose story I told earlier, replied, 'So do I,' to her patient who lay awake thinking of death, she did so not from a need to unburden herself, but rather because she could tell, as a skilled and sensitive professional, that this would be a good way of showing him that he was not alone in his fear, and that he would learn from her example that it could safely be acknowledged and talked about. That she subsequently felt more at ease with other dying patients confirms, I think, that the risk inherent in self-disclosure can be outweighed by its benefits.

Another lesson – also learned by the doctor, previously mentioned, whose bad day was brightened by the gift of chocolate – is that concealing our emotions, trying to suppress the Inner Physician, takes significant effort. In the long term, the cumulative effect of unnecessary defensiveness is burnout, that cancer of the professional soul, when altruism is sabotaged by exhaustion. What makes for long-term job satisfaction, on the other hand, is knowing that we can deal with anything and everything the patient presents. Whether or not the patient's stated problem completely matches one of the biomedical templates installed by our professional training, the Inner Physician will always have something useful to offer.

* * * * *

---

152 BBC television sitcom (1975–79), set in a seedy Torquay hotel owned by Basil
Fawlty (played by John Cleese) and his bossy wife Sybil (Prunella Scales).

The format I have used in Figures 10.9 and subsequently has placed the public-to-public consultation between the patent's stated problem and the doctor's exclusively medical resources above the more covert interactions between inner patient and Inner Physician. Reducing this complexity to diagrammatic form and putting the surface consultation at the top may unfortunately have given the impression that the deep consultation is somehow inferior, less sophisticated, more primitive compared with the high-value high-status exchanges between doctor and patient at the biomedical level. Such a portrayal would sit well with the traditional view of the history of medicine as the subjugation of the irrational by the intellect. It would also chime with simplistic readings of developmental neurology that depict the evolution of the human brain as the progressive (though precarious) domination of the reptilian brain and limbic system by the neocortex, or of the non-dominant right hemisphere by the dominant left. And it tends to reinforce the popular opinion that the cleverness of the specialist is superior to the wisdom of the generalist. The corollary of this 'top-down' view is that the Inner Physician is at best a minor contributor to the real business of medicine, and at worst an impediment, a distraction to be suppressed if hard-nosed science is to prevail in the consulting room.

All this would be to misunderstand the nature of emergence.

Emergence is a 'bottom-up' phenomenon. Complexity emerges from interconnected simplicities. High-level phenomena are the result of lower level connectedness, not of pre-planned design. The world wide web emerges from the interconnectedness of computers, consciousness from the interconnectedness of neurones. The full power of medicine is manifest only when we can contemplate unrestricted connections between every sector of the minds of both doctor and patient.

It is, I'll allow, less risky to confine ourselves to the purely biomedical domain and to paddle only in the shallow waters of physical problem-solving. That way, the only danger to the patient is of misdiagnosis or mismanagement, and to the doctor a malpractice suit. To be sure, once our personal selves and private emotions become engaged in the clinical encounter, there is the potential for manipulation and game-playing, deviousness and entanglement, at which prospect it would be understandable to take fright. But the risk of these aberrations is there anyway, whether we recognise it or not, and will not disappear if we simply deny or ignore it. The alternative – to flip Crichton's switch and ban the Inner Physician from the consulting room – would be to close the door on empathy, on insight, on compassion, on plain ordinary human kindness.

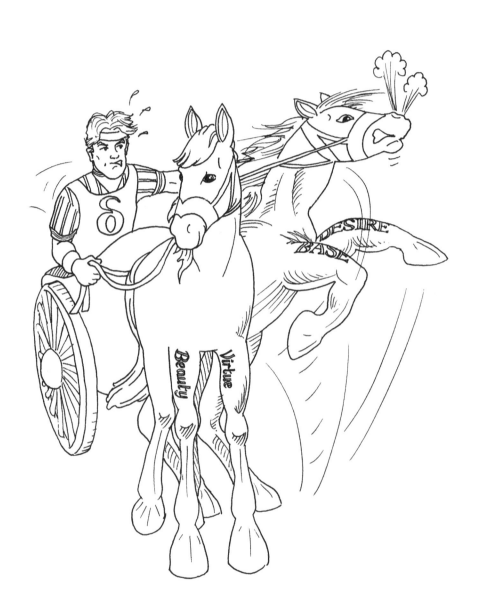

Chapter 11

The Greeks had a word for it

Everyone who wills can hear the inner voice. It is within everyone.
Mahatma Gandhi (1869–1948)
Leader of the Indian independence movement

If you don't take care of that little inner voice, you will really not be very worthy of being with someone else, because you won't be the best version of you.
Kimora Lee Simmons (b. 1975)
American businesswoman

The Inner Physician is nothing more than a special case of the 'inner every-body'. We all have an inner life of memory and imagination, thoughts and feelings, shaped by past experience and set in resonance by the people and situations we encounter in daily life. We all also carry on inside our heads a silent running commentary in which we talk to ourselves in the role of participant observer of our own lives. The medical profession, unfortunately, has tended to ignore these subjective truths in its lemming-rush to scient-ism. Moreover, the scientism with which most of medicine is besotted is the now-outmoded mechanistic Newtonian kind that failed to understand the observer effect and the crucial role of the participant observer in creating what we take to be objective reality.

If it is indeed the case that an inner life and an inner voice are universals in human experience, then we should expect to find them recognised and documented in cultures and periods other than our own. And if these intra-psychic processes are as important as I believe them to be, then we might expect them to confer some survival benefit on every human society and the individuals it comprises. They are; and they do.

Few would challenge the claim that much of what passes for European culture – its values, its institutions and its notions of what it means to be civilised – was conceived in classical Greece, and in the Athens of the fifth and fourth centuries BCE in particular. In her book *Introducing the Ancient Greeks*,[153] Edith Hall lists 10 characteristics of the collective Greek personality that made their influence so enduring. The Greeks were:

- *sea-farers*, who exploited but respected the forces of nature. As explorers, they were
- *inquisitive* and
- *open to new ideas.* Highly
- *individualistic,* the Greeks were
- *competitive* and
- *suspicious of authority*, but nevertheless
- *appreciative of talented people.* In their relations with their fellow citizens they were
- *elaborately articulate*
- *witty* and
- *addicted to pleasure.*

All except possibly the first and last of these could fairly be said to describe most GPs today. And I can think of a good few whose fondness for sailing and fine dining would score them a perfect 10 out of 10.

All of this is by way of excuse for invoking one of my favourite ancient Greeks, the philosopher Socrates, in support of my thesis. Socrates was born in Athens around 470 BCE, the son of a stonemason and a midwife, and died there in 399 BCE at the age of 71, put to death by hemlock. He was arguably the greatest of all philosophers, uncompromising in his pursuit of reason, truth and insight. He was also a maverick, intensely irritating and one of my heroes.

By all accounts, Socrates was no oil painting to look at. Squat, snub-nosed and pot-bellied, he was as ugly as his wife Xanthippe was ill-tempered. Nevertheless, he was a popular, charismatic and highly effective debunker of sloppy thinking. Socrates' persistent questioning of establishment figures, often to the point of their humiliation and on a scale that ultimately provoked the authorities into executing him, gave rise to his nickname 'μύωψ' (myops),

---

153 Hall E. *Introducing the Ancient Greeks: from Bronze Age seafarers to navigators of the Western mind.* London: W.W. Norton, 2014.

the gadfly, whose sting could goad people into a frenzy. Socrates liked nothing more, of a sunny day, than to go down to the agora, the main square in Athens, and wait for a crowd to gather. His audience assembled, he would then light upon some unsuspecting victim, perhaps an aspiring politician or a junior member of an influential family, and ask him a seemingly innocuous question, such as, 'Meno, you're a fine upstanding young man, cut out for leadership; tell me, what do you think "virtue" is?' Meno rattles off examples of virtuous behaviour in a man, in a woman, an old man, a child … 'Yes yes,' Socrates interrupts. 'These are all good illustrations. But isn't there some underlying principle, which we call "virtue", common to them all?' Before long, Socrates' remorseless questioning shows Meno's argument to be circular, and reduces the hapless would-be politician to a spluttering admission of ignorance. Resentfully, Meno rounds on his tormentor. 'Okay, clever Dick, *you* tell *me* what virtue is!' Whereupon Socrates shrugs his shoulders: '*I* don't know; the only thing I know is that I know nothing.' And he saunters off.

Classical scholars are entitled to cringe at the way I have distorted Plato's account of Socrates' dialogue with Meno in this cameo. But I hope it gives a sense of how Socrates, and his method of philosophical enquiry, could provoke an interlocutor to within a whisker of physical violence.[154] Imagine such intellectual embarrassments taking place so publicly, so frequently, and to the chagrin of so many prominent figures, all at the hands of an eccentric old man whose previous exemplary military career had nevertheless earned him considerable popular respect, and it is easy to understand how, in sheer exasperation, the Athenian establishment arranged for capital charges to be laid against him. Some time in late 400 BCE, an indictment was lodged in the name of Meletus, an obscure young poet, alleging that 'Socrates is a wrongdoer in not recognising the gods which the city recognises, and introducing other divinities. Furthermore, he is a wrongdoer in corrupting the minds of the young.'

For most of the 30-odd years he spent philosophising, Socrates walked a fine line, pushing his interlocutors in discourse to the limits of their understanding and tolerance but seldom beyond them. In this way he was able to stretch their intellects, and his own, just so far as kept the discussion productive. He

---

154 Readers of a certain age may be reminded of the famous interview on BBC television's *Newsnight* programme of 13 May 1997, when Jeremy Paxman asked an evasive Michael Howard, the outgoing Home Secretary, the same question – 'Did you threaten to overrule Derek Lewis, the head of the Prison Service?' – 12 times without securing a straight answer. Younger readers will easily find the episode on YouTube.

must have had the ability to read a situation with great shrewdness, judging when to push and when to ease off according to the responses he was getting. How did he do this? In the speech he made in his own defence when on trial for his life before a jury of 500 fellow citizens, Socrates explained.

'You may be wondering,' he told them, 'why I confine my advice to private individuals, and have never ventured to meddle in affairs of state. The reason, as you have often heard me say, is that I am subject to a divine or supernatural experience. It began in my early childhood – a sort of inner voice which comes to me; and when it comes, it always warns me to think again about whatever I was just about to do or say. But it never actually *makes* me do anything I had not been contemplating.'[155]

The word Socrates uses for his inner voice is 'δαιμόνιον' (daimonion), usually translated as 'a little spirit' or 'a divine sign'. To his enemies, it must have appeared that Socrates was claiming to be in direct communication with a god unrecognised in the official pantheon; hence the inclusion of sacrilege on the list of charges against him. But it is clear that this was emphatically *not* what Socrates believed. It is also clear – Socrates being the epitome of rationality – that his daimonion was not the delusional 'voices' of the schizophrenic.

Socrates' daimonion, it seems, was a cautionary inner voice that would sometimes intrude into his consciousness, modifying or aborting a proposed course of action. When he speaks of his daimonion, Socrates is reporting moments when his own internal dialogue became so insistent that it could not be ignored or gainsaid. It would warn him, in effect, *Uh-oh! Look out, here comes trouble.* The daimonion is a composite voice: more than the voice of conscience, it is on occasion the voice of hunch, intuition and insight, the voice of emotion and emotional sensitivity. Sometimes it is a kind of internal mentor, the voice of his own self-imposed standards, asking of Socrates himself the same searching questions he liked to pose to others. At times it alerts him to people or events from his own past having some relevance to the present. At others it serves to draw his attention to the language of the body, his own and that of his interlocutor. In a word, it is the voice of resonance. As the scholar James Hans puts it, the daimonion is Socrates' personal 'manifestation of our constant, subconscious attention to all the antennae we employ to take in the cues of the world'. It is, Hans continues, 'our most important

---

155 This is a paraphrase of excerpts from Plato's account of Socrates' 'apology' (the defence speech he made at his trial), written about 40 years after Socrates' death.

guide every day of our lives, even if most of us are seldom aware of its tutelary presence'.[156]

If we draw the obvious parallels between Socrates' daimonion – his inner philosopher – and the Inner Physician, the interest for us here is to see what Socrates can teach us about how attentiveness to the inner voice can help strike an effective balance between intellect and intuition, between hard logic and fuzzy pragmatism. Let us begin with one of the best accounts of the daimonion in action, Phaedrus's conversation (I nearly wrote 'consultation') with Socrates on the subject of love, as described by Plato.

Strolling one day in the countryside, Socrates encounters Phaedrus, a rather shallow follower of fashion. Phaedrus has recently been impressed by a speech about love by the famous orator Lysias, which he relates to Socrates. The gist of Lysias's argument is that friendship, even casual sex, is preferable to romantic love, on the grounds that romantic attachment leads to jealousy and gossip, and limits the pool of potential partners.

Socrates is not impressed with Lysias's powers of rhetoric, and tells Phaedrus that he, Socrates, could make a much better speech on the same subject. Romantic love, he suggests, is a form of madness, driven by irrational desire, whereas friendship, being more dispassionate, can be cultivated in pursuit of worthier and more rational goals. Romantic love can easily become too possessive, stifling the individuality and development of the loved one. Feeling that he has given a superior demonstration of oratory, Socrates prepares to break off the conversation and depart.

It is at this point that Socrates feels the familiar jolt of his daimonion, urging him not to leave yet. He realises that he does not believe his own argument; in using the skills of rhetoric merely to show off his prowess as an orator, he has betrayed one of his own core ideals, the pursuit of truth. He has out-Lysiased the second-rate Lysias in a purely technical exercise in eloquence, and in so doing has committed what, in the words of T.S. Eliot many centuries later, is '... the greatest treason: To do the right deed for the wrong reason'.[157] Socrates, while his speech may have been made with tongue in cheek, perceives that the admiration it has evoked in the naïve Phaedrus

---

156 Hans J.S. *Socrates and the Irrational*. Charlottesville, VA: University of Virginia Press, 2006, p. 195.

157 These lines are from *Murder in the Cathedral*, a verse drama by the poet T.S. Eliot, chronicling the assassination in 1190 of Thomas Becket, Archbishop of Canterbury, at the instigation of King Henry II. The 'treason' referred to is Becket's temptation to seek martyrdom for the sake of glory.

is genuine. This he cannot allow. It was ever a part of Socrates' mental discipline to be 'the self observing the self', monitoring his own performance and motives, and what he has so far said has set his internal 'hypocrisy' template resonating. Chastened by a sense that he has let himself down, Socrates tells Phaedrus that he needs to atone for this blasphemy by making a further speech, one that will lead to a very different conclusion.

This time, what Socrates has to say is far more worthy of a man of his perspicacity. He argues that romantic love may indeed be a form of madness, but it is *divine* madness, a gift from the gods. He offers an analogy in which he likens the soul – the essence of what it is to be human – to a chariot drawn by two horses. One horse is manageable, attracted to beauty and virtue. The second is hard to control, fickle and motivated by base desires; its wilfulness is something the charioteer must control as he struggles to steer his chariot towards celestial glory. The best form of love, Socrates concludes, is romantic love, when the impulsiveness of carnal lust is gentled and harnessed to the quest for human fulfilment.

The analogy of the two-horse chariot is intended not just for Phaedrus's ears but for his own as well. Socrates knows, though had temporarily forgotten, that human beings are always under tension from conflicting mental forces. He needed to remind himself that his own formidable intellect must be tempered with self-awareness, intuition and sensitivity to the feelings of others. And he knows that he can trust his inner voice to alert him if he is in danger of getting the balance wrong. Over the course of his career, Socrates had learned that he could allow the promptings of his daimonion to steer him towards the best thing to do in a situation where several possible courses of action presented themselves. He was willing on some occasions for it to overrule the conclusions of logic and intellect, and on others for it to stop an over-hasty emotionally driven response in its tracks. So, halfway through the conversation with Phaedrus, Socrates' daimonion whispers *Don't walk away. Do yourself justice; rethink your position.*

Does all this seem unnecessarily arcane, and ancient Athens irrelevantly remote from the consulting room? Not a bit of it. Socrates' detractors, and possibly he himself, used the language of gods and divine forces to describe how his daimonion operated. But we need not. We do not need to see in its workings any supernatural agency, or even anything particularly unusual – merely the normal functioning of an intelligent and articulate mind with well-developed powers of observation and self-observation. And a daimonion, in the form of the Inner Physician, is alive and functioning in every clinician; you are Socrates, and Phaedrus might be any patient. Medicine would be very simple if we were unitary beings and if the problems presented for our attention were one-dimensional. But – alas and Alleluia – things are not like that. We doctors have to find ways of applying our own multiplicity to our patients' complexity. External aids in the form of guidelines and protocols, being generalisations, can never be enough to decide the particular case. Like Socrates, we need a steer from within. Many a medical consultation is a 'Phaedrus in miniature', in which the contribution of the Inner Physician is as crucial as that of his daimonion was to Socrates.

Here is an example.

* * * * *

It's Friday evening, nearly 6 p.m., and your surgery looks as if it's going to run late, as you had to squeeze in an extra patient who insisted that her tennis elbow was an emergency. And you particularly wanted to get home on time tonight, as some friends are coming for a meal. The next patient is Gary, aged 22, a previously healthy young man whom you've seen occasionally when he was at school but who has not consulted you for several years. Fingers crossed, this will be a sports injury, or acne. Something quick, anyway.

'Hello, Gary,' you say cheerily. 'Haven't seen you for a while.'

'Been at Uni,' Gary says. 'Did English literature. Don't know why I bothered.' His voice is flat, his expression morose. 'Actually, I feel a bit silly, coming here. It's not like I'm ill or anything.'

'What's the problem?'

'Oh, you know, Doc. Can't find a job. Stuck back home with mum and dad. Girl stuff.'

Our chariot has two horses. You know perfectly well that what you ought to do is listen, show concern, ask open-ended questions, get this unhappy young man to open up, say 'Tell me about it'. But your friends will be round in an hour, and you need to pick up some nibbles on the way home, and the traffic will be heavy. Damn. Your teeth clench; *Tell me about it* comes out as, 'Are you sleeping?'

'Not really,' Gary says. And before you can ask, 'How's your appetite?', he continues. 'I think I've got depression.'

You feel a flicker of relief. *I've got depression*, he said, not *I'm feeling depressed.* He already sees himself as someone with a medical condition. Good, that will cut down the time it takes to work round to why he needs an antidepressant. Perhaps this won't take too long after all.

The second horse has the bit between its teeth. 'It does sound like that,' you say. 'But, as you know, depression is an illness, and it's something these days we can treat quite easily. I just need to ask you a few more questions …'.

And now you notice. Gary's face is damp with tears. His shoulders heave as, silently, he sobs.

Then it comes, the jolt so familiar to Socrates. Daimonion, Inner Physician – call it what you will, the inner voice of your own standards makes itself heard. The self has observed the self, and has not liked what it has seen. *This is not worthy of you. You are a better doctor than this.* It is '… the greatest treason to prescribe a psychotropic for the wrong reason'. What this young man needs is not a pharmaceutical; not yet, anyway. He needs the box of tissues you push towards him. He needs the consoling touch of your hand on his arm. Above all, he needs your time. From the recesses of your memory comes something you once heard someone say: 'Our values are revealed by the choices we make under pressure'.[158] *What would I rather be,* you ask yourself, *a good doctor or a punctual host?* The friends can manage without nibbles.

'When you're ready,' you say, 'tell me about it.'

* * * * *

It is worth looking a little more closely at how the Inner Physician – the doctor's daimonion – makes its presence known in the consultation.

Perhaps the first thing to appreciate is that we are dealing with something ephemeral, short-lived, dynamic. The Inner Physician expresses itself in fleeting interjections into our stream of consciousness in real time, right now, in the ever-passing present moment. Its messages come in the form of chimes of recognition as something in the patient's narrative or behaviour sets one of our internal associations resonating. It might manifest as an imagined verbal response in the mind's ear, something we might say if we were to speak our thoughts out loud. It could be a silent voice-over as images from memory and imagination flicker in front of our mind's eye. It could be the coming into focus of an unexpected insight, idea or possibility. Or we might notice a sudden physical tension somewhere in the body, or a frisson of emotion. One common experience, alerting us to the fact that the Inner Physician is at hand, is what I can only call (and I don't know how to spell or pronounce it) the 'Nngh! reaction'. *Nngh!* is that noise of frustration or annoyance you

---

158 The 'someone' I heard say this was Robert McKee, a Hollywood screenwriter, whose seminar on story structure I attended many years ago.

might make when the tight lid of a screw-top jar refuses to budge, or the traffic lights change to red just as you thought you would make it through on the amber. You will probably encounter Nngh! in consultations with those patients often referred to as 'heartsink'. Nngh! is the sound of our buttons being pressed; and, as such, it serves to warn us, as Socrates was warned in his conversation with Phaedrus, to be on guard against letting ourselves down in the face of provocation.

The voice of the Inner Physician is sometimes strong and insistent, abruptly dragging our attention away from our 'out loud' conversation with the patient. But more often the inner voice is soft, liminal, on the edge of consciousness, easy to overlook and needing to be actively checked for by periodically swivelling our gaze inwards, scanning our present awareness and taking notice of our immediate thoughts and feelings – the self observing the self. Scan and notice we must, however, for the window of opportunity created by the Inner Physician does not stay open for long. Unlike matters of the intellect, where facts can be checked at leisure and decisions analysed in retrospect, the promptings of the Inner Physician require to be considered without delay, else they subside and lose any usefulness they might have had for influencing our behaviour.

In the speech he made at his trial, Socrates claimed that his daimonion had only an inhibitory effect, warning him *against* something he was contemplating but never itself initiating an action. I suspect he may have been making this distinction for legal reasons; certainly the Inner Physician, our own personal daimonion, can serve both as a warning and as a positive prompt, actively nudging us in some particular direction. We encounter the Inner Physician in inhibitory mode when a voice inside us warns *Take care; don't jump to conclusions; take your time; think.* There are also occasions when it acts rather like the proximity sensors on a car bumper, that beep with increasing insistence the closer we move to something solid. Responding no doubt to subtle cues in the patient's narrative, the Inner Physician sometimes senses when we are in the vicinity of information that matters, something either clinically important or meaningful to the patient. It is that sixth sense that tells us *Pay close attention, prick up your ears, fine-tune your antennae – this could be significant.*

Very often, though, the Inner Physician is in active suggestion mode, as when it:

- picks out a pattern of key clinical features against a background of irrelevance, like the Dalmatian dog in Chapter 10

- spots something anomalous in the patient's presentation, drawing our attention to the detail that doesn't quite fit with an assumption we were making
- detects some minimal cue to latent agenda in the patient's narrative, some verbal or non-verbal nuance that might lead to a deeper understanding
- recognises a barely discernible emotion, either the patient's or our own, set in resonance by something the patient is feeling
- sends a hunch, an inkling or an insight bubbling up from nowhere into our mind
- steers us for no apparently logical reason towards what will prove to be the right response or the right decision.

For all that they seem to come from beyond the boundaries of conscious control, these inner voices should not be thought of as anything irrational. Though the processes leading to its appearance might seem mysterious, the content of what the Inner Physician whispers in our professional ear is firmly rooted in rationality: the knowledge we have accumulated; the events we have experienced; the undeniable emotions we feel; the wisdom we have acquired about how people think and behave; and the values we aspire to lead our lives by.

As Socrates reminds us, we drive a chariot with two horses, not just one. The knack, surely, is to master both and have them pull together as colleagues in the direction we, the charioteer, choose. The ideal, surely, is the collaboration of intellect and intuition, of expert and participant observer. The contribution of the Inner Physician is to challenge and enlighten the logic-slave we might otherwise become; the duty of reason is to check the potential excesses of unrestrained spontaneity. Socrates never allowed his daimonion arbitrarily to overrule the conclusions of rational thought. Its promptings simply became a further piece of evidence to be integrated into a better informed decision. He demanded of himself the full embrace of all his human capacities – rational and irrational, physical and psychological, pragmatic and idealistic. As I said, I think the man was a hero.

* * * * *

Only connect the prose and the passion, and both will be exalted.

E.M. Forster (1879–1970)
English novelist
From *Howards End* (1910)

What Socrates and Forster both realised, and what Gary, overwhelmed with hopelessness, is about to discover is that, when a well-informed intellect is complemented by well-developed self-awareness, the understanding that results can be helpful beyond expectation. The Greeks also had a word for this 'knowledge that really helps' – 'φρόνησις' (phronesis).[159] And phronesis, usually translated as 'practical wisdom', is what generalists are particularly good at.

It has been said that good doctors treat similar problems in similar ways, but the best doctors treat similar problems in importantly *dis*-similar ways. In other words, the suggestion goes, all patients with a given condition should receive the best available (preferably evidence-based) treatment, regardless of which doctor treats them. This is why we have guidelines, protocols and treatment pathways. Consistency is a virtue. But, while guidelines are fine in general for establishing the best thing to do by and large, there is a higher order skill in managing the particularities of an individual patient, knowing the best thing to do for this specific person in these specific circumstances at this specific time. Flexibility, as long as it is evidence-informed, is sometimes a greater virtue. In general practice (and at the most skilful levels of specialist practice) we are in the complex world of 'it all depends'. Phronesis is what it takes to do the right thing in uncertain conditions, when you don't have all the information, and some of the information you *do* have is unreliable or inconsistent.

You are perhaps familiar with Miller's pyramid, a depiction beloved of educationists of how professional competence develops.[160] We begin by acquiring a theoretical knowledge base. Then we go through a stage of learning in principle how to apply it, followed by practising until, on a good day, we can demonstrate satisfactory performance of a new skill. Finally, what we have learned becomes just part of what we routinely do every day. Figure 11.1, if you ignore the cloud around the peak of the pyramid, illustrates this.

But the cloud around the peak represents phronesis, and is supremely important. Nothing we do for patients, no matter how sophisticated, impressive or evidence-based, should be what we *always* do. Deciding whether or not to do what we *could* do, or which of several equally defensible courses of action is the best, is a higher order skill, adding the dimensions of selectivity and judgement to an otherwise prescriptive professional agenda.

---

159 *Phro'*-ne-sis: the stress is on the first syllable. Alice is Billie's sister, but Emma is Ronnie's sis. Phronesis rhymes with 'Ronnie's sis'.

160 Miller GE. The assessment of clinical skills/competence/performance. *Academic Medicine* 1990; **65**(9): S63–7.

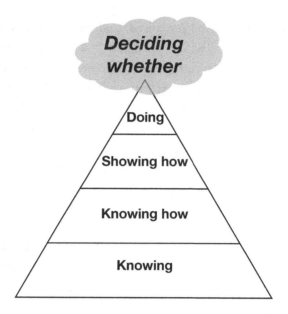

Figure 11.1 Miller's pyramid, upgraded for generalist use.

Phronesis as a concept was first systematically considered by the philosopher Aristotle (384–322 BCE). Aristotle, the son of a physician, was a trainee of Plato, who had been Socrates' pupil and amanuensis. His monumental work *The Nicomachean Ethics* is an exploration of the conditions under which people are happiest and best able to flourish. In it, Aristotle sets out what he thinks it takes to do the best we can in whatever circumstances we find ourselves. As well as the moral virtues of having the right values (hexis) and aspirations to excellence (arete), he lists theoretical knowledge (sophia), scientific knowledge (episteme), practical skills (techne), intuition (nous), and phronesis – applied wisdom. His point was that theory and ethical posturing are meaningless unless they are expressed in actual behaviour.

Phronesis is one of those things more easily recognised than defined. If we must have a definition, I quite like the oxymoronic 'knowing what to do when nobody knows what to do', which seems to capture the paradox inherent in a feature of clinical practice that is commonplace yet mysterious. One essential component of phronesis is to have a solid base of factual knowledge at one's command; in Johari terms, the doctor's 'public' quadrant of medical resources needs to be well stocked. The other is, in situations of uncertainty, somehow to be able to sniff out the key decision-affecting factors that hard-nosed logic alone cannot identify. Phronesis arises from the creative interplay between the rational and the intuitive.

People speak admiringly of 'clinical acumen', which I have heard described as 'the expert's common sense'. But common sense is mainly just decision-making where you can't see the individual steps along the way. An example: an experienced cardiologist feels a patient's pulse, glances at an echocardiogram, turns to a junior colleague and says, 'Right, give a loading dose of clopidogrel'. Impressive though this piece of rapid decision-making may appear, to the cardiologist the process is so familiar as to feel like plain common sense; the patient is clearly in imminent cardiac danger and needs to be prepared for angioplasty. The expert knows where the high-grade decision-affecting clinical information is to be found, and goes straight to it. He then assesses the probabilities of various diagnoses and treatment outcomes, doing Bayesian analysis in his head as easily as lesser mortals multiply two by two. And if I was clever enough and diligent enough, I could learn to do the same. What the cardiologist has done is complicated, but still 100% rational; a protocol could be drafted to represent it – and it does not constitute phronesis as I mean it here.

Others explain phronesis as 'knowing when to break the rules' – in other words, deciding when to prioritise the needs of an individual patient over general principles. At its simplest, this might be no more than writing something vague such as 'neurasthenia' on a sickness certificate rather than the more accurate but socially stigmatising 'depression', in the light of what we know about the patient's personal circumstances. More contentious are those occasions when we prescribe a drug, order a test or make a referral in defiance of local or national policy guidelines. Here the dilemma we face is more one of morality than of clinical management. The issue is not so much knowing what needs to be done in the patient's best interest, but rather of finding the courage to do it. The more clinical freedom becomes ensnared in a net of protocols, targets and financial inducements – all introduced in the interests of quality assurance, but mission-creeping their way into diktat – the more important it becomes for patient-centred doctors to be not just willing to break the rules, but determined to do so. Failure to trust doctors to exercise this kind of judgement responsibly underlies much of the managerial point-missing inflicted on the National Health Service in the name of efficiency.[161] But again, this is not getting quite to the heart of what phronesis is.

Phronesis comes into its own in clinical scenarios of much greater uncertainty, where there are too many factors and not enough facts, and even the

---

161 On the very day I am writing this, 20 May 2015, Nick O'Donohoe, chief executive of Big Society Capital, an independent financial institution with a mission 'to grow the social investment market', has suggested in *The Guardian* newspaper that doctors could be paid for avoiding admitting patients with dementia to hospital. I shudder to imagine the unintended consequences were this no doubt well-intentioned proposal to be implemented.

probabilities come with probabilities, where the territory is uncharted, possibly limitless, and the key features are hard to make out in a fog of ambiguity – in quite a lot of general practice, in other words. A truer understanding of phronesis is better captured in phrases such as 'winging it', 'decision-making off-piste', 'expert improvisation', or (my favourite) 'flying by the seat of one's well-pressed pants'. The 'well-pressed' implies that, though one may be navigating by instinct, one has nevertheless taken the trouble to prepare for the occasion. 'Expert improvisation' suggests a jazz musician picking up material presented by another band member, then allowing himself to express, uninhibited but with practised skill, the resonances it evokes in him. The metaphor of phronesis as jazz is, I think, surprisingly apt; both involve risk-taking within boundaries, those boundaries being elastic if the mood of the moment dictates.

If we want examples of phronesis in action, end of life care presents plenty of situations where a doctor needs to exercise intuitive judgement.

Arthur is 73 and has advanced cancer of the prostate, still being actively treated by the urologists. He trusts that the specialists know what they are doing, and appears to believe that he will be cured. To you, on the other hand, it is evident from his widespread bony metastases and deteriorating blood markers that he is entering the terminal phase of his illness. You explain this to his wife, Margaret, and daughter, Diane, who say, 'Please don't tell Dad he's dying. He couldn't cope with that.' Let us leave aside matters of clinical management – symptom control, coordinating domiciliary services, and so on – all of which can be dealt with by your purely medical knowledge and resources. During the short but precious time that Arthur has remaining there will be several critical points where you will have to make decisions for which no clinical knowledge or protocol will have adequately prepared you. It is at these points that phronesis will be called for and the Inner Physician will come into its own.

How, for instance, will you decide when the time is right to move from curative treatment to palliative care? Arthur's clinical condition will of course be a factor, but so also may be your own preparedness to enter emotionally gruelling territory – and, indeed, your thoughts about mortality, your own included.

How will you explain to Arthur that you, and not the hospital, will be supervising his care from now on? Can you, and do you want to, do this without undermining his trust in the urologists, whose aggressive treatment of his cancer may, you feel, have allowed false hopes to have been built up? Could you contemplate telling a white lie to the effect that 'the specialists have asked me to take over'?

What will you reply when Arthur asks you, 'I am going to be all right though, aren't I?' You will need quickly to assess whether he is in denial and seeking reassurance, or whether he might be hinting that he is finally ready to face bad news. Immediately a moral dilemma confronts you: which is more important, truthfulness or the preservation of hope? The usual broad-brush principles of medical ethics – non-maleficence, beneficence, justice and autonomy[162] – don't help; an ethical case can be made for either. As you sit at the bedside considering your response, you will be looking for guidance in the intonation of his voice, the intensity of his gaze, his facial expression, your memories of previous conversations with him. In reality, practical ethical issues often have to be worked out in real time in that little bubble of concentration where there is only Arthur with his history and experience, and you with yours.

What loyalty, if any, do you owe to the wishes of Margaret and Diane, both of whom are also your patients and who will need your support after Arthur's death? Might it be they, in fact, who are in denial, and not Arthur? One approach might be to invite a discussion with, 'I understand you wanting to make things as easy as possible for him. But I don't know what the right thing to do here is.' How comfortable do you feel with thinking aloud and disclosing some of your own uncertainties to patients or their families?

If Arthur is dying at home, how available are you prepared to make yourself out of hours or when you are off duty? Would you be prepared, for example, to let the family have your private telephone number? How inviolable do you need the boundaries of your personal space to be? Or how much of your personal privacy are you prepared to sacrifice in order to be 'the doctor who was wonderful during Dad's last illness'?

In these challenging circumstances there can be no clear-cut decisions that are definitively 'right' as judged against any objective external standards. There can only be 'what is probably the best thing to do, given that it is me doing it'. Your handling and mine of this these dilemmas may well be broadly similar; you and I do after all have broadly similar medical knowledge and broadly similar cultural and professional values. But our responses will differ in detail because our non-medical selves differ in their particulars. Our widely disparate life experiences have left our Inner Physicians populated with very different repertoires of templates. And so the chords of resonance evoked in you and me by Arthur's case will be uniquely personal. We may well differ

---

162 See, for example, Beauchamp T, Childress J. *Principles of Biomedical Ethics*, 4th edn. Oxford: Oxford University Press, 1994. These authors are usually credited with formulating the 'four principles' ethical framework.

in the accuracy with which we can recognise and interpret the emotional subtext to this family drama; we may have different ideas about what a good death is, and what good doctoring consists of; you and I might draw the boundary between private and professional life in different places. All that can be said is that somewhere beneath the threshold of conscious awareness different associations will be arising, interacting, competing, compromising, until phronesis – the sense of the right thing to do – emerges apparently spontaneously.

* * * * *

Not to be outdone by the ancient Greeks, the Welsh also have a word for something relevant here – 'Cynefin', pronounced kuh-*nev'*-in. The brainchild of Dave Snowden, Honorary Professor at Bangor University, Cynefin was developed in 1999 as an aid to decision-making in business.[163] Cynefin distinguishes four classes of problem where we might be required to act:

- simple
- complicated
- complex
- chaotic.

Each calls for different strategies; the trick is to know which kind of problem you are dealing with.

In the Cynefin framework, summarised in Table 11.1, a 'simple' problem is one with only a single variable, or at least very few. Acute bronchitis would be a good example;[164] the important clinical factor is whether or not there are pathogenic bacteria in the bronchi. The relationship between cause and effect is well understood and linear – A leads to B, which leads to C; bacteria cause inflammation and exudate, which lead to productive cough. The problem is easy to identify, usually from previous experience; you look at the sputum, listen to the lungs, and recognise the signs. The effects of intervention are predictable; if you give an appropriate antibiotic, the condition will improve.

---

163 Snowden D. The social ecology of knowledge management. In: C Despres, D Chavel (eds). *Knowledge Horizons: the present and the promise of knowledge management.* Oxford: Butterworth Heinemann, 2000.

164 I am simplifying the examples in order to illustrate the principles of the Cynefin approach as clearly as possible.

Table 11.1 The Cynefin framework

	Simple	Complicated	Complex	Chaotic
How many variables?	One or few	Multiple but finite	Unlimited, observer-dependent	Unknown
Type of causality	Linear	Linear	Interactive, interdependent	Unknown
Relationship of cause and effect	Known	Knowable in principle	Understandable only in retrospect	Irrational
How is problem identified?	Prior experience, recognition	Systematic analysis	Heuristics, phronesis	Intuition
Effects of intervention	Predictable	Consistent and testable	Inconsistent, possibly emergent	Indeterminate
Appropriate type of response	Standardised	Flexible but comprehensive	Pragmatic, experimental	'Witnessing'

Overall, 'simple' problems can be managed in standardised ways, following established 'best practice' guidelines.

A 'complicated' problem, in Cynefin's terminology, is nothing more than the aggregate of several simple ones – it's just that there are more of them to be dealt with at once. The number of variables might be large, but it is finite. You can tell when, for practical purposes, you have identified them all. Linear causality still operates, so that in principle, through systematic analysis, it is possible to identify all the component sub-problems. The effects of intervening in a complicated system may be hard to predict, but they will be consistent and, if not obvious, can be discovered by testing. Complicated problems are managed by comprehensively addressing each element. Childhood asthma is an example of a 'complicated' problem. The overall clinical picture can be broken down into a number of separate parts, each of which can be treated independently as if it were 'simple': family history of atopy; allergic triggers; management of the acute attack; long-term control; and so on. The best overall treatment is the sum of the best treatments of all the constituent elements – appropriate use of bronchodilator and preventative medications, plus identification of allergens, plus a policy on use of antibiotics, plus documenting the family history.

Traditionally, 'Cynefin-simple' problems have been considered the business of the GP, with 'complicated' ones needing the expertise of the specialist. In a mechanistic world where all health problems could be reduced to physical or chemical malfunctions, such a distinction might be justified, even useful, and the status gradient between specialist and GP forgivable. However, our understanding has moved on. Most generalists and many specialists now recognise that the majority of their patients present problems that the Cynefin framework would classify as 'complex'.

In a 'complex' problem, the number of relevant variables, though not infinite, is unknown and potentially unlimited. The doctor-as-participant-observer has a say in deciding what variables are to be considered. One doctor, for example, may not accept a patient's marital or sexual difficulties as falling within her remit, while another might. Connections between cause and effect are no longer straightforward and linear, but are instead interactive and interdependent. It is not always clear what is cause and what is effect. Indeed, the relevance of some contributory factors may only become apparent in retrospect. In trying to work out what is going on in order to intervene effectively, the doctor may, as in 'simple' and 'complicated' cases, draw upon a conventional biomedical approach. But there will also be a major role for heuristics (rule of thumb) and phronesis (key feature recognition informed by the Inner Physician). The effects of intervening in a complex problem are not always predictable or consistent, and may in fact lead to an entirely unexpected emergent outcome. Overall, in managing complex problems there will always be a pragmatic element of 'let's try this and see what happens'.

Let us return to Gary, the unhappy young man we left in tears earlier in this chapter.

It would be possible to deal with Gary as if his problem were Cynefin-simple. One look at his dejected demeanour and a few quick questions would be enough to confirm his own diagnosis of depression. Depression, some would say, 'is' a malfunction of neurotransmitters, easily treated with antidepressants according to well-established clinical guidelines. Job done.

Few of us would be quite so simplistic. To be sure, a case can be made for a reductionist biochemical approach, but the reality is more complicated. Gary has also mentioned that he is out of work, and has hinted at relationship problems. A more comprehensive approach surely needs to address these psychosocial factors as well. No problem: you can advise him to consult the local Citizens Advice bureau[165] for help with his employment issues, and refer him to the mental health services with a view to obtaining some counselling and possibly cognitive–behavioural therapy. Oh, and the antidepressants too, of course. A complicated job done, or, more accurately, three simple ones.

---

165 Citizens Advice is a voluntary charitable organisation in the UK, giving free, independent, confidential and impartial advice on a wide range of personal, legal and social issues, online and through local bureaux.

However, Gary's depression is more than just complicated; it is complex, and our response should be complex too. Anything else would be to do less than justice to his distress and our professionalism. If, being a good generalist, you pull back and view his situation in its wider contexts, you will soon sense that there is more going on here than is evident at first sight.

'Don't know why I bothered doing English literature,' he has told you, and, 'I feel a bit silly coming here.' He also implied he was not happy 'stuck back home with mum and dad.' These sound like the remarks of someone feeling belittled, under-valued, someone with low self-esteem. The 'Cynefin-complicated' response, involving medication and two referrals, is likely to make Gary feel you are rejecting him, reinforcing his poor self-image. On the other hand, for you to involve yourself with a degree of personal commitment on your part, treating him as worth listening to and welcome to your gladly given attention, can establish a doctor–patient relationship that is potentially healing in its own right. It would set you up in the role of 'good parent'. Would you be happy with this kind of transference? Would you be able to tolerate it, discuss it with him, and in due course draw it to a close? All this depends on your own training, experience and interests, your own personal and professional support systems, and on the degree of insight you have into your own motivations. As in all complex systems, you the participant observer have a degree of control over which variables you will accept as part of the problem.

Why should Gary *need* to cast you in the role of good parent? Have his own parents not been good enough? The intensity of his weeping has taken you by surprise; it seems disproportionate. He is, after all, not the only unemployed graduate having problems with a girlfriend. Is it that these current difficulties have lifted the lid on a reservoir of deeper, older sorrow? Then you remember that his mother, who is also your patient, divorced and remarried some years ago, when Gary would have been in his early teens. The 'dad' he has returned to live with is in fact his step-father …

This is potentially deep water, and we generalists encounter something like it on a daily basis. Can we, are we willing to, do we want to, swim in it? We are of course free to choose not to. The simple and the merely complicated options remain open to us. If diagnosis is insight on the verge of action, the actions that complex insight will bring us to the verge of are themselves complex – for some, possibly, too complex. We are not obliged to say to Gary and all the others like him, 'Tell me about it'. But remember Robert McKee's dictum that 'our values are revealed by the choices we make under pressure'. Our willingness or otherwise to embrace complexity, inevitably bringing parts of our own selves into play, is one of the things that define the kind of doctor we are.

It is the generalist's variable gaze, with its 'zoom and swivel' feature, that is both the cause of our predicament and our means of escaping it.

If we zoom our gaze in close enough to virtually any medical problem we will find something that in Cynefin terms is 'simple' – a faulty enzyme, a blocked duct, an abnormality of cell division. If we lock our gaze at the fixed-focus close-up setting, as the clichéd specialists of old were wont to do, all we will ever see is simple problems. Even that is challenging enough; the human body has 13 organ systems and over 60,000 documented ways in which they can go wrong. No doubt the further research we are always being told is necessary will discover many more. So medicine does need its cohort of specialists who are wonderful at fixing simple problems.[166] The real difficulties begin when we start to pull back and widen our gaze, so that the contexts and interconnectedness of apparently simple problems begin to come into view. The danger then is that we continue to see only the simple, and assume that the bigger picture is nothing more than a complicated mosaic of easy sub-problems that need only to be identified and dealt with one by one. Again, there are many places in medicine where such a thorough, systematic painstaking approach to detail is essential. An operating theatre is one, where it has been shown that the use of checklists can significantly reduce complications and mortality.[167]

The trouble is, checklists are attractive, even addictive, and can lead to what we might call 'the checklist fallacy'. The checklist fallacy is to think that a problem is merely complicated, and can be solved by a 'tick box' approach, when it is in fact complex, and requires fundamentally different thinking that is almost literally 'outside the box'. For a complex problem, as distinct from a complicated one, the best available solution is almost never the sum of the solutions to whatever simple sub-problems can be discerned within it. For confirmation of this, we need only open the medicine cupboard of any elderly person with several coexisting diseases and note the collection

---

166 I need again to make it clear that I am talking about problems that are 'simple' only in terms of the thinking required to understand them in principle, not in terms of the often sophisticated knowledge and skills required to put a solution into practice.

167 In the second of his BBC Radio 4 Reith Lectures, 2014, Atul Gawande, an American surgeon, described a project he led in 2007 under the auspices of the World Health Organization to reduce surgical deaths. He showed in eight cities around the world that introducing detailed checklists for use by all members of the operating team reduced the rate of complications by 35% and mortality by 47%.

of incompatible, cumulatively toxic but mercifully un-swallowed prescribed medications. In complex situations, what is needed is phronesis, not checklists. In phronesis, as we have seen, rational intellect cooperates with the resonating, intuitive Inner Physician, worldly-wise and self-aware, so that the 'best under the circumstances' response that emerges is based on *all* the information available, including that which is discovered when the doctor's gaze swivels inwards.

* * * * *

It will not have escaped your notice, reader, that I have something of a magpie mind. I am attracted by shiny pretty ideas from other people's areas of expertise, and I like to bring them back to my own familiar territory and play with them. You have seen some of my collection already: my Russian dolls, my gobbets of quantum mechanics and catastrophe theory, my *Inchworm* recording, my snippets of Greek philosophy. I have one final trinket to show you, which I stumbled across when reading French mathematician Cédric Villani's book *Birth of a Theorem*,[168] his autobiographical account of work for which he was awarded a Fields Medal in 2010. It is called Markov chain Monte Carlo (MCMC). I have no idea why. But I think MCMC helps us understand how phronesis works and how the Inner Physician goes about its work as an undercover diagnostic agent.

MCMC methods, apparently, model the best way to explore unfamiliar territory where there are no certainties, just possibilities and probabilities. *That sounds like general practice*, I thought. So I read on. The maths of MCMC is quite beyond me. But every dog knows how to do it.

Watch a dog let off the leash into a large open field, and notice how it starts to explore. It will run for a while in no particular direction, attracted by who knows what. Then it will stop and sniff a small area in great detail, before running on in another apparently random direction. It repeats this cycle – run, stop, sniff – a number of times, gradually building up, we can only suppose, a 'scent map' of the field's key features of canine interest. The dog's track is probably not truly random; it just appears so to us who do not

---

168 Villani C. *Birth of a Theorem: a mathematical adventure*. London: The Bodley Head, 2015. Born in 1973, Villani was appointed Director of the Institut Henri Poincaré in Paris in 2009. He was awarded the prestigious Fields Medal, mathematics' equivalent of the Nobel Prize, in 2010 'for his proofs of nonlinear Landau damping and convergence to equilibrium for the Boltzmann equation'. His book, however, is very readable.

understand the animal's priorities. Presumably it is following some internal logic of its own. Likewise, its choice of places to stop may well not be random either; possibly some doggy daimonion is whispering *Not there, not there; yes, here!* At each stopping point, the dog investigates the immediate neighbourhood with all the analytical powers at its command, largely but perhaps not exclusively olfactory, before moving on to the next.

What the dog is doing is, as I understand it, the essence of an MCMC method. Putting it into more general terms, the best way to make sense of complexity is to be neither completely systematic nor completely haphazard, but a combination of the two. For maximum information-gathering efficiency, one enters the territory at an arbitrary point and follows a random track until something – chance, or some inner prompting – causes one to pause. Once paused, one investigates the local area logically and intensively, gleaning and interpreting as much data as one can, before resuming the random walk and sampling afresh elsewhere.

Figure 11.2 illustrates schematically the MCMC method – the random walk punctuated by episodes of detailed local sampling (shown by the shaded circles). It could equally well be a map of the dog's exploratory run through the field, the shaded circles this time representing successive 'sniff zones'. For our purposes here, Figure 11.2 illustrates how phronesis – a sense of the best thing to do – gradually emerges as a doctor periodically pauses and samples a patient's narrative, mining one small part of it intensively for information and analysing it for meaning, before allowing it to run on.

The medical case is rather more sophisticated than the dog in the field. For one thing, at least in the early part of the consultation, it is the patient who

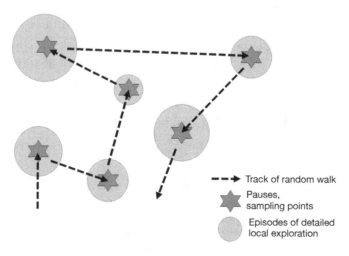

Track of random walk

Pauses, sampling points

Episodes of detailed local exploration

Figure 11.2 Phronesis as Markov chain Monte Carlo method.

sets the direction of the narrative, and, if we have learned our consultation skills diligently, we will not want to interrupt or divert it prematurely. Later in the consultation it may be the doctor who is, so to speak, 'making the running'. At all events, the course of the narrative is never truly random, being governed by the ebb and flow of the patient's or the doctor's agenda.

Second, the decision on when to pause the narrative for more detailed scrutiny can be initiated by either patient or doctor. The patient may stop, having reached the end of a particular section of their story, clearly inviting the doctor to ask questions or choose a new direction. Or the patient may say something so manifestly significant – mention a 'red flag' symptom, perhaps, or hint at some highly sensitive topic – that the doctor will be impelled to explore it there and then. Alternatively, the signal to pause and delve may be given by the doctor's own inner voice, whispering, as Socrates' daimonion did to him, *Whoa! Stop there; this could be interesting.* Throughout the consultation, the Inner Physician will be monitoring the exchanges between patient and doctor, alert to their subtext, detecting the resonances between patient's narrative and doctor's experience, throwing up intuitions and possibilities. Sometimes the Inner Physician's voice becomes so insistent that it must interrupt the consultation and demand that its promptings be considered.

A dog in a field; a mathematician at a whiteboard; a doctor in a room with a patient: three explorers in very different settings, but all trying to make sense of complexity in similar ways. The tactic they have in common is banal but effective: run, stop, sniff. The search for understanding sets them running; intuition tells them when to stop; then logic and intellect do the sniffing.

Gary again: I can imagine two scenarios.

In the first, he declines the antidepressants you suggest, and does not keep his appointment with the counsellor. You hear nothing from him for 3 months. Then one day his mother comes to see you, visibly upset, and shows you an email she has received. It reads: *Peace, everybody. Don't worry, I'm fine. I'm on an ashram here in Bangalore, following my karma. Tell Doc thanks for the advice. Maybe see you in this life or another. Gary.*

'How can I not worry?' says his mother. 'What advice did you give him? He's never said anything about going to India. It doesn't make sense.'

And she's right; it doesn't. Neither of you knows what has led Gary to take this apparently extreme step, nor have you any means of finding out. Was this a rational decision on his part to break free from the confines of an unfulfilling life? A normal, albeit delayed, adolescent search for identity? Is he acting out feelings of aggression towards his family? Is he in denial?

Suicidal? Schizophrenic? Your instincts tell you he will probably return at some point, thinner and wiser and with a girlfriend in tow, but you have no evidence to back up this belief. And what can you do to help? Does he *want* help? You could send him an email yourself, but what would that achieve? All you can realistically do – and it sounds so lame – is be there: be there as a witness to his mother's anxieties as this family saga plays itself out; be there if ever Gary returns and chooses to confide in you; be there to suffer out a gnawing feeling of guilt that you might have done more. You tried to make simple a situation that was complex, and now it has become chaotic.

'Chaotic' is the fourth category of problem described in the Cynefin framework, shown in the right-hand column of Table 11.1. 'Chaotic' problems are beyond rational understanding, beyond control, and beyond constructive intervention; the only appropriate response is to witness them, and await developments.

Here is an alternative scenario.

'Tell me about it,' you say; and he does. He feels useless, a failure. Nothing he wants ever seems to happen – he's wasted 3 years getting a pointless degree, and now he can't even find bar work. The girlfriend he thought was the love of his life – well, that's all over. He's up and running now. All he ever gets from his step-father back at home is don't sit around all day feeling sorry for yourself. You're a waste of space, his mother keeps telling him, like your … 'like my ****ing father!'.

Gary stops. You sniff around: 'Tell me about your father.' His father went off with another woman when Gary was 13. His mother begged him to stay for the sake of the children, but his father said if it was Gary or the new woman in his life, it was the woman every time. He wasn't worth anything then, apparently, and he isn't now. 'Is your father still alive, Doc?', he asks.

You wouldn't mind telling him, but you have a sense that a yes or no reply is not what Gary needs. Rather than answer and move on, you stop and explore. 'Why do you ask?'

'The last I heard of mine, he was in India,' Gary tells you. 'That was years ago. I don't even know if he's still alive. You'd think he'd want to keep in touch with his only son. I mean, it wasn't my fault their marriage failed, it truly wasn't.'

There is another pause. Gary looks as if he is about to weep again, but instead he makes to move the consultation towards a close. 'Anyway,' he says, 'you've got better things to do than waste your time listening to me.'

Your Inner Physician has noticed something. Yes, you probably *have* got other things to do, but the realisation forms in your mind that Gary is trying to provoke you into rejecting him, like his father once did and his mother still seems to, and this will only perpetuate the hurt he feels. Insight is now on the verge of action. 'On the contrary,' you say, 'I'd like to spend some more time talking with you. How about the same time next week?'

This MCMC approach – an example of phronesis in action – is like taking multiple biopsies from Gary's complex narrative, examining the samples under the microscope, and inferring from them a picture of the larger pathology, in this case the lingering effects of a dysfunctional family and parental rejection. Once you have a feel for the big picture, you can trust your existing knowledge and experience to interpret it automatically; the best thing to do will take shape in your mind unforced.

* * * * *

In this chapter I have tried to show how hitching the workings of the subconscious and peripheral parts of the mind to our capacity for rational analysis has been recognised as important for good decision-making for a very long time and in many different contexts. The fictional detective Columbo, played by Peter Falk in the long-running iconic television series of the same name,[169] is one final example, as mathematician Cédric Villani acknowledges. In a 2015 interview,[170] Villani said, 'Doing mathematics' (though he could have said being a doctor) 'is like being a detective. If there are several problems, you have to be like Columbo, use the same two steps he uses. He uses intuition to guess the right problem and the right solution, and then uses logic to prove it.'

---

169 *Columbo* was an American television drama series featuring the unprepossessing Lieutenant Columbo of the Los Angeles Police Department. It ran to 68 episodes between 1971 and 2003. Columbo's hallmark style was the relentless pursuit of hunches backed up by a formidable eye for detail.

170 Interview with Carole Cadwalladr: Cédric Villani: 'Mathematics is about progress and adventure and emotion. *The Observer*, 1 March 2015.

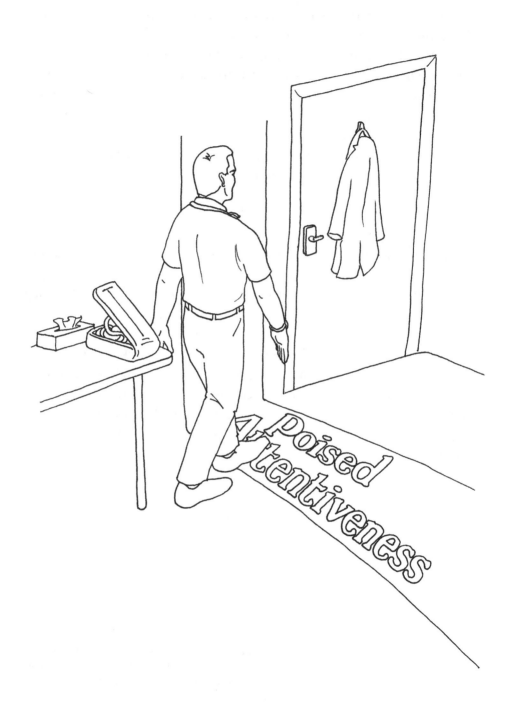

Chapter 12

In praise of innersense

> As with any form of mental self-improvement, you must learn to turn your gaze inward, concentrate on processes that usually run automatically, and try to wrest control of them so that you can apply them more mindfully.
>
> Steven Pinker (b. 1954)
> Canadian psychologist and linguist,
> writing on English sentence structure in
> *The Sense of Style* (2014)

> The perfect man uses his mind as a mirror.
> It grasps nothing, it rejects nothing;
> It receives, but does not keep.
>
> Flow with whatever may happen and let your mind be free.
> Stay centered by accepting whatever you are doing.
> This is the ultimate.
>
> Chuang Tzu
> Chinese Taoist philosopher
> *c.* 360 BCE

This book has taken me longer to write than I expected when I began it. As the writing progressed, I found myself eagerly looking forward to the final chapter – this one. I imagined it as a climax-cum-testament, a culmination and a working-out of lines of thought explored in earlier chapters. But now that the moment has arrived, I'm nervous.

I'm nervous because, in a file labelled *Ending*, I have accumulated a sizeable stash of notes, jottings, excerpts and 'memos to self', all expecting to find a neat place in a well-crafted finale. And I'm not sure whether, let alone how, they all fit together.

I'm nervous, too, because I know I shall want to say that incorporating the Inner Physician into ordinary everyday practice is largely a matter of mindfulness, of being able to control the attention and focus it at will in the present moment. And I'm afraid that this might be off-putting for some readers.

It feels as if I am entering a Cynefin-complex field of my own creation, where instinct tells me that sense lies buried but reason thinks it may be difficult to find. I think I must heed my own advice about how to approach complexity, take my own metaphor seriously, be the dog in the field. Run, stop, sniff.

* * * * *

I opened this book with the cryptic assertion that Britain has a first-class second-rate health service. The NHS is a long way from first rate; it is too under-funded and over-managed, too riddled with perverse incentives and conflicting priorities ever to be that. Too many clinical outcomes are still not good enough. Nevertheless, as second-rate health systems go, the NHS is first class.[171] For this, several factors deserve credit.

One, for sure, is the political courage of its founding politicians, who, by guaranteeing that state-funded medical care was available to all and free at the point of delivery, ensured that society's concern for the health of its citizens was more than mere rhetoric. Another is the calibre and dedication of its clinicians, supported as they are by excellent systems of postgraduate education and by the medical royal colleges. This is not to impugn the calibre and dedication of our non-clinical policy makers and managers; however, many of them come from financial and commercial backgrounds, where the values are those of the marketplace and ought not

---

171 A 2014 report by the Commonwealth Fund, a US think tank, compared health performance indicators in the USA with those in 10 other developed countries, including the UK, Canada, Australia, France and Germany. The UK came top overall, ranking first in measures of quality of care, access and efficiency, and second only to Sweden in equity. The USA came bottom overall. But our NHS was 10th out of 11 in terms of mortality from remediable conditions. For full details, see *Mirror, Mirror on the Wall: how the performance of the US health care system compares internationally* (New York: Commonwealth Fund, June 2014).

to trump, unchallenged, the softer and less assertive person-centred values of the caring professions.[172]

But I believe the most important factor ensuring that that our patients receive first-class medical care is the first-class nature of the medicine we practise. There is a balance to be struck – and I think in Britain we strike the right one – among primary, secondary and tertiary care, between the specialist way of doing medicine and the generalist way, between medicine as applied science and medicine as the art of consolation. These are precarious balances to maintain. The lure of the checklist fallacy, mistaking the complex for the merely complicated, is strong, always threatening to topple the equilibrium towards simplistic, mechanistic, reductionist conceptions of what medicine is about. Ours remains one system of health care not so far hypnotised either by the checklist fallacy or by market forces. But that could change if doctors, particularly generalists, allow themselves to be dehumanised by excluding their Inner Physician from the clinical process. Without the Inner Physician, the generalist's creed that *people are more than the sum of their body parts* is just a slogan. As long as there is a significant cadre that appreciates that science-based consolation calls for the involvement of the whole doctor – trained *and* Inner Physicians – the balance between science and humanity can be preserved. I hope that you, the reader, are one of that number, or that this book might have encouraged you to join it.

The nest of *matryoshka* dolls was the image I chose for the kind of doctor I believe it takes to work in a first-class way. Within the institutions of organised medicine, behind the popular stereotypes, inside every clever specialist, at the heart of each individual doctor is an Inner Physician – an 'amateur within', whose only contribution is to be ordinary and worldly-wise. But that is a huge contribution, not least in situations too complex and unpredictable to be handled by science alone, situations that call for the exercise of a more intuitive judgement. It is certainly possible to practise medicine in the absence of an Inner Physician, or, more accurately, in denial of its presence. But as we unpack each successive doll, it becomes ever clearer that doctors

---

172 Professor Michael Sandel of Harvard University, in his BBC Radio 4 Reith Lectures 2009, proposed the term *market triumphalism* for the belief that market forces are effective in harnessing personal greed to the public good. He suggested that there are some areas, medicine being one of them, where market forces do not belong. 'There are some things money can't buy,' he said, 'and there are some things money *can* buy, but shouldn't. Market triumphalism,' he continued, 'changes the norm, so that care is treated as a commodity, medicine is reduced to a delivery system, and quality is nothing more than cost-effectiveness.'

who are comfortable with the 'professional use of self' are the ones best capable of phronesis. They are the doctors who best know what to do when no one knows what to do. They are the ones whose shrewd and judicious husbandry of resources enables the NHS to do so much with so little. They are the ones of whom patients tend to say, 'I don't like doctors, but I *do* like mine.'

* * * Run, stop, sniff * * *

In many ways, the Inner Physician represents in medicine the same idea that Einstein found he had to introduce into classical Newtonian physics – the observer effect. The observer effect, you will recall, refers to the fact that how we look at something, and the properties of the person doing the looking, change what is seen. Pushing a thermometer into a joint of meat as it roasts slightly lowers its temperature. Taking the temperature of a feverish child doesn't cool the child much, but the act of doing it can significantly alter the behaviour of the attendant family. Sending an assessor into a general practice to report on its performance can have profound effects on how the practice operates, before, during and after the visit.

The observer effect means that the doctor cannot avoid being personally involved in every interaction with a patient. Medicine, being a consensual act between two sentient beings, can never be conducted at arm's length. To be sure, the observer effect can be minimised, by concentrating exclusively on a physical malfunction and turning a blind eye on the patient's psychological, social and cultural dimensions. But it cannot be completely abolished. Even turning a blind eye has its effect on patients, who tend not to like having blind eyes turned on them and react unpredictably to being amputated from the offending part of their body.

Hypertension is a good example of a condition inescapably subject to the observer effect. One might think that, with clear-cut diagnostic criteria and well-evidenced treatment protocols, it can and perhaps should be treated mechanistically. But not so. The well-documented 'white coat effect' is only the beginning. Even disregarding errors of measurement, blood pressure readings vary according to who takes them – doctor, nurse or patient. The threshold for diagnosis may change if the doctor has recently read an article, conducted an audit, or been to a clinical update meeting. Faced with an errant blood pressure, some doctors are ruthless, others more tolerant. A doctor's willingness to diagnose and treat is susceptible to financial pressure from performance-related targets, and even alters according to the time of day; towards the end of a Friday afternoon is a popular time for not identifying time-consuming problems. Management, too, is observer-dependent; compliance with a treatment regime is affected by the doctor's enthusiasm, encouragement, communication skills, and by the degree of mutual respect patient and doctor have for each other.

As we know, a patient's narrative is shaped and co-authored by the doctor to whom it is told. Its final draft, the one that patient and doctor settle on as an agreed basis for action, is substantially influenced by the way the story has been elicited and selectively interrogated; and these influences are themselves reflections of the doctor's own idiosyncrasies and priorities as well as his medical knowledge.

In Chapter 7, I suggested that diagnosis should be thought of as an exercise in hermeneutics, a search for meaning leading to 'insight on the verge of action'. The diagnostic process is one of interpreting two stories: the first being the patient's spoken narrative, and the other the physical story told by the patient's body. By combining the two, we aim to arrive at an account of the presenting problem that makes sense to both patient and doctor. And it matters what *kind* of sense we make, especially to the patient. As we learned from catastrophe theory, a comprehensive understanding of one's own illness is a powerful attractor towards recovery. Our medical training has made us adept at picking out from the narrative and physical texts those cues that make biomedical sense; and sometimes, as in emergency situations, biomedical sense is all that is necessary. But patients need their problems to make other kinds of sense as well – emotional sense, psychological sense, sense in terms of their larger life stories, even existential or spiritual sense. Our formal medical training has *not* made us adept at understanding these dimensions. If we have any ability in this regard, it comes from our accumulated experience *outside* medicine, that is to say, from our Inner Physician.

The prevailing culture in medical research is to treat the observer effect as a problem, a distraction that gets in the way of discovering objective truth. Double-blind trials are designed to factor out the observer effect by aggregating data from multiple observers and subjects, researchers hoping thereby to arrive at the kind of uncontaminated conclusions on which, in the Brave New World of evidence-based medicine, individual clinicians are supposed to base their management of individual patients. Yet at the individual level, which is what concerns us in the consulting room, the Inner Physician's contribution to exploring the full richness of the patient's predicament cannot be ignored. Nor should it be; my contention is that the observer effect, far from being a distraction, is in fact clinically useful, even essential.

In Chapter 10 we saw how, when relatively simple systems interact in complicated ways, the phenomenon of emergence can occur, and unexpected things start to happen. When we accept, as the observer effect insists that we must, that a deep consultation between private, blind and unknown sectors of doctor and patient is taking place in parallel with the surface consultation, then the doctor–patient relationship takes on emergent properties. This is the lesson of the Balint movement, which can be thought of as an investigation of the observer effect in general practice.[173]

The Balint approach is sometimes misrepresented as a method or style of conducting a consultation. In fact, it is an exploration of phenomena that arise in every doctor–patient relationship, whether or not the doctor intends or recognises them. The essence of the Balint method is, through guided self-examination in a trusted small group setting, for the doctor to become aware of the emotional and transference dimensions of the relationship, and to use that awareness to unlock complex or frustrating cases. As they become comfortable with the Balint approach, doctors consistently make two discoveries, which often come as something of an epiphany:

1   the doctor's feelings can act as an instrument of diagnosis, and
2   the doctor–patient relationship potentially has therapeutic properties.

Each is a manifestation of the Inner Physician at work.

It is not uncommon for a doctor to feel frustrated, stuck, helpless, angry, intimidated, hopeless – the list is long – when dealing with a patient with a complex problem or a challenging way of presenting it. Balint's gift to us is the realisation that these feelings are not simply unpleasantnesses to be endured, but are reflections, experiences by proxy, of something real in the patient's own life. Once recognised as such, they become easier to bear, and are as diagnostically valuable as, say, an irregular heartbeat or an abnormal

---

173 Michael Balint (1896–1970) was a Hungarian psychoanalyst who moved to the UK in 1938 and worked mainly at London's Tavistock Institute of Human Relations. In the 1950s, together with his wife Enid, he developed the 'Balint group', a small group of GPs that meets regularly over extended periods under the leadership of a trained psychoanalyst to discuss challenging patients presented by group members. The emphasis is on the doctor–patient relationship and its emotional subtext, rather than clinical aspects of the case. The work of the early Balint groups is described in the classic book *The Doctor, His Patient and the Illness*, first published in 1957 (revised edition: London: Pitman Medical, 1968). The Balint movement remains active in the UK and worldwide. For further information, see www.balint.co.uk.

blood test. Making use of these insights is a matter of personal style. But it can be helpful to respond with a remark along the lines of, 'When you tell me about your problem, I get a feeling of xxx, and I wonder whether that's something you yourself have felt,' or 'I seem to be reacting a bit like your (parent, child, best friend); does that makes any sense to you?'

In their book *Six Minutes for the Patient*[174] the early Balintians described something they called 'the Flash', which was a moment sometimes encountered in even a brief consultation when there was 'a peculiar intense flash of understanding between the doctor and the patient'. Puzzling or troubling aspects of the case would suddenly fall into place, often resulting in a seismic refashioning of how they both perceived the patient's problem. In the language I have used in this book, the Flash would be triggered by a particularly strong instance of narrative resonance, such that a recognition of transactions taking place in the deep consultation would break through into the doctor's consciousness. If the insight was a shrewd one, it would come as a relief and a revelation, when discussed, to both doctor and patient.

Some GPs are sceptical of, even opposed to, the suggestion that concerning themselves with these transference and counter-transference issues might be part of their everyday work. 'I haven't the skills for this,' they protest, 'and I certainly haven't the time.' My response would be that deeper layers of the consultation are inevitably present, whether or not they are acknowledged; ignoring them in the short term probably stores up delays and frustrations in the long term, and the skills needed to work with them are not particularly sophisticated. All it takes is a willingness to lend an ear to the voice of one's Inner Physician, and the courage to act on its promptings. Which is better and more satisfying medicine, I would ask – to subject a patient with medically unexplained symptoms to an endless round of fruitless investigations and referrals, or to grasp the nettle and say, gently and respectfully, 'I wonder if your body is trying to tell us something we haven't properly understood yet'?

Formal psychoanalysis and psychotherapy, which are the specialties making full use of the observer effect, are indeed beyond the remit of the generalist. But it would be a shame to forgo the potential of even the most humdrum doctor–patient relationship to be a force for healing. Ask any patient who has ever unburdened himself or herself to you; to be comprehensively understood and accepted by a doctor unafraid to engage at many levels is intrinsically therapeutic, and a much appreciated source of consolation.

---

174 Balint E, Norell JS (eds). *Six Minutes for the Patient*. London: Tavistock, 1973.

*** Run, stop, sniff ***

In this book I have made much of what I have termed 'narrative resonance' – the ringing of an internal bell when some significant feature in a patient's story chimes with a sufficiently similar template in the Inner Physician, previously laid down by the doctor's own personal history. It would seem that we can diagnose only what we are primed to recognise; can recognise only what we know already; can empathise only with situations we ourselves have experienced.

What a chastening thought. Were it the whole truth, I, being male, could have no conception of what it is like to give birth or undergo hysterectomy. You, if you are female, would be incapable of appreciating the distress of a boy with cystic acne or a man going bald. I, being now in my sixties, should (if memory serves) be able fully to identify with the problems of the child, the adolescent, the adult, the middle-aged – been there, felt that. You, if you are young, could have no idea what it means to grow old and to wonder whether every fleeting symptom might be the calling card with which death announces its imminent arrival.

If it were really the case that empathy is contingent upon first-hand personal experience, there are three possible responses. One: who needs empathy? It is (some would say) an unnecessary luxury; medicine needs to be no more than applied bioscience, and medical schools can install all the diagnostic templates required for that purpose. Two: only the diseased, the elderly or the tragic should be allowed to be doctors; everyone else is too naïve to be of value. Or three: perhaps there are more ways of populating the Inner Physician with templates than just through personal experience.

And of course there are. The important element seems to be story. Stories seem to be a universal programming language for the human brain, one of the ways that have evolved for transferring socially important information between individuals. Bees have their waggle dance; human beings have story-telling. Stories are how other people's experiences make their way into our own minds, where, through the power of imagination, they take root and begin to function as if those experiences were our own. In the consulting room, for the purposes of narrative resonance, second-hand or imaginary stories are almost as good as autobiography.

Stories can be factual, mythic or fictional; and all are clinically useful for building up the Inner Physician's store of templates. Most familiar to us are the facts of our own biographies and those of the people closest to us, our families and friends. There are probably few of life's great vicissitudes that have not been experienced, and recounted to us, by someone in our immediate circle. Even if we ourselves have no first-hand knowledge of birth, illness, death, love, marriage, divorce, we usually know someone who has, from whom we can learn to imagine and thus to empathise. Other rich sources of 'insight by proxy' are our patients, and those we hear about from other doctors. The attraction of swopping clinical anecdotes with colleagues is that the exchange leaves us better equipped to resonate with similar cases of our own.

Other stories are mythic, legends, the stories of heroes, instilling values against which we can match ourselves. When Socrates, one of my own heroes, realised that by fobbing off Phaedrus with a second-rate argument he was letting himself down, he judged that his behaviour fell short not of any objective standard but of his own internalised ideal of how a man true to himself should behave; and his daimonion called *Stop!* The novelist E.M. Forster is to me another hero, for his insistence that nothing is more precious than human relationships.[175] I hope that we all have role models. Role models are our real-life heroes, people we know in the flesh but to whom we attribute mythic, heroic status, with the power to improve us by their example. Myths, heroes, role models all install templates that resonate not only with someone else's behaviour but, more importantly, with our own.

It has become almost a cliché to claim that the arts, particularly the narrative arts of the novel, poetry, theatre and film, have a role in fostering the sensitivity of doctors in training. Many university Departments of Medical Humanities and postgraduate training schemes publish their reading lists and run their seminars on 'Literature and empathy'.[176] Fiction (so conventional wisdom has it) puts us inside the minds of other people and lets us see the world through their eyes. And certainly fiction in its various forms allows us to imagine people and situations we could not possibly encounter in real life but which may well on some future professional occasion resonate

---

175 A remark of Forster's that encapsulates his belief in the primacy of the personal, and which moves me to this day, is to be found in his 1938 essay *What I Believe*, written just before the outbreak of World War II, in which he controversially declares, 'If I had to choose between betraying my country and betraying my friend I hope I should have the guts to betray my country.'

176 A comprehensive compendium of medically relevant books, poems, plays and films, compiled by the New York University School of Medicine, can be accessed at http://medhum.med.nyu.edu/.

with a patient's predicament. It can be entertaining and instructive to review one's own favourite novels, poetry, plays and films, and to explain, as if to an interested medical student, exactly what they could teach us about the human condition and a doctor's role within it.[177]

But does it work? In a discussion paper in *The Lancet*,[178] Daniel Marchalik laments that too many students show only pseudo-participation in formal humanities teaching sessions, emerging having expressed the required sentiments and claimed to feel the expected emotions, but ultimately un-enriched, their capacity for real-life narrative resonance un-enhanced and their empathic range un-extended. There seems to be something about the passive method of instruction that negates the goal. A more active form of participatory listening, involving deeper levels of the doctor's mind, seems necessary for imagined events, as in a novel, to become templates primed for clinical application. It is as if the author's creativity needs to be mirrored by some creativity of our own. Take Shakespeare's play *Othello*, a testimony to the destructive power of jealousy; watching it, we will be powerfully moved by the corrosive misunderstanding that turns a loving husband into a wife-murderer. But it takes more than a student group visit to the theatre for Shakespeare to bequeath the full strength of his insight to their Inner Physicians, the insight that will allow them, when doctors, to find the right words to console the lady who tearfully confides that her husband is having an affair. Her needs will be better met if the students, having seen the play, had discussed feelings or incidents of jealousy in their own lives, or per-haps considered what would have happened if Desdemona had really been unfaithful, or if Iago had a conscience.

The lesson seems to be that while our personal life experiences, real and imagined, can indeed populate the Inner Physician with the wherewithal for empathic resonance, to make the most of their potential contribution they need to be actively discussed and reflected upon.

That phrase 'reflected upon' resonates in turn with the idea, associated

---

177 My own list would include: most of E.M. Forster's novels, Tolstoy's *Anna Karenina* (for its encyclopaedic understanding of the crises of family life), and some of Jodi Picoult's fictionalisations of ethical dilemmas; Peter Shaffer's play *Equus* (about sexual obsession and the role of psychiatry); Shakespeare's tragedies; and the films *Patch Adams* (about patient advocacy) and *Rain Man* (autism). What would be on *your* list?

178 Marchalik D. The art of medicine: saving the professionalism course. *The Lancet* 2015; **385**: 13 June. Available online: www.thelancet.com/pdfs/journals/lancet/PIIS0140-6736(15)61093-5.pdf.

with the name of Donald Schön, of 'the reflective practitioner' – one who, as a professional responsibility, is committed to reviewing, mulling over and learning from his or her experience and actions.[179] Reflective practice means taking clinical events as they happen, and from them creating an educational story. What I am advocating here is an extension of reflective practice beyond a purely medical context, and opening up, at least in part, other areas of our lives and minds to the same dispassionate scrutiny. In Chapter 10, drawing upon the Johari model, I suggested that we could perhaps increase our usefulness to patients by co-opting some of our personal history, emotional responses and personality traits into our therapeutic repertoire through self-awareness and judicious self-disclosure. Applying the same principle, reflective practice for the Inner Physician means creating a narrative that links experience (real or imagined), emotion, meaning and behaviour into a coherent story ready for our patients to set in resonance.

If I were presumptuous enough to offer advice on how we might best prepare the Inner Physician for its clinical role, it would be this.

- Widen our concept of continuing professional development to include furthering an interest in the arts and humanities, as well as keeping medically up to date.
- Cultivate the habit of reflecting on how our own life experiences and values impinge on our clinical practice, preferably in discussion with colleagues we trust.
- Participate in professional forums such as Balint groups, mentorship schemes, young practitioner groups, case discussion groups and trainers' workshops, and use them as opportunities for self-disclosure, self-examination and self-acceptance.
- Experiment with controlled self-disclosure in our consultations, testing out its usefulness with patients and finding our own limits.

* * * Run, stop, sniff * * *

So far, so static. Much of what I have written describes what the Inner Physician is, what it can contribute to the clinical encounter, and how it can be brought to a state of readiness, like an athlete on his mark. The Inner Physician:

---

179 Schön DA. *The Reflective Practitioner: how professionals think in action*. New York: Basic Books, 1983.

- is everything we are, except what we have learned about medicine; the expert minus the expertise; the amateur within
- underlies the observer effect that distinguishes the generalist from the specialist way of doing medicine
- comprises our repository of memories and associations ready to be set in resonance by the patient's narrative
- is particularly attuned to the non-physical aspects of the patient's illness
- complements our clinical knowledge in making comprehensive multidi-mensional diagnoses
- can make itself heard as an 'inner voice' or daimonion
- has a major role in phronesis, the competent management of complexity
- can be the key to making sense of a multi-layered consultation.

The remaining task is to consider how this potential energy is converted into kinetic energy, so that we can use it to make a practical difference to how a consultation unfolds in real time. I believe that it is a question of getting ourselves into the right mindset. The Inner Physician works just fine if we don't get in its way. But it is hard *not* to get in its way. What that right mindset is, and how we can access it, occupies the remaining pages of this book.

> To hear the inner voice, we need to be in solitude, even in crowded places.
>
> A.R. Rahman
> Indian musician (b. 1967)

What was remarkable about Socrates was not that he had an inner voice – we all have one of those. Nor was it that he factored its promptings into his decision-making – we all do that, though we often only realise the fact in hindsight. Socrates' strength was that he was able to hear his inner voice amidst the din of the outside world and the chatter of his own thoughts. And he was able to make use of the wisdom of that inner voice in real time, in time to meld its insights with the workings of his rational intellect into actions that did full justice to both. One aspect of expertise is to be able to tell what matters from what does not, to discern meaning against a background of confusion. By that light, Socrates was an expert user of his own mind.

As we begin a consultation with a patient, the inside of our head can be a noisy place. We try to appear calm, welcoming, professional – but inside, our thoughts are often in uproar. As we listen to what the patient tells us, we are on the alert for clinically significant information. At the same time we know we must look carefully for hints of a subtext of hidden agenda or unexpressed concerns. In addition we have our own agenda, medical (*When did I last check the blood pressure?*) and personal (*I'm already late; please let this be quick*). Random thoughts flit in and out to distract us further – *I must remember to phone the dentist. Is there enough milk in the fridge?* Our attention is at the mercy of memory and imagination, being tossed hither and yon in space, and backwards and forwards in time. *Concentrate*, we tell ourselves; and that thought itself becomes a further distraction. Against this hubbub, one might suppose, it would be no use for the Inner Physician to try whispering in our mind's ear; it would need to shout itself hoarse.

What we need is a way to improve the signal-to-noise ratio by reining in the wandering mind and gaining better control of what we pay attention to.

So, by contrast, imagine a focused state of awareness in which your attention is fully taken up with what is happening here and now, in the room and in your mind right now, right this moment. You are concentrating on what *is*, not what *was* or what *might* be. You are noticing what actually *is* going on, not what should be – things as they actually *are*, not as you would *like* them to be. For the time being, you are uncritically allowing your thoughts and sensations just to register as they come and go, without analysing or interpreting them. Think of your attention as being on a threshold, or a place of pivot. From it, you could direct your attention outwards, onto your patient, onto what is being said and done by the person in front of you. Alternatively, you could turn the gaze inwards, and notice the thoughts and feelings arising in your own mind and body. It could go either way.

The best term I have come up with to refer to this condition of being ready for anything is 'poised attentiveness'. Poised attentiveness is the mental equivalent of the state of a top tennis player about to receive serve. The ball might come either to the backhand or the forehand, so the player, up on the balls of the feet, covers both possibilities, uncommitted until the service ball is struck, at which point commitment becomes total.

Ideally, I think poised attentiveness should be the consulting mind's default setting, the condition it returns to after excursions either outwards or inwards. Poised attentiveness establishes a vantage point from which you will immediately detect something happening in both the external and internal worlds. Or, more accurately, something happening in *either* the external *or* the internal world, for one cannot do both at once. I am reminded at this point of Forster's dictum, quoted as the epigraph to Chapter 4, to the effect that 'truth … [is] only to be found by continuous excursions into either realm.' In other words, the poised gaze is gently oscillating, not static, alternately scanning the reality offered by the patient and one's own internal landscape.

Poised attentiveness is the state of mind – quiet enough and vigilant enough – in which the voice of the Inner Physician is most clearly heard without its having to shout. You are undistracted by external irrelevancies or internal chatter. Background noise is stilled; you are alert to the arrival of signals, wherever they originate. If what your patient presents is significant, you will notice it. And if the Inner Physician should give voice, or a chord of narrative resonance should softly chime, you will hear it.

There is nothing mysterious or unfamiliar about what I am calling poised attentiveness. It is the state you start from whenever you are about to become engrossed in something you are good at, whether that 'something' is painting a picture, mowing the lawn or making love. It is the state from which musicians and other creative artists launch their best performances. You already have the skills; all you have to do is to let go of the fear that it might not go well if you just let go. Sportsmen speak of 'being in the zone', or 'living in the moment'. In the Zen tradition, it is sometimes called 'walking the razor's edge'. Half the world nowadays seems to call it 'mindfulness'.

Mindfulness is currently big business. In a very few years an entire industry has grown up, marketing mindfulness as a universal remedy for everything from depression to missed sales targets, and including that condition endemic amongst the moderately dissatisfied, 'stress'. Nonetheless, evidence is mounting that the self that can observe the self is indeed a happier self. The fact that mindfulness has lately become fashionable does not detract from its value as a psychological stabiliser. The benefits of taming the undisciplined mind, so that it becomes capable of stillness and of not being hijacked by every passing thought, have been appreciated by many traditions over many centuries, notably the Buddhist tradition of meditation, to which today's exponents of mindfulness gladly acknowledge their debt.

When you are in a state of poised attentiveness, your attention is focused on whatever you happen to be noticing, inwardly and outwardly, without trying to steer your thoughts in any particular direction. Thoughts of *Why?* or *How?* are suspended. There is just a mild curiosity as you track the flow of one moment to the next: *Now I am aware of this ... oh, and now this ... and now this.* The ever-astute E.M. Forster captures the feel of this present-centredness when, in his unfinished novel *Arctic Summer*,[180] he writes of 'fixing your eyes on the piece of rope that is moving through your hand rather than on the coil you have built up and the tangle you are diminishing'.

---

180 Forster EM. *Arctic Summer.* London: Hesperus Press, 1980.

Two Zen stories

Think about a piece of music – some great symphony. We don't expect it to get steadily better as it develops, or that its whole purpose is to reach the final climax. The joy is found in listening to the music in each moment.

Alan Watts (1915–73)
British populariser of Eastern philosophy

Master Seung Sahn encouraged his students just to do what they were doing. He would say, 'When eating, just eat. When reading the paper, just read the paper.'
A student once discovered Seung Sahn eating while reading the paper. Seung Sahn said, 'When eating and reading the paper, just eat and read the paper.'

Seung Sahn (1927–2004)
South Korean Zen master

'That sounds boring,' I think I hear you say. 'What's more,' I hope I hear you say, 'this is a medical consultation, supposedly for the patient's benefit, where problems have to get sorted out; it's not a meditation session where the doctor can sit in some kind of trance, just letting things come and go!' And you would be right on both counts.

As to 'boring': were one able to sustain poised attentiveness unswervingly for 10 minutes at a time, one would already be a meditation master. Although techniques vary, most training in meditation involves sitting still with the intention of maintaining mindfulness for extended periods. In the early stages, boredom is a problem. As one becomes more adept, one sometimes experiences in meditation a falling away of lines of distinction between self and other, between external and internal … That, however, is another journey, for another book and another author. In the context that concerns us here, and as we shall see, the amount of consultation time spent in poised attentiveness is too short to get boring.

The question implicit in the second objection – 'How does it help the patient for a doctor to be able to do poised attentiveness?' – is crucial.

Assume for now that, just before the patient enters the room, you can rein in your wandering mind and put aside distracting thoughts, so that you are fully present and in your very best state of alertness – the tennis player about to receive serve. The consultation begins. Before long, something the patient says will take your interest, or some line of thought of your own will occur to you, and will seize your attention, wrench it from its poised position, and shift it either outwards or inwards. For a while then your attention will follow wherever it is led. If outwards, you will engage with the patient and their narrative, listening and questioning as seems appropriate. If inwards, your attention will shift away from the patient, and instead you will follow your own train of thought in silent soliloquy.

In either event, an interesting phenomenon soon occurs. There comes a moment when, instead of just thinking, you suddenly become *aware* that you are thinking. You suddenly catch yourself in the act of thought. With a slight jolt of self-consciousness, you realise what it was that your mind was just doing. Your perspective abruptly shifts so that you temporarily become 'the self observing the self'; your awareness of the consultation's content is replaced by awareness of its process. And then, having noticed the fact that you were thinking, you set that thought aside and return to the state of poised attentiveness from which, a little while ago, you had wandered. This cycle – *poised attentiveness → attention shift, external or internal → realisation → return to attentiveness* – repeats continually throughout the consultation. It constitutes, I think, the 'continuous excursions into either realm' described by Forster. Between excursions there is a brief period where you return to your default mindfulness. Figure 12.1 attempts to depict this cycle graphically.

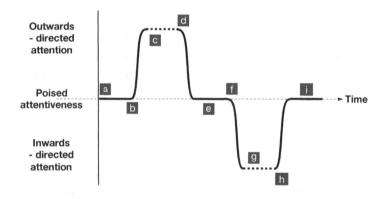

Figure 12.1 '… continuous excursions into either realm'.

You begin the consultation in a state of poised attentiveness (a). At (b) your attention shifts wholly out onto the patient, with whom you engage for a time (c), until at (d) you become self-aware and notice what you are doing in process terms (e.g. *I'm asking a lot of closed questions*). This realisation returns you to a period of poised attentiveness (e). At (f) your attention shifts again, this time inwards; you think, for example, *Could this be asthma? I need to ask about family history.* After a period (g) you realise (h) that you have not been listening to the patient and had been lost in thought, which brings you back again to your default poised attentiveness (i).

The periods of attentiveness between excursions form oases of stillness, gathering points where you can re-establish a degree of serenity. It is at these times that you are most receptive to the promptings from your subconscious mind. This is when you are most likely to be able to identify whatever narrative resonances have been occurring: clinical possibilities generated by your medical knowledge, or intuitions and hunches arising from the Inner Physician. These are the silences in which the daimonion's soft voice can be heard, when insights are likely to appear, and when, through phronesis, you will have your clearest sense of the right thing to say or do.

One final diagram (Figure 12.2) will, I hope, give a sense of how this works in practice.

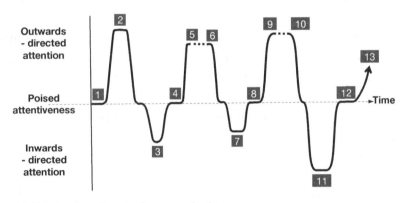

Figure 12.2 Attention flow in the consultation.

The consultation begins with the doctor, ideally, in the default setting of poised attentiveness (1). Being a good doctor, she pays her best quality attention to the patient's opening remarks (2). But, unfortunately, she latches too soon onto some clinical feature in the patient's narrative, causing her prematurely to medicalise the patient's problem and to switch off from what the patient is telling her. At (3) she is preoccupied with her medical thoughts about red flag symptoms and possible investigations. Luckily, she realises (4) that her concentration had lapsed, and she refocuses on the patient (5), this time resisting any temptation to force the consultation in any particular direction. At (6) she detects something like a warning cough from her Inner Physician, causing her to disengage. Turning her attention inwards (7), she is aware that she has picked up cues suggesting that the patient is secretly afraid of having a serious neurological disease. She pauses to choose her words carefully (8), then raises this possibility with the patient (9). The patient is relieved that these concerns have been recognised and acknowledged, and a fruitful conversation ensues until (10), when again the doctor experiences a jolt of narrative resonance. 'Let me just think about this for a moment,' she says, and at (11) does so. On reflection she realises that there is a danger that she could over-investigate this patient under the guise of reassurance; she considers a number of alternative strategies. At (12) she gathers her thoughts, checks that she does indeed feel happy with what she is about to propose, and at (13) moves into the action-planning phase of the consultation.

I hope we have a sense here of a competent patient-centred doctor at work, cleanly and elegantly varying her gaze between close-up detail and wide-angle context. She is able to focus her attention more or less at will on external and internal sources of information. She steers the consultation with a light touch, informed simultaneously by her clinical training and by the gut feelings we now know to be the contribution of her Inner Physician. Periodically she can centre herself, drawing her attention back to the present moment and allowing herself the time and mental space to register whatever resonances the patient's narrative has evoked in her.

Not least, our idealised doctor – I recognise her now as Emily, whom we met in Chapter 1 – was able to begin her consultation already in a state of poised attentiveness, alert and energised and open to all possibilities. If we were to ask her how she achieves that state, I wonder what she would tell us. Perhaps she has had some formal training in a meditation method or a mind–body technique such as autogenic training.[181] Perhaps she has read a book or attended a seminar about mindfulness,[182] and has been practising at home until it becomes something she can easily incorporate into her working routine. She might have learned how to do a '1-minute meditation' or a 'body scan'. Or perhaps she has just evolved her own centring ritual, such as taking a few deep breaths, counting to 10, and looking at the photograph of her favourite landscape she keeps on her desk for the purpose. I suspect Emily would also tell us that there is no one ideal method of quieting the mind.

---

181 Autogenic training: a mental technique for relaxing and restoring healthy functioning to the body. See, for example, Bird J. *I Could Do With Some of That: the power of autogenics*. Sunbury-on-Thames: Legends Publishing, 2015.

182 See, for example, Williams M, Penman D. *Mindfulness: a practical guide to finding peace in a frantic world*. London: Piatkus, 2011.

It begins by knowing that it is possible, and that it matters; after that, we explore on our own.

All these physicianly virtues – insight, empathy, perceptiveness, judgement, the acumen with which clinical knowledge is deployed – arise of themselves. Like the best decisions, they emerge unbidden and fully formed from the quieted mind. The poet Seamus Heaney once said that poetry showed 'the way consciousness can be alive to two different and contradictory dimensions of reality and still find a way of negotiating between them.'[183] I am sure he was right; certainly his words provide a good description of our work as medical generalists, which is to be alive to the multiple dimensions of suffering and to find a way of negotiating between them. Luckily, we don't have to be poets for this synthesis to occur. It is enough just to be human. Negotiating uncertainty is what our brains are good at. It is enough just to make ourselves consciously aware of all the relevant information, whether it comes from the external or the inner world, and then trust our inbuilt mental processes to do the synthesising. If Socrates could do it, so can we all.

* * * * *

I had thought perhaps to close with the famous speech from Shakespeare's *Hamlet* in which Polonius advises his son Laertes, who is about to leave home for university in France:

> *This above all: to thine own self be true,*
> *And it must follow, as the night the day,*
> *Thou canst not then be false to any man.*

These powerful words, penned by one of the greatest generalists of all time, express something I believe to be true; namely, that it is by cherishing our own integrity that we best prepare ourselves to be at the service of others.

This would be a fitting note on which to conclude; and if, having read on to my own preferred ending, you feel you would like this one better, then feel free to ignore what follows and consider my book now to be done.

But Polonius has not quite captured the thought I want to end on, which is slightly more dangerous. E.M. Forster, in his usual tentative and modest way, seems to catch more exactly the notion that transformative encounters between human beings require the deepest levels of *both* parties to be engaged.

---

183 Heaney S. *The Redress of Poetry: Oxford lectures*. London: Faber & Faber, 2002.

Forster's novel *Arctic Summer*, begun in 1911 and abandoned after 80 pages, tells of an encounter between intellectuals Martin and Venetia Whitby, who are holidaying in Italy, and a young army officer, Lieutenant Marsh. Marsh has come to Italy in search of a 16th century wall fresco possibly depicting one of his ancestors. Venetia rubbishes his quest, telling him it is out of date and irrelevant to modern life. Marsh is so chastened by her scorn that he abandons his search. Martin thinks his wife has been too hard on the young man, and tells her so. (And here you must make a leap of imagination, recasting the Whitbys as doctors and the lieutenant as patient.)

Venetia: 'I think I've given him something to think about. Most work is done indirectly. Educationists admit as much. They try to drop knowledge into the subconscious stratum of the child's mind.'

Martin: 'But here's my argument with educationists. I maintain that such knowledge must itself be dropped subconsciously. A child, even a young lieutenant, is a sharper subject than you school ma'ams suppose. He sees through you. You try to touch his depths without using your depths, and it can't be done. One subconsciousness must call to another. Which is a clumsy way of saying there must be affection.'

Touching a patient's depths without using your own can't be done. That one subconsciousness must call to another has been my theme throughout this book. But affection? Of a doctor for a patient? Not love, of course, nor even fondness. Not attraction, not involvement, not entanglement. And certainly not intimacy. But affection – concern softened with platonic warmth?

Would that be so unthinkable?

Index

Page numbers in *italics* refer to tables and figures.